# Color Atlas of

# PEDIATRIC DISEASES

## with Differential Diagnosis

# Color Atlas of

# PEDIATRIC DISEASES

## with Differential Diagnosis

### CLAUS SIMON, M. D.

University Children's Clinic
Kiel, West Germany


### MICHAEL JÄNNER, M. D.

University Dermatology Clinic
Hamburg, West Germany

*translated by*

## JAKE BARICKMAN

*Adapted and edited by*

## ROGER F. SOLL, M. D., F. A. A. P

Assistant Professor of Pediatrics
University of Vermont
College of Medicine
Burlington, Vermont

B.C. DECKER INC • Toronto • Philadelphia 1987
F.K. Schattauer Verlag • Stuttgart • New York

Publisher

**B.C. Decker Inc**
3228 South Service Road
Burlington, Ontario   L7N 3H8

**B.C. Decker Inc**
320 Walnut Street
Suite 400
Philadelphia, Pennsylvania   19106

Sales and Distribution

| | |
|---|---|
| United States and Possessions | **The C.V. Mosby Company**<br>11830 Westline Industrial Drive<br>Saint Louis, Missouri   63146 |
| Canada | **The C.V. Mosby Company, Ltd.**<br>5240 Finch Avenue East, Unit No. 1<br>Scarborough, Ontario   M1S 4P2 |
| United Kingdom, Europe and the Middle East | **Blackwell Scientific Publications, Ltd.**<br>Osney Mead, Oxford OX2 OEL, England |
| Australia | **Harcourt Brace Jovanovich**<br>30–52 Smidmore Street<br>Marrickville, N.S.W. 2204<br>Australia |
| Japan | **Igaku-Shoin Ltd.**<br>Tokyo International P.O. Box 5063<br>1-28-36 Hongo, Bunkyo-ku, Tokyo 113, Japan |
| Asia | **Info-Med Ltd.**<br>802–3 Ruttonjee House<br>11 Duddell Street<br>Central Hong Kong |
| South Africa | **Libriger Book Distributors**<br>Warehouse Number 8<br>''Die Ou Looiery''<br>Tannery Road<br>Hamilton, Bloemfontein 9300 |
| South America (non-stock list representative only) | **Inter-Book Marketing Services**<br>Rua das Palmeriras, 32<br>Apto. 701<br>222-70 Rio de Janeiro<br>RJ, Brazil |

CIP - Short title entry of the German library:

Simon, Claus:
Color Atlas of Pediatrics
C. Simon, M. Jänner
Stuttgart; New York: Schattauer, 1981

ISBN 3-7945-0496-8

English edition:
Color Atlas of Pediatric Diseases
adapted and edited by R.F. Soll

ISBN 1-55664-005-6

© 1981 by F.K. Schattauer Verlag GmbH, Stuttgart, Germany
© 1987 by B.C. Decker Inc • Toronto • Philadelphia

Library of Congress catalog card number:  87–71151

Printed in West Germany

10  9  8  7  6  5  4  3  2  1

# FOREWORD

The color figures of this atlas demonstrate symptoms of illnesses observed mostly in the medical treatment of children, as well as in other specialties of medicine. Therefore, the atlas will be of interest not only to pediatricians and general practitioners, but also to midwives, surgeons, and other specialists. Medical students can use the book as a supplement to a basic text, which will allow them to become familiar with diseases rarely dealt with in clinical instruction. The figures chosen for their rarity of symptoms seemed most valuable; other figures were chosen with certain instructional points in mind. A comprehensive discussion of every conceivable symptom was not our intent and would have made the atlas unnecessarily cumbersome and expensive. Rather, the accompanying text consists of short descriptions of each figure and offers possible differential diagnoses. Only those figures illustrating rarer diseases receive a more detailed discussion along with important points for clinical diagnostic interpretation. The carefully compiled index facilitates the location of illustrated symptoms as well as diseases; this can be important with regard to differential diagnosis. For the most part, the figures originate from the Photography Department at the University of Kiel Children's Clinic, directed by Ms. Herta Dibbern, whom we thank in particular for her assistance. Other photographs were made available to us courtesy of the Dermatology Clinic at the University of Hamburg and other clinics and institutes of the University of Kiel (Orthopedics, Dermatology, Ophthalmology, Otolaryngology, Craniofacial Clinic, as well as the Institute for Human Genetics and the Pathology Institute). We owe a debt of thanks to the doctors there as well as to many colleagues at other institutions who have loaned us photographs, especially Dr. O. Braun (City Children's Clinic of Pforzheim) and Professor V. von Loewenich (University Children's Clinic in Frankfurt/Main). Finally, we thank our publisher, F. K. Schattauer, and in particular Professor P. Matis, for their openness to our objectives and for their active support.

Kiel, September 1981

C. Simon
M. Jänner

# Preface to the English Edition

Much has been said about the relative worth of pictures over words. Perhaps nowhere is this cliche more true than in the practice of medicine where the recognition of the disease process is essential to diagnosis and treatment. It was, therefore, a pleasure to help with the English edition of Drs. Simon and Jänner's *Color Atlas of Pediatric Diseases*. The excellent photographs and accompanying text should aid in the recognition of a broad range of pediatric problems.

In preparing the English edition, I would like to thank Jake Barickman for the translation of the German text, Brian Decker for his advice, Nancy Moreland for her expert preparation of the manuscript, and both Nancy and my wife Roberta for their patience.

Roger F. Soll, M.D
April, 1987

# CONTENTS

Living with an illness is a task that many people, including children, must face. The value judgments of the healthy must not apply to the ill. Illness is a part of human existence and, even when prolonged, should not be perceived as a defect. On the contrary, an illness can raise a person's esteem when one rises above suffering and shapes one's life according to one's own standards.

C. Simon
M. Jänner

# 1. Diseases of the Newborn

**Figure 1  Hydrops Fetalis 2° Rh-Incompatibility (Erythroblastosis Fetalis):** Generalized edema and ascites without jaundice in a 2-hour-old newborn whose 35-year-old Rh-negative mother had already given birth to two children with symptoms of Rh-incompatibility. Erythroblastosis fetalis can occur through trans placental passage of anti-D antibody in sensitized mothers. The infant was profoundly anemic at birth. Peripheral blood smears revealed an increase in nucleated red blood cells (erythroblastosis) and reticulocytosis. Cord bilirubin was 3.7 mg% and direct Coombs test was strongly positive. The infant was treated with exchange transfusion.

**Differential Diagnosis:** Previously, erythroblastosis fetalis was the most common cause of hydrops fetalis. With the widespread use of RhoGAM in recent years, fewer cases due to isoimmunization are seen and non-immune causes of hydrops fetalis are increasing in frequency. Hydrops fetalis can occur in conditions where there is increased intravascular hydrostatic pressure either from primary myocardial failure (cardiac malformation or arrhythmia), high output failure (anemia or arteriovenous malformation) or obstruction of venous return (neoplasm). Decreased plasma oncotic pressure seen in liver failure or congenital nephrosis can present as hydrops. Increased capillary permeability (seen with anoxia or congenital infection) and obstruction of lymph flow (seen in Turner's syndrome) may also represent causes of hydrops.

### References

1. Holzgreve W, et al. Investigation of non-immune hydrops fetalis. Am J Obstet Gynecol 150(7):805, 1984.
2. Holzgreve W, Holzgreve B and Curry CJR. Non-immune hydrops fetalis: Diagnosis and management. Semin Perinatc 9(2):52, 1985.
3. Machin GA. Differential diagnosis of hydrops fetalis. Am J Med Genet 9:341, 1981.

**Figure 2  Kernicterus 2° Rh-Incompatibility:** Erythroblastosis fetalis led to kernicterus in this 6-day old newborn. Peak bilirubin level was 36 mg%. The early signs of lethargy and loss of Moro reflex were followed by rigidity and opisthotonos. Death occurred on the eighth day due to respiratory complications.

**Differential Diagnosis:** Opisthotonos may also occur in connection with intracranial bleeding (infratentorial) and bacterial meningitis. Neck stiffness and opisthotonos have also been observed in connection with retropharyngeal abscess due to the severe pain.

### References

1. Lucey JF. Bilirubin and brain damage—a real mess. Pediatrics 69:381, 1982.
2. Turkel S, et al. A clinical pathologic reappraisal of kernicterus. Pediatrics 69:267, 1982.
3. Turkel SB, et al. Lack of identifiable risk factors for kernicterus. Pediatrics 66:502, 1980.

**Figure 3  Bronze Baby Syndrome:** Grayish-brown discoloration of the skin in a 10-day-old premature infant with hyperbilirubinemia after treatment with phototherapy. This side effect of phototherapy is noted in infants with an elevated direct reacting bilirubin. Natural skin color was completely restored after 4 months. The exact cause of the discoloration is unknown. Other side effects of phototherapy include loose stools, skin rash, hyperthermia, and dehydration.

### References

1. Clark CF, et al. The "bronze baby" syndrome: post postmortem data. J Pediatr 88:461, 1976.
2. Kopelman AE, et al. The "bronze baby" syndrome: a complication of phototherapy. J Pediatr 81:466, 1972.

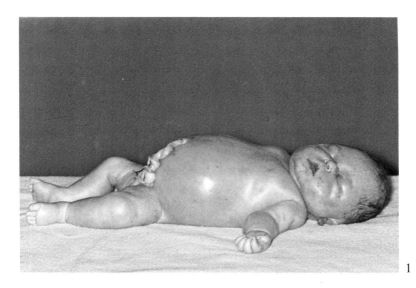

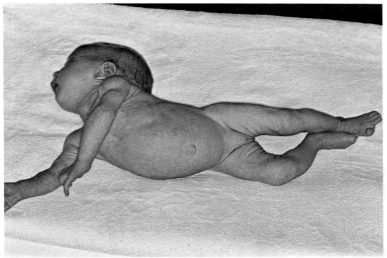

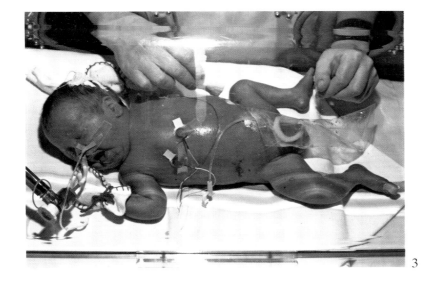

# 1. Diseases of the Newborn

**Figure 4** **Infant of Diabetic Mother:** Macrosomic infant (birthweight 5,200 g) born to a diabetic mother whose blood glucose was poorly controlled during pregnancy. Polyhydramnios is frequently seen during pregnancies complicated by diabetes.. The infant is remarkable for a puffy, plethoric appearance. Polycythemia was noted (hematocrit 75 percent). Dextrose infusions given immediately after birth and early enteral feedings successfully prevented hypoglycemia.

**Diagnosis:** Macrosomic infant prone to hypoglycemia due to the effect of maternal diabetes. Intrauterine growth retardation is possible if there is uteroplacental insufficiency due to long standing diabetes with vascular involvement. Infants of diabetic mothers have a higher incidence of asphyxia, birth injury, metabolic imbalance, respiratory distress, and congenital anomalies.

**Differential Diagnosis:** Macrosomia may be seen in Beckwith-Wiedemann syndrome (macrosomia with macroglossia, see p 56), cerebral gigantism (Sotos' syndrome) or as a variant of normal. Hypoglycemia (blood glucose less than 30 mg%) may be seen with intrauterine growth retardation, erythroblastosis fetalis, galactosemia, leucine sensitivity, and glycogen storage disease. Resistant hypoglycemia may be caused by nesidioblastosis or islet cell adenoma.

## References

1.  Hayworth JC, Dillig LA. Relationship between maternal glucose tolerance and neonatal blood glucose. J Pediatr 89:810, 1976.
2.  Kitzmiller JL, et al. Diabetic pregnancy and perinatal morbidity. Am J Obstet Gynecol 131:560, 1978.
3.  Miller E, et al. Elevated maternal hemoglobin $A_1C$ in early pregnancy and major congenital anomalies in infants of diabetic mothers. N Engl J Med 304:1331, 1981.
4.  Pagliara AS, et al. Hypoglycemia in infancy and childhood. J Pediatr 85:365, 1973.

**Figure 5** **Congenital Nephrotic Syndrome (Infantile Microcystic Disease):** Two-week-old boy with generalized edema (especially noticeable on the eyelids), which has steadily increased since birth. Laboratory tests revealed proteinuria and hypoproteinuria as well as low serum complement levels. Renal biopsy demonstrated cystic dilation of the proximal tubules. Since congenital nephrosis is always resistant to steroid treatment, therapy was limited to restriction of sodium intake and provision of adequate nutrition. The child died 6 months later of severe pneumonia. For Differential Diagnosis of edema in the newborn, see Figure 1, p 2.

## References

1.  Kaplan BS, et al. The nephrotic syndrome in the first year of life: is a pathologic classification possible? J Pediatr 85:615, 1974.
2.  Strauss J, et al. Nephrotic syndrome: etiopathogenic and therapeutic considerations. Nephron 38:75, 1984.

**Figure 6** **Turner's Syndrome:** Two-day-old infant (birthweight 2,600 g) with extensive edema of the dorsum of the foot, loose skin (Cutis laxa), low posterior hairline, widely spaced nipples and deep-set hypoplastic finger and toenails. Karyotype was 45, XO. The swelling of the soft tissue in the dorsum of the foot and the hand is lymphedema and occurs in about 40 percent of cases. Turner's syndrome is also associated with short stature, cardiac abnormalities (coarctation of the aorta), cubitus valgus, renal abnormalities, and ovarian dysgenesis.

**Differential Diagnosis:** Noonan's syndrome may share many of the features of Turner's syndrome, but individuals have a normal karyotype and may be of the male sex. Cardiac abnormalities (pulmonary stenosis) are more common with Noonan's syndrome. Congenital hereditary lymphedema (Milroy's disease) is usually restricted to the lower extremity, and may be progressive.

## References

1.  Brook CGD, et al. Growth in children with 45XO Turner syndrome. Arch Dis Child 49:789, 1974.
2.  Collins E and Turner G. The Noonan syndrome. J Pediatr 83:441, 1973.
3.  Palmer CG, et al. Chromosomal and clinical findings in 110 females with Turner syndrome. Hum Genet 35:35, 1976.

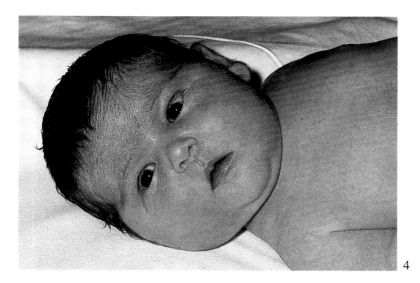

4

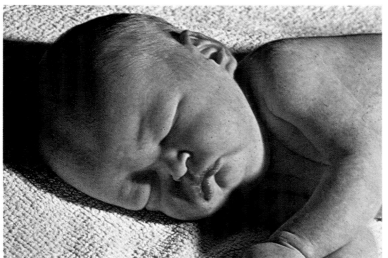

5

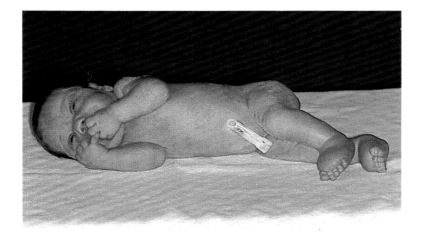

6

# 1. Diseases of the Newborn

**Figure 7  Intrahepatic Biliary Hypoplasia:**  Conjugated hyperbilirubinemia in a 2-month-old boy. Finding included jaundice due to an elevated direct reacting bilirubin (4 mg%), acholic stools, hepatomegaly, an failure to thrive. Associated facial, cardiac, or vertebral anomalies (Alagille-Watson's syndrome) were nc seen in this case. The child became increasingly jaundiced after birth. Laboratory investigations reveale an elevated total and direct bilirubin as well as elevated transaminases and gamma glutamyl transferase The etiology is unclear. Diagnosis or intrahepatic biliary hypoplasia was confirmed by liver biopsy. Histc logical examination revealed interlobular bile duct proliferation. The outcome in these children is varie the disease may slowly progress toward biliary cirrhosis or may stabilize without obvious progression. Cor jugated hyperbilirubinemia may also occur in extrahepatic biliary atresia, choledochal cyst, neonatal hepa titis, congenital infections, and metabolic disorders including galactosemia and alpha$_1$-antitrypsin deficienc

## References

1.  Andres JM, et al. Liver disease in infants; Part I: Developmental hepatology and mechanisms of liver dysfunction. J Pedia 90:686, 1977.
2.  Andres JM, et al. Liver disease in infants; Part II: Hepatic disease states. J Pediatr 90:864, 1977.
3.  Ferry GD, et al: Guide to early diagnosis of biliary obstruction in infancy: review of 143 cases. Clin Pediatr 24:305, 198

**Figure 8  Physiologic Jaundice (Icterus Neonatorum):**  Mild jaundice in a 3-day-old baby girl. Jaur dice was first noted on the second day of life and resolved by day six. Indirect bilirubin reached a pea level of 6.8 mg%. Mild elevation of indirect bilirubin is common in the newborn due to the immaturit of hepatic enzymes and increased enterohepatic circulation. Pathologic conditions causing hyperbilirubine mia in the newborn can be differentiated from physiologic jaundice by their early onset (before 24 hours, persistence beyond 1 week, and greater elevation of either the total or direct bilirubin. Differential diagnc sis includes fetal-maternal blood group incompatibility (isoimmunization), closed space hemorrhage, in paired hepatic uptake (Gilbert's syndrome) or impaired conjugation (Crigler-Najjar syndrome).

**Figure 9  Extrahepatic Biliary Atresia:**  Cirrhosis of the liver and ascites (due to portal hypertension) i an 8-month-old boy. Other physical findings included hepatosplenomegaly. Diagnosis of extrahepatic biliar atresia was confirmed by documenting interrupted bile flow and performing a liver biopsy to rule out a intrahepatic process. The child underwent a hepatic portoenterostomy (Kasai procedure) at 4 months age. The operation was unsuccessful. The child went on to develop severe conjugated hyperbilirubinem and cirrhosis of the liver. Despite supportive care, the child died at 1 year of age.

**Differential Diagnosis:**  Conjugated hyperbilirubinemia (see Figure 7). Severe abdominal distension ma be seen in ileus, intra-abdominal tumors, hemoperitoneum or fecal impaction. Ascites may be seen in cor gestive heart failure, malnutrition, malignancy, nephrotic syndrome or other protein losing states, pancreatit and urinary obstruction.

## References

1.  Balistreri WF. Neonatal cholestasis. J Pediatr 106:171, 1985.
2.  Hansen RC, et al. Bile ascites in infancy. Diagnosis with [131]I-rose bengal. J Pediatr 84:719, 1974.
3.  Kasai M, et al. Follow-up studies of long-term survivors after hepatic portoenterostomy—survivors for after "non-correctable biliary atresia. J Pediatr Surg 10:173, 1975.

**Figure 10  Alpha$_1$-antitrypsin Deficiency:**  Five-month-old boy with abdominal distension, hepatomeg ly, ascites, and cirrhosis. The alpha$_1$-antitrypsin level in serum specimens was low. Typical PAS-positiv granules were detected in the cytoplasm of hepatocytes on liver biopsy. Children who are homozygotes f this disorder (pi type ZZ) may develop liver disease, but the majority present with pulmonary complication

## References

1.  Moore JO. Alpha-$_1$-antitrypsin deficiency. N Engl J Med 299:1045, 1099, 1978.
2.  Moroz SP, et al. Liver disease associated with alpha-$_1$-antitrypsin deficiency in childhood. J Pediatr 88:19, 1976.

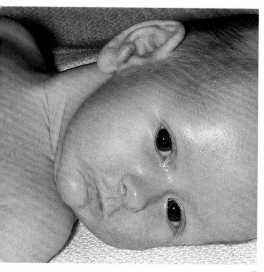
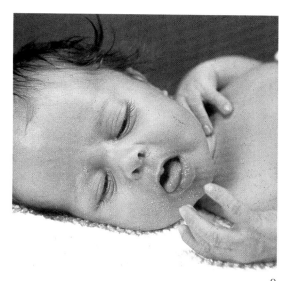

7

8

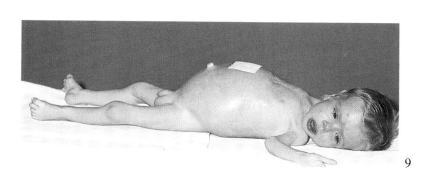

9

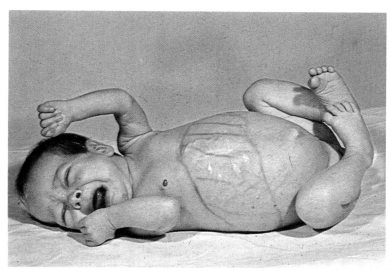

10

# 1.  Diseases of the Newborn

**Figures 11–13   Prematurity:**   Nine hundred gram premature infant born at 28 weeks gestation, pictured in Figures 11 and 12 on the second day of life. Physical findings include thin red skin with little subcutaneous fat, ample lanuginous hair, large head relative to body size, and soft pinna due to a lack of cartilage. Figure 13 demonstrates the infant at 97 days of age weighing 3 kg. No striking neurological sequelae were noted at this time. The child was discharged and sent home.

**Differential Diagnosis:**   Infants of low birth weight are not all premature. The dysmature infant achieves a birth weight lower than that expected for the corresponding gestational age. These infants may have dry peeling skin, little subcutaneous fat, and meconium staining. Although the weight is low, head growth may be normal. These infants do not usually show signs of immature organ development.

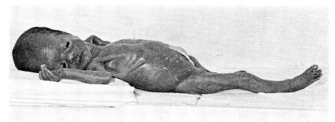

11

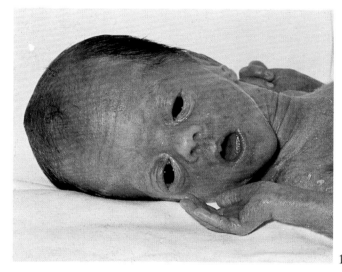

12

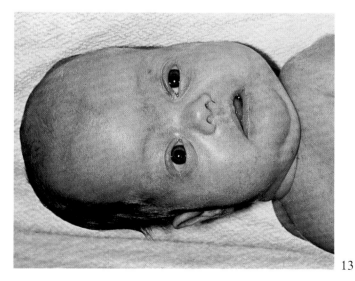

13

# 1. Diseases of the Newborn

**Figure 14  Feto-fetal Transfusion Syndrome:**  Feto-fetal transfusion syndrome seen in prematurely born identical twins. The syndrome is due to vascular anastomosis in the monochorionic placenta. Of greatest pathologic significance is the arteriovenous anastomosis (due to the pressure differential). Transfusion syndrome may complicate 15 percent of identical twin pregnancies. Discordance, defined as a 20 percent difference in birth weight or a difference in hemoglobin of greater than 5 mg per deciliter, may result between the twins. These twins were discordant. The pale donor twin had a hemoglobin of 20.7 mg per deciliter. The donor twin had hypovolemia, respiratory distress, and anemia at birth, requiring blood transfusions. The recipient twin developed hyperbilirubinemia and required phototherapy. Polycythemia may also be seen in uteroplacental insufficiency, delayed cord clamping, and materno-fetal transfusion.

## References

1.  Bryan EM. The intrauterine hazards of twins. Arch Dis Child 61:1044, 1986.
2.  Galea P, Scott JM and Goel KM. Feto-fetal transfusion syndrome. Arch Dis Child 57:781, 1982.

**Figure 15  Dysmaturity:**  Two-day-old newborn noted to be underweight (2.8 kg) relative to length (4 cm). Findings included decreased subcutaneous fat, dry desquamating skin with poor turgor, and meconium stained skin and nails. Numerous causes can be considered including placental insufficiency, fetal alcohol syndrome, prenatal infection, and chromosomal abnormalities.

## Reference

1.  Ting RY, et al. The dysmature infant. J Pediatr 90:943, 1977.

**Figure 16  Postmaturity:**  Postmature 1-day-old newborn (birthweight 3.3 kg, length 58 cm) born 2 weeks after expected date of confinement. Findings included dry desquamating skin, decreased subcutaneous fat, "washerwoman's" hands, long nails, and yellow discoloration of both nails and skin due to meconium staining. Additional signs include absence of lanugo and vernix caseosa.

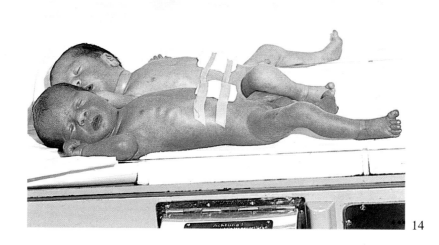

14

15

16

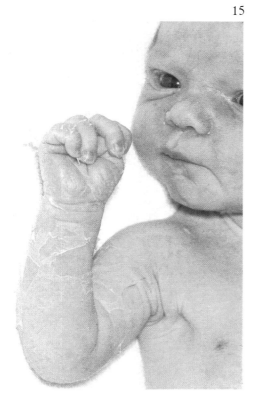

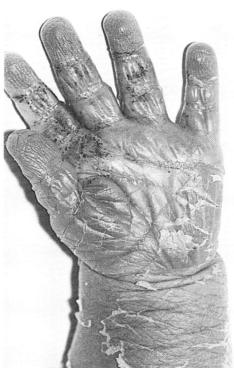

# 1. Diseases of the Newborn

**Figure 17  Isoimmune Thrombocytopenia:**  Petechial and purpuric skin lesions in a 1-day-old girl. Lesions were observed over the face and body of the infant. No signs of prenatal viral infection or bacterial sepsis were noted. Thrombocytopenia was noted on peripheral blood smear, but no other laboratory abnormalities were seen. The cause of thrombocytopenia was the transplacental passage of maternal isoantibodies directed against the child's platelets. The most common platelet antigen involved in isoimmune thrombocytopenia is the Pl$^{A1}$ antigen, present in 98 percent of the general population. Intracranial hemorrhage, the major risk of thrombocytopenia in the newborn, was not seen in this case. Over the first month of life the infant's platelet count gradually normalized, and no more skin lesions appeared. Other causes of thrombocytopenia in the newborn include maternal autoimmune thrombocytopenia, inherited disorders of platelet production (thrombocytopenia with absent radius, Wiskott-Aldrich syndrome), prenatal or postnatal infection, maternal medications, or consumption in a cavernous hemangioma (Kasabach-Merritt syndrome).

## Reference

1.  Gill FM. Thrombocytopenia in the newborn. Semin Perinatol 7:201, 1983.

**Figure 18  Birth Trauma:**  Severe birth trauma seen in a 6-day-old newborn. Pictured are the superficial skin hemorrhages over the extremities and torso. This infant experienced severe fetal distress in utero (slow, irregular fetal heart rate) and evidence of asphyxia postpartum (cyanosis, bradycardia, respiratory distress, cardiogenic shock) which led to death on the ninth day. Autopsy revealed an infratentorial hemorrhage as well as pulmonary hemorrhage with edema and atelectasis of both lungs.

**Figure 19  Sepsis Neonatorum:**  Sepsis due to *E. coli* in a 2-day-old boy born after prolonged rupture of membranes. Petechial skin lesions were the first diagnostic sign in this infant. Other clinical signs of sepsis include poor feeding, lethargy, hypothermia, respiratory distress, and apnea. Bacteria were isolated from both the blood and cerebrospinal fluid. Although thrombocytopenia was noted, the typical findings of disseminated intravascular coagulation were not seen. The infection apparently began in utero due to maternal chorioamnionitis. Coagulation problems in the newborn can also be caused by vitamin K deficiency, hepatic dysfunction, or hereditary coagulation disorders.

## Reference

1.  Siegel JD, McCracken GM, Jr. Sepsis neonatorum. N Engl J Med 304:642, 1981.

**Figure 20  Birth Trauma:**  Ecchymotic skin lesions in a 1-day-old premature infant born after face presentation. Of note is the deep blue discoloration and swelling of the face.

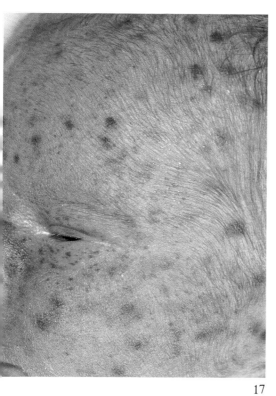

17

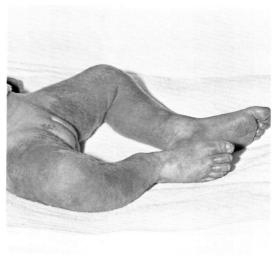

18

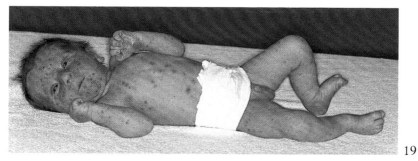

19

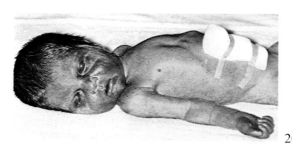

20

# 1. Diseases of the Newborn

**Figure 21  Birth Trauma:**  Pseudoparalysis of the legs due to traumatic epiphyseal fracture after difficult delivery (abnormal presentation). Radiograph demonstrates lateral shift of both femoral epiphyses. Patellar and Achilles tendon reflexes were absent. The infant died on the sixth day of life due to a large subdural hematoma. Epiphyseal fracture of the femur with extensive subperiosteal hematomas was confirmed on autopsy.

Traumatic proximal epiphyseal fracture must be distinguished from traumatic or congenital hip joint subluxation. In epiphyseal fracture, the radiograph reveals typical callus formation after 1 week; callus formation is not seen in subluxation. Fracture of the shaft of the femur can be easily ruled out. Genuine paralysis (complete or incomplete paraplegia) is possible, due to traumatic vertebral fracture and damage to the spinal cord. Pseudoparalysis of Parrot noted with congenital syphilis, can present with similar symptoms. Other conditions which may appear as reduced spontaneous movement include muscular hypotonia caused by Werdnig-Hoffman disease or the temporary hypotonia caused by intracranial hemorrhage.

**Figure 22  Umbilical Cord Furrows:**  Umbilical cord furrows with skin ulcerations in the flank of a prematurely born twin. The skin lesions were caused by the binding of the hip of one twin with the umbilical cord of the other that had died utero. Because of uterine myomatosis in the mother, the delivery was done by cesarean section. The skin lesion healed over time, requiring antibiotic treatment due to secondary bacterial infection.

**Differential Diagnosis:**  Similar skin lesions may be seen with amniotic bands. Intrauterine rupture of the amnion may cause entrapment in these fibrous bands, leading to skin lesions or, in severe cases, amputation of the extremity. (See Figures 75 and 83).

**Figure 23  Hematoma of the Umbilical Cord:**  Large hematoma of the umbilical cord resulting from rupture of umbilical vein. The hematoma was present at birth and removed surgically on the 2nd day. Other wise, the pregnancy followed a normal course and delivery was without complications.

**Differential Diagnosis:**  Congenital omphalocele, umbilical cord tumors, such as angioma, enteroteratoma, dermoid cysts, myosarcoma, and persistence of the omphalomesenteric duct or urachus.

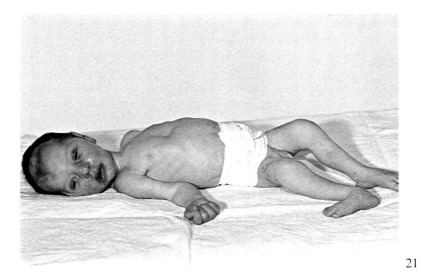

21

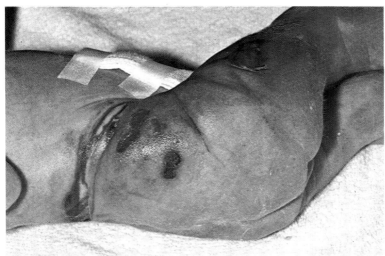

22

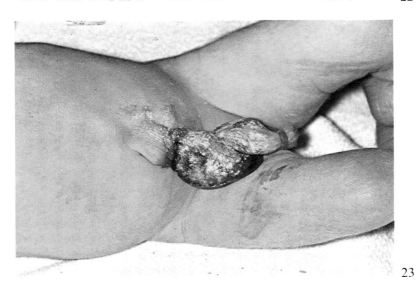

23

# 1. Diseases of the Newborn

**Figure 24  Congenital Facial Paresis:**  Facial paresis in a 1-day-old newborn with multiple deformities (dysplastic pinna and tympanic canal, bilateral radial aplasia, and congenital heart disease). When the infant cried, only the non-paralyzed side of the face would move. On the affected side, the forehead was smooth, the eye could not be closed, the nasolabial fold was absent, and the mouth drooped. The other cranial nerves were intact. Meningitis and encephalitis were ruled out. The facial paresis was probably attributable to traumatic damage to the peripheral nerve at birth. Complete recovery from the paresis was noted later in the course. No single syndrome that encompassed the other deformities was identified.

In cases of traumatic facial paresis, it is frequently only the mandibular branch that is affected. In central facial paralysis, the two lower branches are affected, allowing for movement of the forehead. With central lesions, there are usually other signs of brain damage (e.g., simultaneous abducent paralysis). In Möbius' syndrome (malformation of the cranial nerve nuclei), facial paralysis starts at birth, but is usually bilateral and incomplete. Abducent paralysis of one or both sides is always present. Children affected with Möbius syndrome have a noticeably expressionless face and a constant flow of saliva. Other deformities are often present including micrognathia, talipes equinovarus, and Poland sequence (absence of pectoralis muscle). Older children can have facial paralysis due to tumors of the brain stem, basilar skull fracture, acute or chronic otitis media or Bell's palsy (idiopathic). Facial paresis is seen in Melkersson's syndrome (p 198) associated with edema of the lids.

**Figure 25  Congenital Facial Faresis:**  Congenital facial paresis in a 3-day-old boy. The right corner of the mouth hung down and flattening of the nasolabial cleft was noted. The temporofacial branch was intact, because the right eye could be closed and the forehead could move symmetrically. In this case, only the fibers supplying the cervicofacial branch were damaged due to birth trauma (forceps delivery). With greater trauma, the entire nerve could be affected.

Similar facial appearance occurs in asymmetric crying facies which is caused by unilateral absence or hypoplasia of the angular depressor muscles. In this syndrome, the nasolabial fold is normal and the affected side will not move when the infant cries. The syndrome may be associated with cardiovascular abnormalities.

## Reference

1.  Miller M, Hall JG. Familial asymmetric crying facies. Am J Dis Child 133:743, 1979.

**Figure 26  Subgaleal Hemorrhage:**  Subgaleal hemorrhage in a 1-day-old infant born with the aid of vacuum extraction. Edematous swelling, subcutaneous hematoma, and skin abrasion was noted over scalp. There was no evidence of skull fracture or intracranial bleeding. Subgaleal hematoma occurs between the periosteum and the epicranial aponeurosis. The hematoma often goes beyond the cranial suture line and may spread over the entire scalp. Significant blood loss may occur.

**Differential Diagnosis:**  A cephalhematoma lies subperiosteal, and is confined by the cranial sutures. Caput succedaneum refers to edematous or ecchymotic swelling of the scalp, and may cross over suture lines.

## Reference

1.  Plauche WL. Subgaleal hematoma: a complication of instrumental delivery. JAMA 244:1597, 1980.

**Figure 27  Cephalhematoma:**  Cephalhematoma in a 9-day-old infant. Of note was a spherical fluctuant mass over the right parietal bone, which did not cross the sagittal suture. No other scalp was defect noted. There was no radiographic evidence of parietal skull fracture. Calcification of this lesion occurred, giving the lesion an "egg shell" feel.

**Differential Diagnosis:**  Other extracranial hematomas, including caput succedaneum and subgaleal hemorrhage, must be excluded. Encephalocele may present in a similar area and can be differentiated by pulsation during crying and by radiographic studies demonstrating a skull defect.

## Reference

1.  Zelson C, et al. The incidence of skull fractures underlying cephalhematomas in newborn infants. J Pediatr 85:371, 1974.

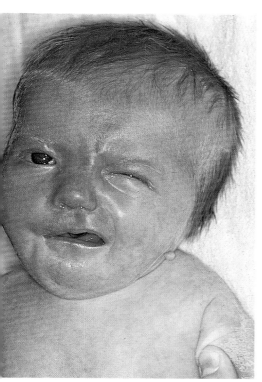

24

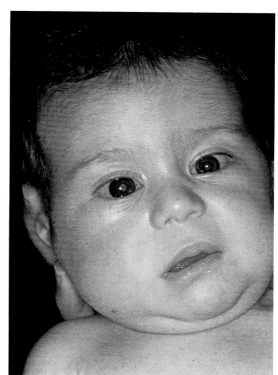

25

26

27

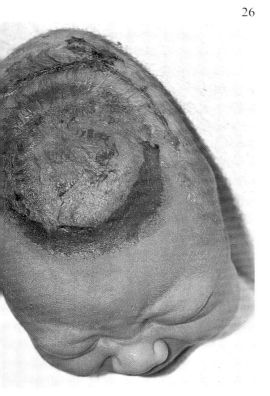

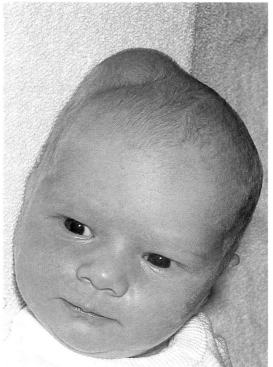

# 1.  Diseases of the Newborn

**Figure 28  Omphalocele:**  A walnut sized omphalocele in a 6-week-old boy. An omphalocele involves the herniation of abdominal contents through a defect at the base of the umbilical cord. The defect is covered only by peritoneum, without overlying skin. Intestinal contents were noted in the hernial sac. The child was treated conservatively with frequent brushing of the hernial sac with a 2 percent Merthiolate solution leading to epithelialization and shrinking of the hernial sac, retraction of the bowel contents, and closure of the hernial opening. Malrotation was diagnosed by barium enema, but was not associated with any clinical manifestations. Conservative therapy is successful in only some of the cases of omphalocele, others require surgical correction.

### References

1.  Knight PJ, et al. Omphalocele: A prognostic classification. J Pediatr Surg 16:599, 1981.
2.  Seashore JH. Congenital abdominal wall defects. Clin Perinatol 5:61, 1978.

**Figures 29 and 30  Omphalocele:**  One-day-old infant with omphalocele. The omphalocele lay at the base of the umbilical cord, covered only by peritoneum fused with amniotic membrane. Liver, spleen, and bowel could be seen through the thin membranous covering. Malrotation, frequently associated with omphalocele, was recognized after radiographic examination. Due to the size of the omphalocele, immediate operative repair was not undertaken. With conservative treatment (brushing the surface of the omphalocele with 2 percent Mercurochrome solution), the hernial sac gradually decreased in size and the everted viscera returned to the abdomen. Within 4 weeks, the hernial sac had shrunk to half the original size and was fully epithelialized (Figure 30). Treatment with organic mercurial antiseptic is controversial since infants may develop potentially toxic levels of mercury. Surgical correction of malrotation was not necessary.

**Differential Diagnosis:**  Omphalocele must be distinguished from umbilical hernia that occurs with incomplete closure or weakness of the umbilical ring, and is often combined with diastasis recti. An umbilical hernia is covered with skin, protrudes when the child cries, and can be easily reduced.

### Reference

1.  Fagan DG, et al. Organ mercury levels in infants with omphaloceles treated with organic mercurial antiseptic. Arch Dis Child 52:962, 1977.

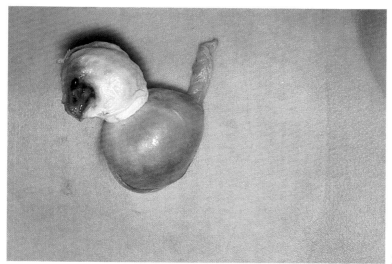

28

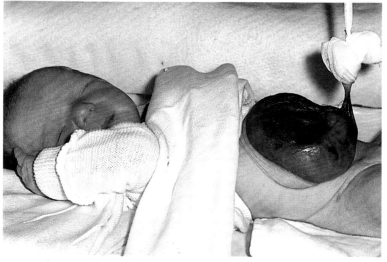

29

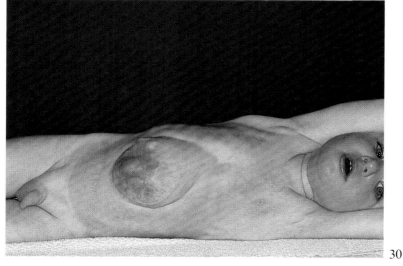

30

# 1. Diseases of the Newborn

**Figure 31 Harlequin Skin Changes:** A 5-day-old newborn with harlequin skin changes (due to vasomotor instability). The child is pictured lying on one side. The left lateral aspect of the child is pale; the right side is deep red. The color change lasted only a few minutes and disappeared when the child's position was changed. Sometimes the skin changes were noted only on the torso or face. Movement of the infant would occasionally cause a generalized temporary redness.

**Figure 32 Cutis Marmorata:** Cutis marmorata with harlequin skin changes in a 2-week-old newborn. The lightly reticulated skin became pale on the right side when the infant lay on the left; the left side became livid and red. The opposite changes were noted when the infant lay on the right side. The infant was referred to the clinic because of unilateral "cyanosis", when in fact the child had cutis marmorata. When the child was picked up, the color change disappeared. Congenital heart disease was ruled out. By the time the child was four weeks old, this phenomenon could no longer be detected.

**Figure 33 Cutis Marmorata:** Cutis marmorata in a 4-month old child. A fine reticulated network of superficial vessels could easily be appreciated due to the paucity of subcutaneous fat. The relatively frequent finding of cutis marmorata may later become idiopathic livedo reticularis (gray-blue skin discoloration with characteristic vascular network). Livedo reticularis may first present with exposure to the cold, but later may become a more permanent finding. Frequently it begins on the arms and legs, but it can also spread to the torso. Livedo reticularis may occur secondary to vascular disease such as periarteritis nodosa or systemic lupus erythematous.

**Figure 34 Cutis Marmorata Telangiectasia Congenital:** Congenital cutis marmorata telangiectasia (congenital livedo reticularis) in a 6-week-old girl. Dilated superficial capillaries and veins were noted from birth. The skin appears as a reticulated network with white insulae. The constantly visible light red marking of the skin increased with crying and became livid with cooling. The affected skin seemed thinner than normal due to a deficiency of subcutaneous fat. These skin changes were found predominantly on the legs, face, and back.

Congenital livedo reticularis usually persists throughout life, but may improve with increasing age. Some patients will develop small areas of superficial ulceration. Nevi araneous (p 138) and angiokeratomas can also be present.

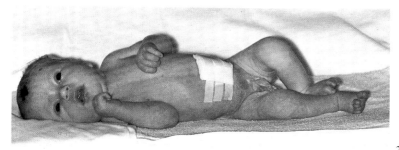

31

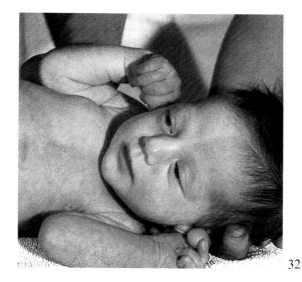

32

3

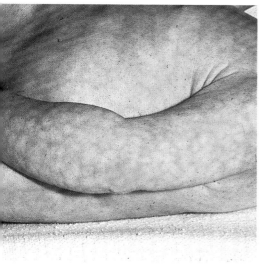

34

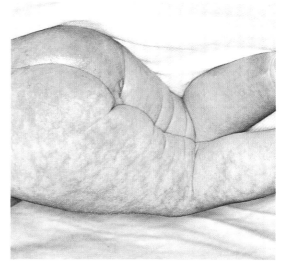

21

# 1. Diseases of the Newborn

**Figure 35  Cavernous Hemangioma:**  Cavernous hemangioma (strawberry nevus) in a 5-month-old gir
The soft, spherical, compressible growth was noted over the right parietal bone, measuring 3 × 4 cm. Th
mass was reddish-blue in color and nonpainful. Radiograph demonstrated normal cranial bones underneat
the lesion. By age 4 years the hemangioma had spontaneously disappeared.

The vast majority (90 percent) of cavernous hemangiomas are noted within the first month of life; th
remainder develop within the first 9 months. They may go through a growth phase during the first 6 t
9 months, but then will begin a period of involution by 1 to 2 years. After 5 years, 50 percent have involu
ed; after 7 years 70 percent disappear. During the growth phase, complications may occur if the hemangi
ma impinges on vital structures. Larger lesions can cause thrombocytopenia and hemorrhag
(Kasabach-Merritt syndrome). Steroids may be used to induce involution.

### Reference

1.  Finn ML, et al. Congenital vascular lesions: clinical application of a new classification. J Pediatr Surg 18:894, 1983

**Figure 36  Congenital Dermoid Cyst:**  Two-day-old newborn with a cystic growth in the midline of th
head over the parietal bone. The lesion was notable for the localized reddening of the surrounding sca
and a central tuft of hair. The mass grew slowly over a two week period and required surgical remova
Histologic examination revealed a cyst comprised of an outer surface of squamous epithelium and containi
hair, fatty material, and keratin. Dermoid cysts usually develop from sequestered cells in embryonic rest
Dermoid cysts are most common in the area of the eyes, nose, mouth, or neck.

Differential diagnosis includes meningoencephaloceles. These lesions are associated with an underlyi
bony defect and as a rule are pulsatile.

**Figure 37  Cutis Aplasia:**  Congenital cutis aplasia in an 8-month-old boy. At birth, the child had a sha
ply delineated solitary skin defect with granulation tissue. The lesion crusted and healed within a few week
leaving an oval, hairless, atrophic gray scar (1 × 2 cm) located at the vertex, displaced from the midlin
No other malformations were noted. Trisomy 13 (Patau's syndrome, p 58) was ruled out.

Differential diagnosis includes traumatic skin lesion from the birth process (forceps marks). Other po
sibilities include nevus sebaceous (p 140, 144) and certain forms of alopecia including oculomand
bulofacial syndrome (abnormal cranium, microphthalmia, cataracts, micrognathia).

**Figure 38  Scalp Abscess:**  Abscess of the parieto-occipital scalp in an 8-day-old prematurely born i
fant. The infant was delivered by cesarean section after prolonged rupture of membranes and maternal an
nionitis. The abscess was successfully treated by surgical incision and drainage followed by antibiotic therap
Skin abrasions caused by forceps marks or scalp electrodes for fetal monitoring may often be the site
similar lesions. The parietal area is a frequent site for scalp abscesses, and often these lesions are bilatera
The infection is usually caused by staphylococcus.

### Reference

1.  Balfour MM, et al. Scalp abscesses following fetal blood sampling or monitoring. J Pediatr 79:344, 1971.

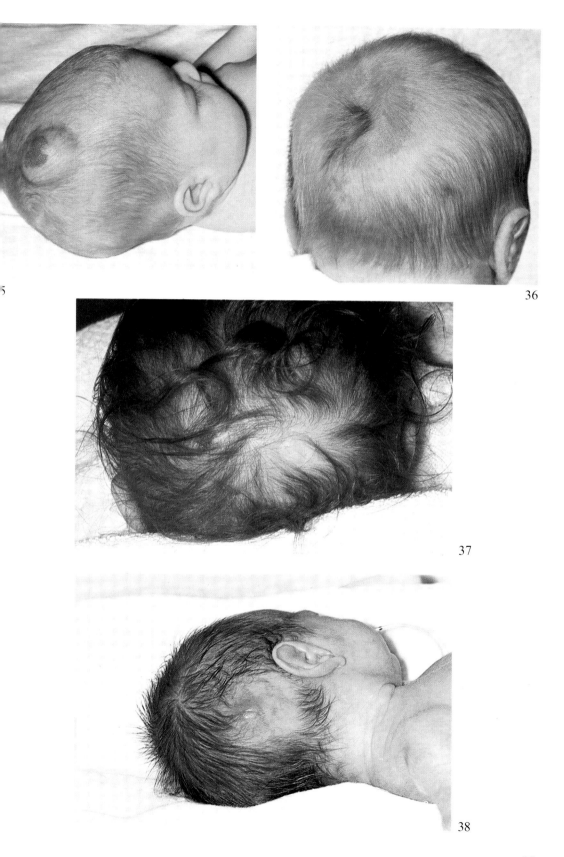

35

36

37

38

# 1. Diseases of the Newborn

**Figure 39  Milia:**  Numerous tiny, yellow papules on both sides of the cheeks, as well as the nose, upper lip, and chin of a 7-day-old boy. Milia are small, superficial inclusion cysts containing keratin. They occur in 40 percent of all newborns. In addition to the face, milia may be found over the upper body and limbs but seldom on the genitals. They disappear by the third or fourth week. Persistent and numerous milia may be seen in orofacial-digital syndrome Type 1 (cleft palate, flat midface, brachydactyly).

**Figure 40  Mongolian Spot:**  Mongolian spots in a 6-month-old Korean girl. Several oval, poorly defined gray-blue pigmented spots of varying size were noted in the lumbosacral area. Mongolian spots occur relatively frequently in Oriental and African infants (80 percent), while the frequency in the European Caucasian population is only 1 to 5 percent. They are usually located on the flanks and shoulders and fade during childhood. They seldom persist into adulthood. Unlike mongolian spots, the blue nevus (p 144) is slightly raised, is located on the arms, legs or face, and lasts throughout life.

### Reference

1.  Cordova A. The mongolian spot: a study of ethnic differences and a literature review. Clin Pediatr 20:714, 1981.

**Figure 41  Erythema Toxicum:**  Erythema toxicum in a 1-day-old girl. Numerous, irregularly defined erythematous areas (0.5 to 3.0 cm in diameter) were noted over the torso as well as the arms and legs. With pressure, the erythema faded and the underlying skin appeared slightly thickened. After a few hours, the rash could no longer be detected.
  The cause of erythema toxicum is unknown. Erythema toxicum is relatively frequent in full term infants, but seldom seen in prematures infants. The rash may be present at birth, but usually begins on the first or second day of life and is rarely seen after the 14th day of life. In more severe cases, the erythema evolves into a papular, vesicular exanthem. The rash will usually disappear within 2-4 days.

**Figure 42  Erythema Toxicum:**  Erythema toxicum in a 2-day-old full term girl. Small vesicles and pustules on an erythematous base were noted over the torso and the extremities, but spared the palms of the hand and soles of the feet. Wright stain of the contents of the vesicles demonstrated eosinophils and no bacteria.

**Differential Diagnosis:**  Staphylococcal skin infection can be ruled out. In staphylococcal infections, neutrophils and bacteria may be demonstrated in the pustule. Miliaria crystallina (caused by superficial blockage of the secretory ducts of sweat glands) could be confused with erythema toxicum. Miliaria crystallina can be recognized by characteristic tiny diaphanous retention "cysts" which can easily be wiped away. Miliaria rubra (caused by deeper blockage of the sweat gland ducts) is associated with red "pinhead" sized papules over the torso which are pruritic and somewhat painful. Candidal skin infections may be acquired congenitally from ascending maternal colonization or infection. In generalized cutaneous candidiasis, a scaly erythematous rash as well small pustules are noted on an erythematous base. The palms and soles are also affected. Candida albicans is detected microscopically or through culture. If systemic disease is present, the disease is usually fatal.

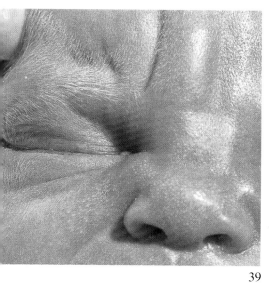

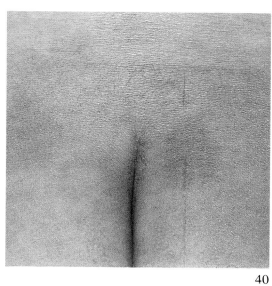

39

40

41

42

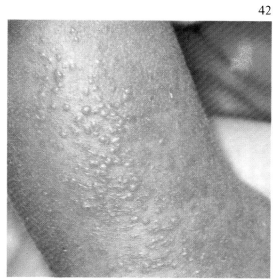

# 1.  Diseases of the Newborn

**Figure 43  Congenital Syphilis:**  Three-week-old girl with diffuse erythematous maculopapular rash over the soles of her feet and legs due to congenital syphilis. The rash was also noted on the torso, arms, and palms of the hands. Areas of the rash were consistent with a bullous eruption. Hepatosplenomegaly was noted. Serologic testing was positive for syphilis in both the mother and child. The infant was treated with penicillin G for 2 weeks.

**Differential Diagnosis:**  Since the appearance of the rash in congenital syphilis can be extremely variable, many different skin diseases must be ruled out including bullous impetigo, pemphigoid, exfoliative dermatitis, dermatitis herpetiformis, epidermolysis bullosa, intercontinentia pigmenti syndrome, urticaria pigmentosa, acrodermatitis enteropathica and congenital bullous ichthyosiform erythroderma.

### References

1.  Esterly NB, Solomon LM. Neonatal dermatology II. The blistering and scaling dermatoses. J Pediatr 77:1075, 1970.
2.  Oppenheimer EH, et al. Congenital syphilis in the newborn infant: clinical and pathological observations in recent cases. Johns Hopkins Med J 129:63, 1971.

**Figure 44  Congenital Syphilis:**  Six-week-old child with an erythematous rash which formed vesicles and bullae on the toes and the soles of feet. The infant had no other symptoms except serous coryza (snuffles). The mother was not tested during her pregnancy, but subsequent serologic testing was positive in both the mother and child. The child was successfully treated with penicillin G.

**Differential Diagnosis:**  Syphilic dactylitis (osteochondritis of the hand) must be differentiated from tuberculous dactylitis, dactylitis associated with sickle cell anemia or coccidioidomycosis as well as distal dactylitis with blister formation due to streptococcal infection.

**Figure 45  Congenital Syphilis:**  Although asymptomatic at birth, this 4-week-old girl slowly developed hepatomegaly and direct hyperbilirubinemia. Radiographs demonstrated typical bony changes (an area of periosteal calcification at the tibial diaphysis and a translucent band under the metaphyseal plate).

**Differential Diagnosis:**  Hepatomegaly and direct hyperbilirubinemia occur in biliary atresia, choledochal cysts, other prenatal or postnatal infections, galactosemia, and alpha$_1$-antitrypsin deficiency.

**Figure 46  Congenital Syphilis:**  Fifteen-year-old girl with abnormal dentition. The teeth had the typical changes associated with congenital syphilis (Hutchinson's teeth, barrel shaped upper incisors with halfmoon shaped indentations due to a defect in the enamel). The girl also had defective hearing and chorioretinitis. The diagnosis of congenital syphilis was not recognized until the girl was 13. After serologic confirmation the girl was treated with penicillin G for 15 days.

**Differential Diagnosis:**  Tooth anomalies are present in:
1.  Ectodermal dysplasia
2.  Intercontinentia pigmenti
3.  Cleidocranial dysplasia (Scheuthauer-Marie-Sainton syndrome)

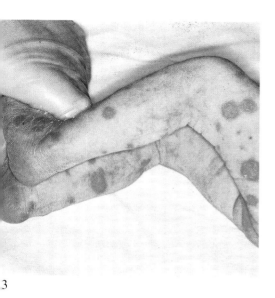

3

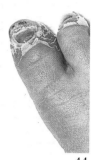
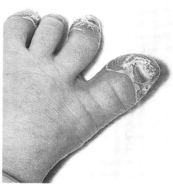

44

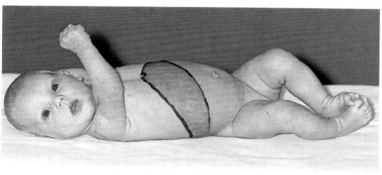

45

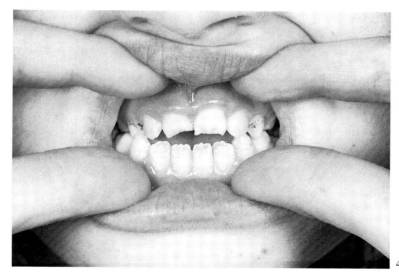

46

# 2. Congenital Anomalies

**Figure 47  Brachycephaly:**  Flattening of the occiput (brachycephaly) in a 3-week-old boy with Down syndrome. Brachycephaly also occurs in Brachmann-de Lange Syndrome, hypochondroplasia, cleidocranial dysplasia, Apert's syndrome, Carpenter's syndrome, or other clinical situations where there is premature closure of the coronal suture.

**Figure 48  Apert's Syndrome:**  Apert's syndrome (acrocephalosyndactyly) in a 5-day-old newborn. Physical findings included turribrachycephaly (due to bilateral congenital coronal craniosynostosis) and facial dysmorphism (protruding forehead, small nose, maxillary hypoplasia, high arched palate). Soft tissue syndactyly of both the hands and feet was noted. Osseous syndactyly of the 3rd and 4th phalanges was demonstrated radiographically. No other anomalies were noted. The child underwent early operative treatment even though there were no symptoms of increased intracranial pressure. Surgical correction of the syndactyly began at 6 months of age. Although mental retardation may be frequent, mental development was normal in this case. Apert's syndrome follows an autosomal dominant pattern of inheritance. The parents of this child are unaffected, therefore this case was due to a new mutation. Acrocephaly (turricephaly) also occurs in:
1. Other acrocephalosyndactylic syndromes such as Saethre-Chotzen syndrome, Oral-Facial-Digital syndrome Type II (Mohr's syndrome), and Pfeiffer's syndrome.
2. Acrocephalopolysyndactylic syndromes such as Carpenter's syndrome.
3. Crouzon's syndrome (craniofacial dysostosis) associated with craniosynostosis, midface hypoplasia and exophthalmos.

**Figure 49  Microcephaly:**  Congenital microcephaly in a 6-month-old boy. The cranium was small (OFC 39 cm), the fontanel closed, and the ears low set. The child had convergent strabismus. This child was severely mentally deficient. The underlying cause of the microcephaly was unclear.

Congenital microcephaly occurs with intrauterine infections (rubella, toxoplasmosis, cytomegalovirus), with chromosomal abnormalities (such as cri du chat syndrome, Wolf-Hirschhorn syndrome, trisomy 13), with toxic drug effects (fetal alcohol syndrome, fetal aminopterin syndrome), and with Fanconi pancytopenia syndrome.

**Figure 50  Anencephaly:**  A 6-day-old newborn with anencephaly (just prior to death). The infant had a major congenital skull and CNS defect including the absence of the skull bones, cranial vault, and incomplete development of the brain. Facial features include protruding eyes and prominent nose. Malformation of other organs may occur including adrenal hypoplasia, and genitourinary abnormalities. Children with anencephaly are frequently stillborn or die within a few days after birth.

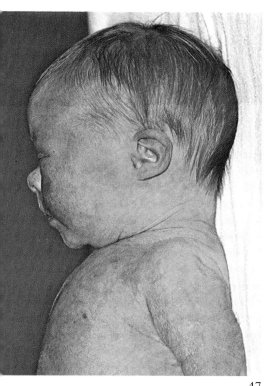

47

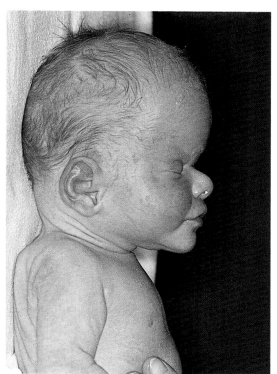

48

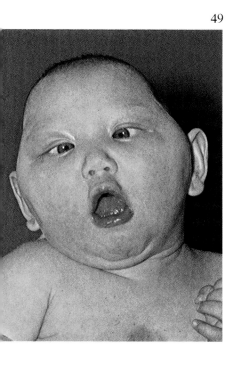

49

50

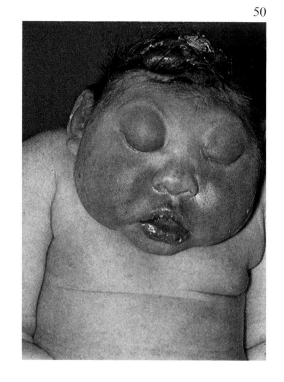

# 2. Congenital Anomalies

**Figure 51** **Cleft Lip and Palate:** Complete unilateral cleft lip, alveolar process and palate in a 1-week-old newborn. The nose was flattened and the right nostril shifted laterally. Cleft palate occurs when the lateral palatine process fails to fuse with either the median palatine process, the nasal septum or the primary palate. Because of difficulties with feeding, gavage feedings were initially used. After the infant was seven weeks old, bottle feeding was possible. In the second week of life, the infant developed acute otitis media, a frequent complication of cleft lip and palate. Other complications include failure to thrive, pneumonia due to milk aspiration, recurrent otitis media, abnormal dentition requiring orthodontic procedures, and problems with speech.

**Figure 52** **Cleft Lip:** Incomplete unilateral cleft lip in a 4-week-old boy. The upper lip was indented to the left of the philtrum, but the defect did not extend into the alveolar process or palate. Defects are described as "complete" if the cleft reaches the nostril on the affected side. Unilateral cleft lip occurs when the maxillary process on the affected side fails to merge with the medial nasal elevations. Cleft lip may occur in conjunction with clefts of the alveolar process or palate. Isolated cleft palate (either the soft palate, hard palate, or both) occurs more frequently in females and is frequently associated with other abnormalities. Isolated cleft palate is a frequent finding in the Robin sequence.

## Reference

1. Hanson JW, Smith DW. U-shaped palatal defect in the Robin anomalad: developmental and clinical relevance. J Pediat 87:30, 1975.

**Figures 53 and 54** **Cleft Lip, Alveolar Process and Palate:** Child with complete unilateral cleft lip, alveolar process and palate seen before (Figure 53, age 4 months) and after (Figure 54, age 8 months) corrective surgery. Cleft lip and alveolar process with or without cleft palate occurs in approximately 1:1,000 births and is more frequent in males. Cleft lip and palate occur in conjunction with many syndromes including trisomy 13 (Patau's syndrome), trisomy 18 (Edwards' syndrome), Wolf-Hirschhorn syndrome (partial deletion of the short arm of chromosome 4), cri du chat syndrome (partial loss of the short arm of chromosome 5) and certain of the ectodermal dysplasia syndromes including ectrodactyly-ectodermal dysplasia-clefting syndrome (EEC syndrome).

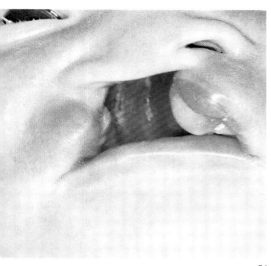

51

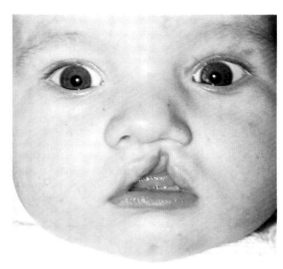

52

53

54

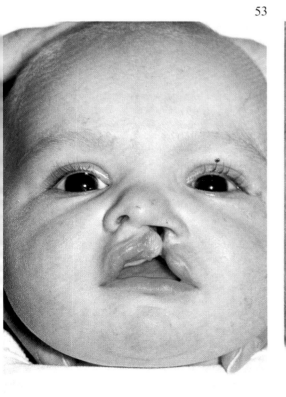

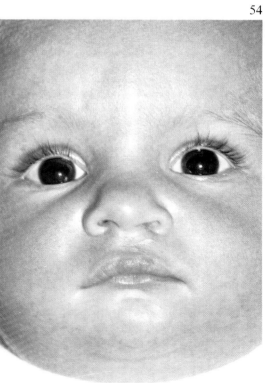

# 2. Congenital Anomalies

**Figure 55 Lateral Cleft:** Congenital lateral or transverse facial cleft of the mouth in a 2-week-old boy. The asymmetrical mouth with the right lateral cleft is due to malformation of the mandibular arch (failure of the lateral maxillary and mandibular processes to merge). The defect may be unilateral or bilateral and is associated with deformities of the outer ear, hypoplasia of the mandible or maxilla and median cleft palate.

**Figure 56 Oblique Facial Cleft:** Four-week-old boy with a unilateral (left) oblique facial cleft or orbitofacial fissure extending from the left upper lip to the medial aspect of the orbit. Oblique facial clefts are often bilateral and may involve the orbit, leading to colobomas or microphthalmia. The deformity may involve the nose, the tear ducts, the ears or the central nervous system. Surgical correction may involve several stages.

**Figure 57 Ankyloglossia:** A 4-week-old boy with ankyloglossia (tongue tie). The lingual frenulum is shortened and lies close to the tip of the tongue. Movement of the tongue may be limited. Generally, this anomaly is of no pathologic importance. Surgery, if necessary, should not be performed before the child is 8 months old.

**Figure 58 Microstomy:** Two-week-old girl with microstomy (small mouth). Congenital microstomy is due to excessive merging of the maxillary and mandibular processes of the mandibular arch. In this case, microstomy was an isolated finding. Congenital microstomy is seen in Ruvalcaba's syndrome, Hallermann-Streiff syndrome, and craniocarpotarsal dysplasia. Acquired microstomy may occur in older children with progressive scleroderma (as a result of hardening and shrinking of the skin surrounding the mouth).

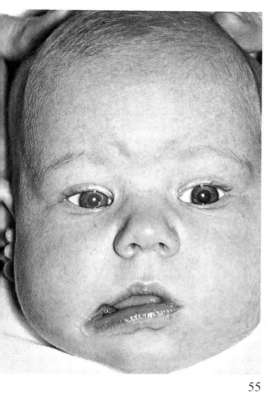

55

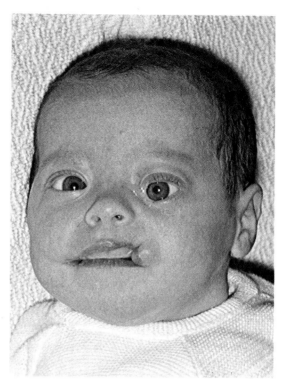

56

57

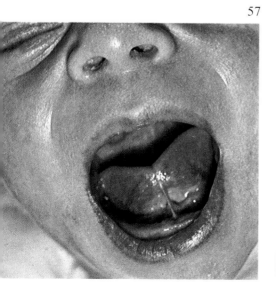

58

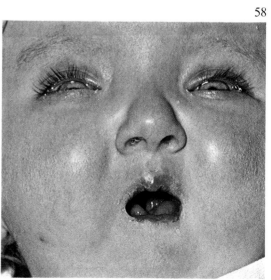

# 2. Congenital Anomalies

**Figure 59  Exophthalmos:**  Unilateral exophthalmos due to a retrobulbar cavernous hemangioma in a 5-month-old girl. In the few weeks prior to presentation, the parents noted enlargement, prominence and limited motion of the right eyeball. Sonography and computerized tomography were used to locate the tumor. Because of imminent danger to the optic nerve, the retrobulbar hemangioma was removed surgically using a transfrontal approach.

## Differential Diagnosis of Unilateral (or Bilateral) Exophthalmos Includes:
1.  Intraorbital tumors such as rhabdomyosarcoma, metastatic neuroblastoma, dermoid cyst, teratoma, glioma of the optic chiasm, intraorbital glioma, orbital cyst, leukemia.
2.  Inflammatory processes such as orbital cellulitis, thrombophlebitis.
3.  Malformations such as anterior meningocele or encephalocele, and vascular anomalies.
4.  Trauma leading to basilar skin fracture, fracture of the orbital wall, and retroorbital hemorrhage.
5.  Orbital pseudotumor (unilateral chronic inflammatory process amenable to steroid therapy).

### Reference
1.  Oakhill A, et al. Unilateral proptosis. Arch Dis Child 56:549, 1981.

**Figure 60  Torticollis:**  Congenital muscular torticollis in a 10-year-old girl. Shortening of the right sternocleidomastoid muscle caused the head to tilt toward the affected side and turn toward the opposite side. A rope-like hardening of the sternocleidomastoid muscle was noted. Over time, the face became increasingly asymmetrical. The cause of the torticollis, which has persisted since 1 year of age, was unknown. Unlike torticollis secondary to strabismus (ocular torticollis), correction by means of active or passive physical therapy was not possible; surgical release was required.

**Differential Diagnosis:**  Torticollis persisting from birth may be due to malformation of the cervical vertebra (e.g., with Klippel-Feil syndrome). Acquired torticollis may occur after fracture or dislocation of the cervical vertebrae, or in association with pharyngitis, cervical lymphadenitis, intraspinal tumors, and juvenile rheumatoid arthritis.

### References
1.  Ferkel RD, et al. Muscular torticollis. A modified surgical approach. J Bone Joint Surg 65A:894, 1983.
2.  Maxwell RE. Surgical management of torticollis. Post Grad Med 75:147, 1984.

**Figure 61  Facial Hemiatrophy:**  Five-year-old boy with atrophy of the right side of the face (absent subcutaneous tissue, musculature and bone). Atrophy developed gradually over the course of a year. Facial asymmetry was clearly evident when the boy opened his mouth. There was no sign of hyper- or hypopigmentation of the skin on the affected side of the face (Russell-Silver syndrome) or alopecia (Hallerman-Streiff syndrome). The cause in this case was unknown.

**Differential Diagnosis:**  Facial hemiatrophy occurs in conjunction with scleroderma (frontoparietal involvement "en coup de sabre," p 114) and with inflammation or traumatic injury to the mandible. Hemihypertrophy of half of the face or body persists from birth onward. Unilateral mandibular hypoplasia is easily ruled out.

**Figure 62  Hemihypertrophy:**  Left-sided hemihypertrophy in an 8-year-old girl. As an infant, she was incorrectly diagnosed as having congenital hip dislocation. From birth onward, enlargement of the entire left side of the body occurred, so that at the age of 8, the left leg was 4 cm longer than the right leg, the left arm was 2 cm longer than the right arm, the mass of the left side of the body was obviously greater, and a right convex scoliosis of the spine was noted. (Scoliosis can be corrected by use of orthopedic shoe which adjust for the discrepancy in leg length). Hemihypertrophy may be associated with aniridia, neoplasms, genitourinary abnormalities, hemangiomas, and nevi. In this girl, a cavernous hemangioma of the right upper lip and a small capillary hemangioma above the sacrum were noted; otherwise, no anomalies were detected.

**Differential Diagnosis:**  In Klippel-Trenaunay-Weber syndrome there is usually no true hemihypertrophy but localized hypertrophy of a limb or its parts. Angiography (to detect vascular anomalies which occur in Klippel-Trenaunay-Weber syndrome) was not performed in this case. Hemihypertrophy is found in Beckwith-Wiedemann syndrome (in about 15 percent of cases) and in Russell-Silver syndrome (skeletal asymmetry with prenatal growth disturbance, and abnormal sexual development).

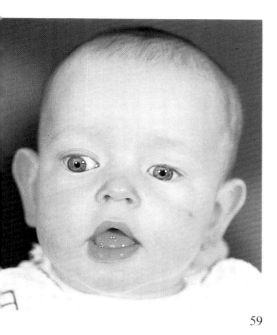

59

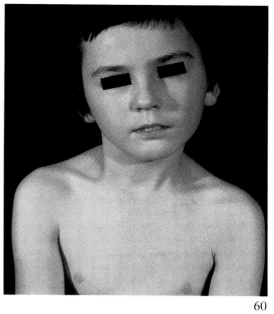

60

61

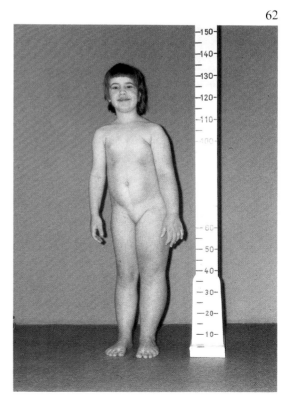

62

# 2. Congenital Anomalies

**Figures 63 and 64   Robin Anomaly (Pierre Robin Syndrome):**   Two-month-old boy with micrognathia (Figure 63, hypoplasia of the mandible) and glossoptosis (retraction of the tongue, which may lead to stridor and upper airway obstruction). No cleft palate was noted. The child had problems with upper airway obstruction; nutritional intake was poor, the child vomited frequently, and failed to grow appropriately. Due to respiratory difficulty, the child had to lie prone and be fed by a gavage tube. After several months, the problem improved due to growth of the mandible. In certain circumstances, the tongue tip may be sutured forward or tracheotomy may be required.

**Differential Diagnosis:**   Micrognathia and glossoptosis may be part of Smith-Theiler-Schachenmann syndrome (along with hypoplasia of tracheal cartilage) as well as hypoglossia-hypodactylia syndrome (in combination with limb anomalies). Micrognathia also occurs in conjuction with mandibulofacial dysostosis (see Figure 65), certain deletion syndromes (including cri du chat syndrome, Wolf-Hirschhorn syndrome, antimongolism 21q-), trisomy 18, Bloom syndrome (see p 38) and Brachmann-de Lange syndrome.

### Reference

1.   Lewis MB, Pashayan HM. Management of infants with Robin anomaly. Clin Pediatr 19:519, 1980.

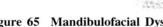

**Figure 65   Mandibulofacial Dysostosis (Treacher-Collins or Franceschetti-Klein Syndrome):**   Six-month-old child with mandibulofacial dysostosis. Findings included downward slanting palpebral fissures (antimongoloid), coloboma of the lower eyelid, hypoplastic malar bones, hypoplasia of the mandible, deformities of the auditory canal as well as conductive hearing loss. Other cases may include malformation of the outer and middle ear, large beak-like nose, micrognathia, and deformities of the eye. Intelligence is usually normal. Plastic or orthodontic surgery may improve appearance.

**Differential Diagnosis:**   Downward slanting palpebral fissures (so called "antimongolism") may be seen with partial deletion of the long arm of chromosome 21, with G-monosomy, and other syndromes including Coffin-Lowry syndrome, Soto's syndrome, and Apert's syndrome.

### Reference

1.   Herring SW, et al. Anatomical abnormalities in mandibulofacial dysostosis. Am J Med Genet 3:225, 1979.

**Figure 66   Potter Syndrome:**   Bilateral renal agenesis in a 2-day-old male infant. Birthweight was 2,100 g. Of note was the typical "Potter" facies: wrinkled facies (with a prominent skin fold extending from the inner corner of the eye laterally to the cheek), wide set eyes, beak-like nose, and low-set dysplastic ears. Oligohydramnios (decreased amniotic fluid) was noted at birth, and the infant was anuric until he expired on the second day of life. The autopsy demonstrated bilateral renal agenesis with agenesis of the ureters, a rudimentary bladder, and bilateral pulmonary hypoplasia, confirming the diagnosis of Potter syndrome. No anomalies of the spine or lower extremities were noted.

**Differential Diagnosis:**   Physical findings virtually identical to those seen in bilateral renal agenesis may occur in any situation where amiotic fluid is severely decreased (oligohydramnios sequence).

### Reference

1.   Thomas IT, Smith DW. Oligohydramnios, causes of the non-renal features of Potter's syndrome, including pulmonary hypoplasia. J Pediatr 84:811, 1974.

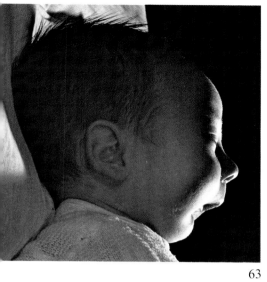

63

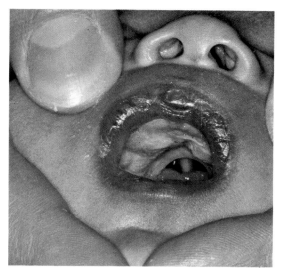

64

65

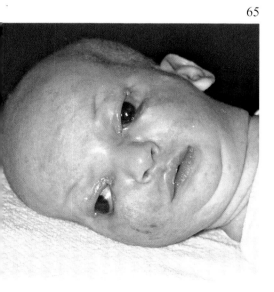

66

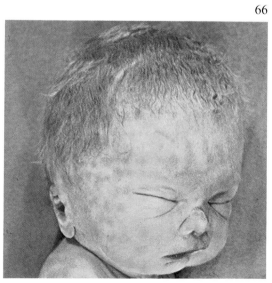

# 2. Congenital Anomalies

**Figure 67  William's Syndrome:**  William's syndrome (idiopathic hypercalcemia syndrome) in a 10-month old mentally retarded child. Findings included "elfin facies" (full cheeks, slightly upturned nose, depressed nasal bridge, long philtrum, prominent lips) and growth deficiency. Postnatal growth was poor due to anorexia and obstipation. Microcephaly (OFC 29 cm) and muscular hypotonia were noted. Metabolic abnormalities included hypercalcemia, decreased serum alkaline phosphatase and decreased renal function (elevated BUN, decreased creatinine clearance). Cardiac catheterization demonstrated supravalvular aortic stenosis. Clinical and laboratory improvement was noted after one year on a low calcium diet.

1.  Aarskog D, et al. Vitamin D metabolism in idiopathic infantile hypercalcemia. Am J Dis Child 135:1021, 1981.

**Figure 68  Brachmann-de Lange Syndrome:**  Brachmann-de Lange syndrome in a 15-year-old girl. Mental retardation was noted since early childhood and epilepsy was diagnosed since age 5. The child had the typical face seen in Brachmann-de Lange syndrome; synophrys, downward slanting palpebral fissures, low hairline, long eyelashes, long philtrum, and down turning of the corners of the mouth. Other findings include microcephaly, mental retardation, and limb abnormalities (small hands and feet, short digits, single flexion creases, and limb reduction).

### Reference

1.  Opitl JM. The Brachmann-DeLange syndrome. Am J Med Genet 22:89, 1985.

**Figure 69  Sturge-Weber Syndrome:**  Sturge-Weber syndrome (encephalotrigeminal angiomatosis) in a 4-month-old boy. Of note was a nevus flammeus (port wine nevus) on the left side of the face in the distribution of the trigeminal nerve (ophthalmic distribution). At 6 months of age, right-sided spastic hemiplegia was noted (contralateral to the hemangioma). Glaucoma may occur secondary to choroidal angioma, but intraocular pressure was normal in this case. Radiographs of the skull revealed unilateral, curvilinear, double contoured lines of calcification in the cerebral cortex. These radiographic findings are pathognomonic of Sturge-Weber syndrome.

### Reference

1.  Andriola M, Stolfi J. Sturge-Weber syndrome. Am J Dis Child 123:507, 1972.

**Figure 70  Bloom's Syndrome:**  Bloom's syndrome in a 7-year-old girl. Findings included telangiectatic erythematous lesions in a butterfly-shaped distribution over the face (noted since 1 year of age). Lesions were also noted on the volar surface of the arm. The rash was photosensitive; sunlight intensified the erythema causing blister formation particularly on the eyelids or mouth. Short stature and dolichocephaly were present; intelligence was normal. The syndrome is an autosomal recessive trait causing defective chromosomal repair (increased exchange in homologous chromatids). Parents and siblings were unaffected.

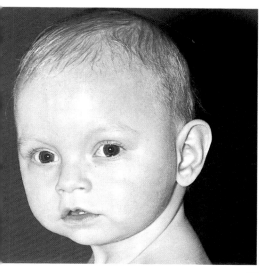

67

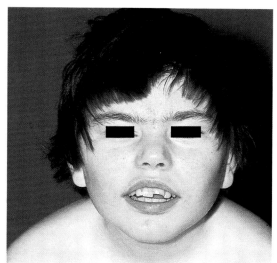

68

69

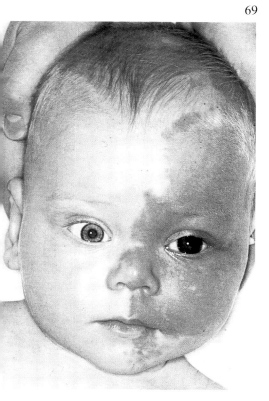

70

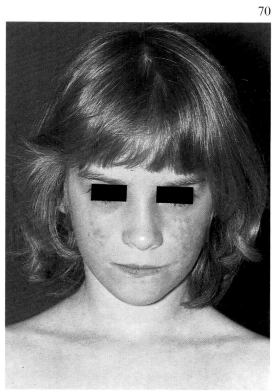

# 2. Congenital Anomalies

**Figure 71  Talipes Equinovarus:**  Bilateral congenital clubfoot (talipes equinovarus) in a 3-month-old boy. Findings included inversion and adduction of the forefoot, inversion of the heel, and plantar flexion of the foot. The foot cannot be dorsiflexed to the neutral position and the heel is fixed in the varus deformity. Congenital clubfoot is a structural deformity which has a familial predisposition and occurs more often in male children. The skeletal changes observed radiographically occur because of medial and plantar deviation of the anterior talus. Clubfoot is associated with congenital hip dysplasia, spina bifida, as well as other neuromuscular conditions. Early treatment is warranted in cases of talipes equinovarus. Conservative management consists of manipulation and casting; if not successful, surgical treatment is necessary.

**Differential Diagnosis:**  Talipes equinovarus must be differentiated from talipes calcaneovalgus and metatarsus varus (or metatarsus adductus). In the two latter conditions, the foot can be dorsiflexed and the heel is in valgus (when observed from behind). Both are considered positional defects.

### References

1.  Pokrassa MA, Rodgveller B. Talipes equinovarus: current concepts. J Am Podiatry Assoc 71:472, 1981.
2.  Wenger DR, Leach J. Foot deformities in infants and children. Pediatr Clin North Am 33(6):1411, 1986.

**Figure 72  Talipes Equinovarus:**  Talipes equinovarus (clubfoot) in a 2-day-old newborn with an open thoracolumbar meningomyelocele. The infant was paralyzed from the level of T8 downward, and had progressive hydrocephalus, as well as other malformations. No operative repair was performed. The child died at 2 months of age due to increased intracranial pressure. In spina bifida aperta (with meningomyelocele) neurologic defect may lead to paralysis of the lower limbs, dislocated hips and talipes equinovarus. Without treatment, increasing deformity may occur. Specific therapy for clubfoot may be conservative (braces or support devices) or operative (tendon release or transfer, arthrodesis, or osteotomy).

**Figure 73  Pes Cavus:**  High arched foot (pes cavus) and claw-like big toe in an 8-year-old girl with progressive neuromuscular atrophy associated with Charcot-Marie-Tooth disease. This motor neuropathy first became noticeable when the child developed an abnormal gait and progressive muscle wasting of the lower legs. The child's mother and aunt both suffered from the disease, which is inherited as an autosomal dominant. The diagnosis was confirmed by electromyography (demonstrating decreased nerve conduction velocity) and muscle biopsy.

**Differential Diagnosis:**  The development of pes cavus may be seen in other neurologic disorders including Friedreich's ataxia.

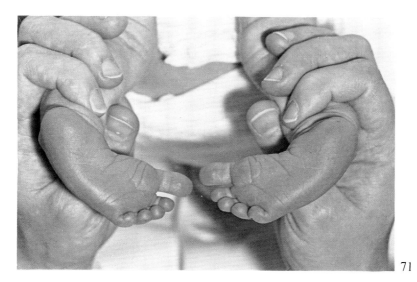

71

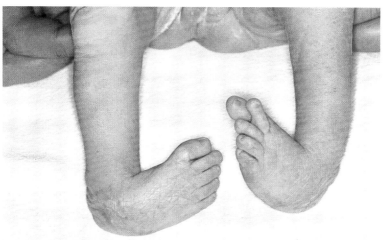

72

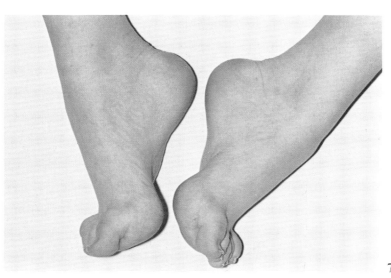

73

# 2. Congenital Anomalies

**Figure 74  Polydactyly:**  Polydactyly (specifically, hexadactyly) with cutaneous syndactyly of the foot in a 6-month-old girl. The fifth and sixth toes of the left foot were shortened and joined by connective tissue and skin. There was also cutaneous syndactyly of the third and fourth fingers of the left hand. The cause in this case was not clear.

**Differential Diagnosis:**  Polydactyly is relatively frequent and may occur in conjunction with a number of syndromes, including the short rib-polydactyly syndromes (chondroectodermal dysplasia or Ellis-van Creveld's syndrome), Bardet-Biedl syndrome, Goltz's syndrome, and trisomy 13. The extra digit may be complete or incomplete (with or without bony structures).

**Figure 75  Amniotic Band Disruption Complex:**  Autoamputation and furrows of the fingers in a 1-day-old newborn. These findings probably originated during fetal development due to amniotic bands. Cutaneous syndactyly developed between the second and third finger. The infant died at 2 days of age due to other severe malformations.

Amniotic bands may cause major disruptions in the newborn that lead to defects in the extremities (constriction or amputation) or to craniofacial disruption. Disruption from amniotic bands may be differentiated from genetic causes of craniofacial or limb anomalies by the lack of symmetry of these lesions.

### References

1. Higginbottom MC, et al. The amniotic band disruption complex: timing of amniotic rupture and variable spectra of consequent defects. J Pediatr 95:544, 1979.
2. Jones KL, et al. A pattern of craniofacial and limb defects secondary to aberrant tissue bands. J Pediatr 84:90, 1974.

**Figure 76  Osteogenesis Imperfecta:**  Osteogenesis imperfecta in a 4-week-old boy. Findings included shortened, deformed upper and lower extremities (due to multiple fractures of the long bones), impressionable cranial bones and blue sclera. Radiographic studies revealed deformities of long bones due to multiple fractures, generalized osteopenia, and thinning of the calvarium. This is an example of one of the congenital osteogenesis imperfecta syndromes, in which collagen synthesis is disturbed leading to imperfect formation and calcification of bone.

### Reference

1. Sillence DO, et al. Clinical heterogeneity in osteogenesis imperfecta. J Med Genet 16:101, 1979.

**Figure 77  Klippel-Trenaunay-Weber Syndrome:**  Klippel-Trenaunay-Weber syndrome (unilateral enlargement of an extremity associated with vascular anomalies) in a 2-month-old boy. Findings included gigantism of the entire right leg, associated with capillary hemangioma on the back (confined to the left side, stopping at the midline), and varicosities of the left leg (not shown). Differences in the length of the long bones of the leg was evident radiographically. Follow-up examination at age 10 years demonstrated continued leg length discrepancy (3 cm difference). In order to prevent scoliosis, special shoes (to compensate for the discrepancy in leg length) were recommended.

### Reference

1. Kuffer FR, et al. Klippel-Trenaunay syndrome, visceral angiomatosis and thrombocytopenia. J Pediatr Surg 3:65, 1968.

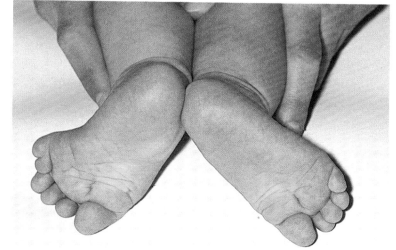

74

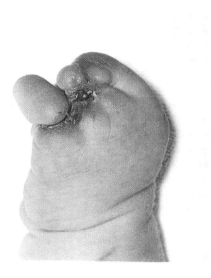

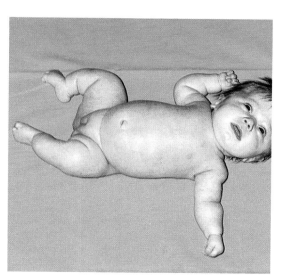

76

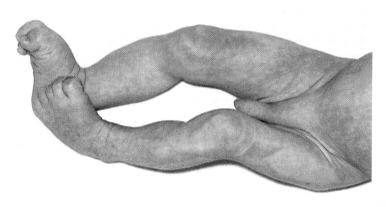

77

# 2. Congenital Anomalies

**Figures 78–80 Fanconi's Pancytopenia Syndrome:** Fanconi's pancytopenia syndrome in a 3-year-old boy. The child had multiple congenital anomalies including hypoplastic thumbs, hypoplastic radius, hypogenitalism, microsomia, microcephaly, and abnormally dark skin pigmentation. Laboratory investigations revealed pancytopenia (anemia, neutropenia, and thrombocytopenia), evidence of chromosomal breaks and elevated fetal hemoglobin (Hb F). Radiologic examinations demonstrated bilateral radial hypoplasia with absence of the first metacarpal. Bone marrow failure leading to pancytopenia typically appears after age 7 years.

**Differential Diagnosis:** Hypoplasia or aplasia of the radius or thumb also occurs in conjunction with:
1. Thrombocytopenia absent radius syndrome
2. Aase's syndrome (hypoplastic anemia-triphalangeal thumb syndrome)
3. Holt-Oram syndrome (with atrial or ventricular septal defect)
4. Nager's syndrome (acrofacial dysostosis)
5. VATER association (associated with vertebral, gastrointestinal or renal anomalies)
6. Thalidomide embryopathy

Hypogenitalism (hypoplasia of the external genitalia) is also seen in Laurence-Moon-Biedel's syndrome, Prader-Willi syndrome, Fröhlich's syndrome, Klinefelter's syndrome, Smith-Lemli-Opitz's syndrome, Leopard's syndrome (multiple lentigines syndrome), and hypophyseal dwarfism.

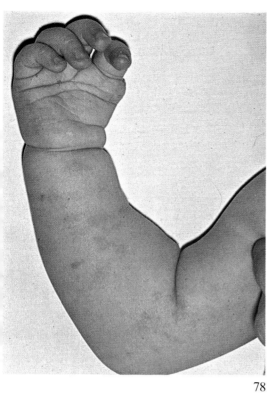

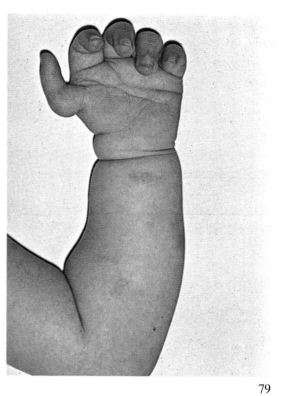

78

79

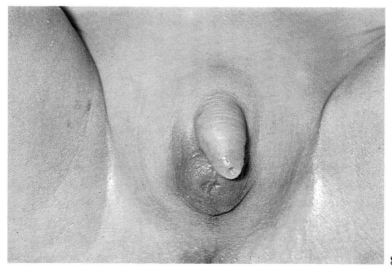

80

# 2. Congenital Anomalies

**Figure 81  Smith-Lemli-Opitz Syndrome:**  Smith-Lemli-Opitz syndrome in a 1-year-old boy. Findings included osseous and cutaneous syndactyly of the third and fourth fingers of the left hand. Further features typical of this syndrome included microcephaly, facial dysmorphism (ptosis, broad upturned nose, and low-set ears), hypogenitalism (hypospadias, cryptorchidism), and severe mental retardation. Other malformations of the hand may include single palmar crease, brachydactyly, clinodactyly, and polydactyly (particularly ulnar hexadactyly). Syndactyly occurs frequently in conjunction with other syndromes including:
1. Apert's syndrome (acrocephalosyndactyly)
2. Carpenter's syndrome (acrocephalopolysyndactyly)
3. Poland anomaly (with ipsilateral aplasia of the pectoralis muscle)
4. Oculodentoosseous dysplasia (with microphthalmia, abnormal tooth enamel)
5. Cryptophthalmos syndrome

## Reference

1. Cherstvos ED, et al. The pathological anatomy of the Smith-Lemli-Optiz syndrome. Clin Genet 7:382, 1975.

**Figure 82  Clubhand:**  Clubhand in a 3-year-old child. Of note was the absence of the radius and thumb of the right forearm and hand; the left forearm was also shortened due to an ulnar defect, and movement at the elbow joint was restricted.

    Clubhand may be a unilateral or bilateral defect, and may be seen as an isolated finding or in combination with other anomalies (cleft lip and palate, costal or vertebral defects) or in certain syndromes (p 44, 50) Different conservative and operative procedures have been developed which must be carried out in a timely fashion if function is to be preserved.

**Figure 83  Amniotic Band Disruption Complex:**  Bilateral amputation of the distal fingers and toes in a 12-day-old child. Of note were partial ring shaped indentations and cutaneous syndactyly. These findings suggest that amniotic bands caused intrauterine amputation of the distal fingers and toes. The child had no other deformities and had full normal mental development. Surgical treatment to correct the syndactyly was needed in order to improve function of the hands. For references see Figure 75.

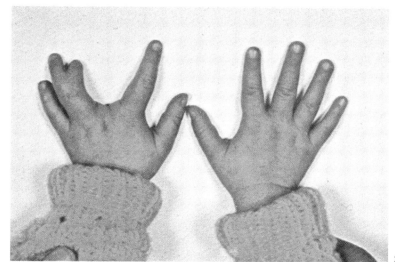

81

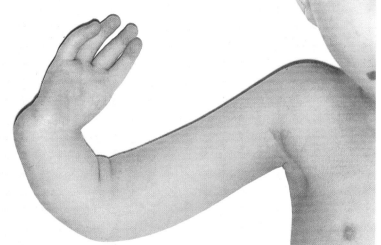

82

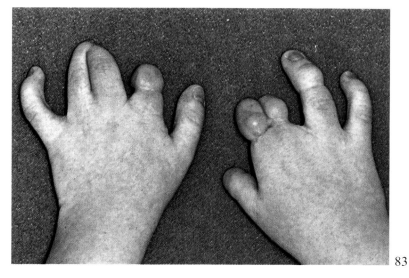

83

# 2.   Congenital Anomalies

**Figure 84   Phocomelia:**   Complete phocomelia in a 2-week-old newborn. The infant had a severe limb defect in which both arms were absent bilaterally (the hands emerged directly from the torso). Malformation of both hands was also noted (three phalangeal bones and three metacarpal bones only). The remainder of the skeletal exam was normal and no further anomalies were noted. The cause of the deformities in this case was unknown. Phocomelia is a limb reduction defect in which there is concurrent lack of the humerus, radius, and ulna in the upper extemity, or absence of the femur, tibia, and fibula in the lower extremity. Sophisticated prosthetic devices are required if these children are to have a functional life. Phocomelia is seen in conjunction with thalidomide embryopathy.

**Figure 85   Partial Hemimelia (Peromelia):**   Partial hemimelia (congenital shortening of the limbs resembling amputation) in a 1-day-old new born. The forearms and hands, as well as the feet, are missing bilaterally. Sophisticated prosthetic devices were required.

**Figure 86   Amelia:**   Amelia (lack of the entire limb structure) in a 2-week-old newborn. The upper extremities were completely absent and both femurs were hypoplastic. The cause in this case was unknown. Extensive training to improve the grasping function of the foot, as well as an arm-hand prosthesis was required.

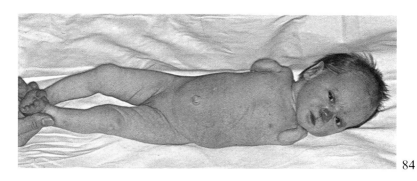

84

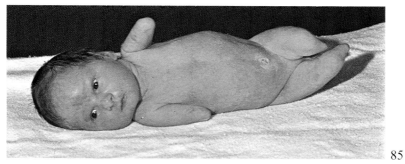

85

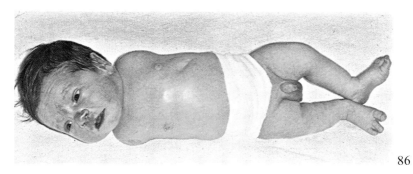

86

# 2. Congenital Anomalies

**Figure 87  Cutaneous Syndactyly:**  Partial unilateral cutaneous syndactyly of the fourth and fifth finger of the left hand in a two-month-old girl. This was the sole deformity in this case and surgical correctio was accomplished at 1 year of age.

In the event of osseous syndactyly, earlier operative repair would be advisable since persistence of th bony deformity can lead to secondary changes of the joints. Syndactyly is the most frequent form of han deformity. It is often bilateral and may be combined with polydactyly, brachydactyly, ring-shaped indentation or congenital finger amuptations. Syndactyly of the index and middle finger is more frequent than syndac yly of the fourth and fifth fingers. Severe syndactyly (total fusion) is seen in Apert's syndrome. Syndactyl also occurs with other syndromes (see p 46) including Poland's anomaly (unilateral syndactyly and ipsilater absence of the pectoralis major muscle).

**Figure 88  Club Hand:**  Six-month-old boy with bilateral clubhand. Of note was radial deviation of th hand, shortening of the forearm and hypoplasia of the thumb. Radiographs demonstrated partial absenc of the radius. No further anomalies were noted. Initially the hands and lower arms were placed in a brace After the child's first year of life, operative correction (involving repair in several stages) took place.

Clubhand can be either unilateral or bilateral, and stems from a complete or partial absence of th radius. Other bone or muscular anomalies are associated. Clubhand may be associated with cleft lip an palate, vertebral or costal anomalies, urogenital deformities, Franceschetti-Klein syndrome (see p 36), Fan coni's pancytopenia syndrome (see p 44), and thrombocytopenia (TAR syndrome).

**Figure 89  Polydactyly:**  Polydactyly (in this case, hexadactyly) in a 6-year-old girl. There was a hypoplasti sixth digit on the ulnar side of the left hand with partial syndactyly. This rudimentary finger was remove surgically. In polydactyly, the additional digit may consist solely of soft tissue, may contain bone, or ma be complete (including a metacarpal bone). The extra digit is usually found on either the radial or ulna side of the hand. Double thumb or triple phalangeal thumb may be seen. Polydactyly occurs with certai syndromes including Ellis-van Crefeld syndrome, Bardet-Beidl syndrome, Carpenter's syndrome, and tris my 13 or 18.

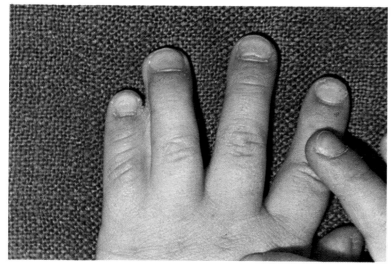

87

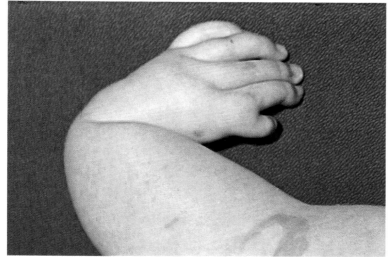

88

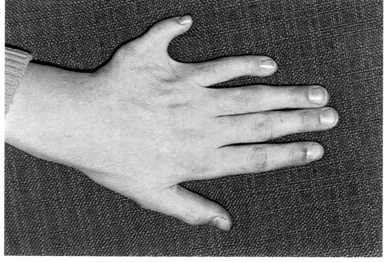

89

# 2. Congenital Anomalies

**Figure 90  Cleidocranial Dysostosis:**  Cleidocranial dysostosis in a 7-year-old girl. Findings included hang ing, narrow shoulders, narrow pectus, and abnormal shoulder movement due to the bilateral absence of the clavicles. The cranium was notable for frontal bossing and a large open fontanel. Skull radiograph demonstrated widening of the cranial sutures. In addition, the child had delayed ossification of the pubic bone. The hands had short distal phalanges and a long second metacarpal bone. Except for a minor gait problem, the child had no further disorders.

**Figure 91  Pectus Excavatum:**  Pectus excavatum in a 3-year-old boy. The lower third of the sternum is abnormally depressed. There is no obstruction to breathing. Operative correction of pectus excavatum is controversial and should be undertaken only if lung function is restricted. Pectus excavatum may occur in conjunction with Marfan's syndrome, homocystinuria, and Coffin-Lowry syndrome.

## Reference

1.  Pyerite RE and McKusick VA. The Marfan syndrome: diagnosis and management. N Engl J Med 300:772, 1979.

**Figure 92  Joint Contractures:**  Bilateral flexion contracture at the knee and hip with compensatory lordosis of the lumbar spine in a 5-year-old boy. These findings have been noted since the age of 1 year. The contrac tures are probably the result of cerebral palsy, specifically spastic diplegia. Other causes, such as neuromus cular disease or skeletal dysplasia, were ruled out.

Contractures in children with cerebral palsy are due to the predominantly flexed posture assumed b these children. Treatment involves intensive physical therapy with stretching exercises and operative cor rection if necessary.

## Reference

1.  Diamond M. Rehabilitation strategies for the child with cerebral palsy. Pediatr Ann 15:320, 1986.

**Figure 93  Congenital Hip Subluxation:**  Bilateral congenital hip subluxation in a 9-year-old boy. The child walked with a waddling gait and was noted to have severe lordosis of the lumbar spine. Subluxation of the hip was unfortunately identified late in this case. Therapy should be instituted as soon as possible Therapy may consist of either conservative (casting) or operative measures to correct the subluxation and osseous malformation.

**Figure 94  Hemihypertrophy:**  Hemihypertrophy (partial gigantism) of the left leg of a 9-year-old girl The girl was treated for a seizure disorder and mental retardation (due to encephalopathy). On physical examination, the left leg was 2 cm longer, the pelvic stance was slanted, and scoliosis of the lumbar spine was noted. There were no nevi or other vascular abnormalities. Funduscopic examination of the eye was normal. No Wilms' tumor could be detected. The discrepancy in leg length was treated with appropriate orthopedic shoes.

**Differential Diagnosis:**  Partial gigantism may have the following causes:
1.  Congenital malformations such as congenital hip subluxation and other skeletal diseases.
2.  Specific syndromes such as Klippel-Trenaunay-Weber syndrome or Beckwith-Wiedemann syndrome
3.  Infections such as osteomyelitis.
4.  Arthritic processes (juvenile rheumatoid arthritis)
5.  Trauma such as fracture or damage to the epiphyseal plate.
6.  Neuromuscular conditions such as cerebral palsy or poliomyelitis.
7.  Tumors such as neurofibromatosis, Wilms' tumor.
8.  Avascular necrosis of the femoral head

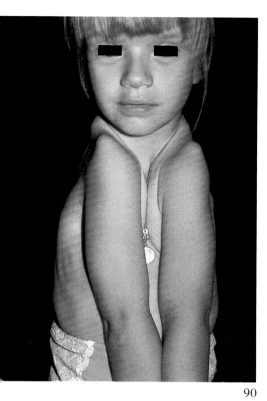
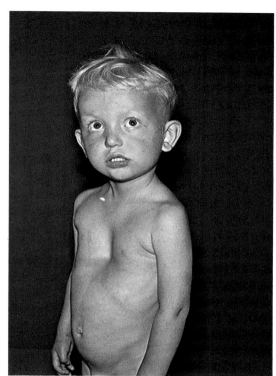

90

91

92

93

94

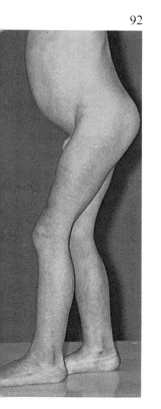
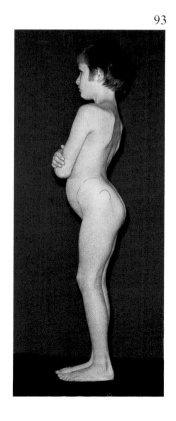
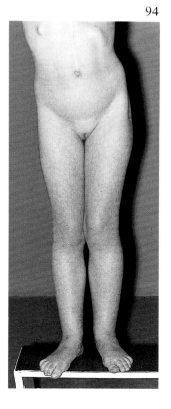

# 2.  Congenital Anomalies

**Figure 95  Fetal Alcohol Syndrome:**  Fetal alcohol syndrome in a 2-month-old girl. Intrauterine grow retardation (birthweight 1,200 g) had been noted. Physical findings included microcephaly and dysmorph facial features. The face was remarkable for short palpebral fissures, hypoplasia of the midface, hypoplast philtrum, and thin vermilion border of the upper lip. The prenatal history was remarkable for considerat alcohol abuse by the mother during the pregnancy. The hospital course was unremarkable. Many of the children may have serious developmental delays, behavioral disorders, or continued failure to thrive.

### Reference

1.  Clarren SK, Smith DW. The fetal alcohol syndrome. N Engl J Med 298:1063, 1978.

**Figures 96–98  Fetal Hydantoin Syndrome:**  Fetal hydantoin syndrome in a 13-year-old girl whose moth had taken anticonvulsants regularly during pregnancy. The findings included craniofacial abnormaliti (microcephaly, low broad nasal bridge, short upturned nose, and hypertelorism), nail and digital hyp plasia, and failure to thrive. Mental retardation is also a part of this syndrome. In this case, the girl ha a seizure disorder requiring anticonvulsant therapy.

### References

1.  Hanson JW, et al. Risks to the offspring of women treated with hydantoin anticonvulsants with emphasis on the fetal hydanto syndrome. J Pediatr 89:662, 1976.
2.  Hill RM, et al. Infants exposed in utero to antiepileptic drugs. Am J Dis Child 127:645, 1974.

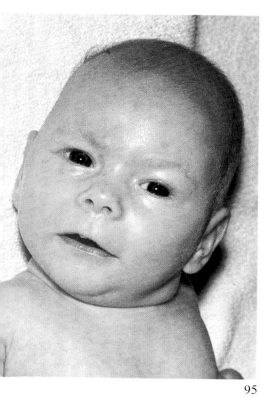

95

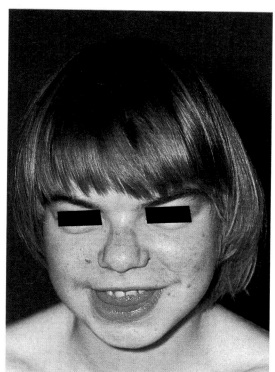

96

97

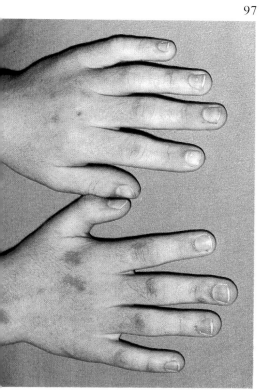

98

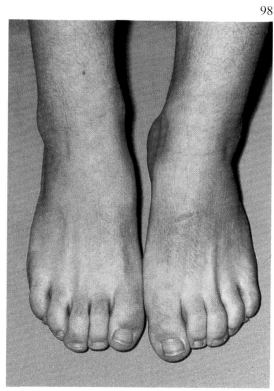

# 2. Congenital Anomalies

**Figure 99  Down Syndrome:**  Down syndrome (trisomy 21) in a 4-year-old boy. Findings include a broad, flat face with small orbits and downward slanting palpebral fissures. The ears were small and low set. The tongue protruded forward and the mouth was held open. Congenital heart disease was also noted (ventricular septal defect with severe pulmonary hypertension diagnosed on cardiac catheterization).

**Figure 100  Congenital Hypothyroidism:**  Congenital hypothyroidism in an 11-month-old girl. Of note was myxedema of the face, swollen lips, macroglossia, and an abnormally broad nose. The condition was noticed due to developmental delay and abnormally quiet behavior. Laboratory examination revealed a low thyroxine level (T4) and a high thyroid stimulating hormone level (TSH).

Macroglossia is seen in Down syndrome as well as Pompe's disease (Type II glycogenosis) and Beckwith Wiedemann syndrome (see p 202).

### Reference

1.   Fisher DA, Klein AH: Thyroid development and disorders of thyroid function in the newborn. N Engl J Med 304:701, 1981

**Figure 101  Down Syndrome:**  Down syndrome in a 4-year-old boy. The posture is the so-called "jacknife" phenomenon (caused by muscular hypotonia, weak ligaments, and loose skin).

**Figure 102  Down Syndrome:**  Down syndrome in a 1-year-old girl. The hand findings include a bilateral transverse palmar crease (the so-called "simian crease"), brachydactyly, and clinodactyly.

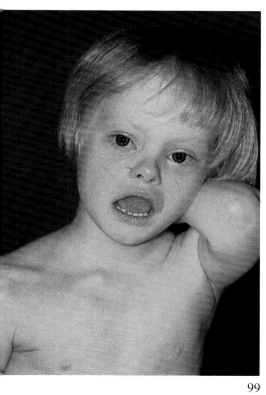

99

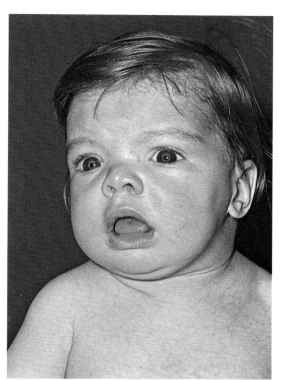

100

101

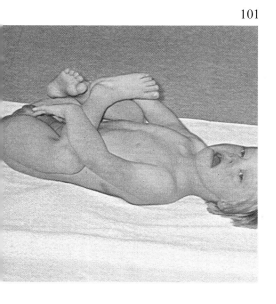

102

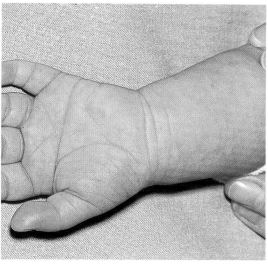

# 2. Congenital Anomalies

**Figures 103–104  Trisomy 13 (Patau's Syndrome):**  Trisomy 13 in a 3-day-old boy, the ninth child of a 40-year-old mother. The child has characteristic craniofacial features of trisomy 13 including microcephaly, sloping forehead, microphthalmia, hypertelorism, and bilateral cleft lip and palate (Figure 103). Several ulcer-like scalp defects were found in the occipitoparietal area (cutis aplasia, Figure 104). In addition, the child had bilateral colobomas, numerous capillary hemangiomas, a transverse palmar crease, polydactyly, a large omphalocele, and congenital heart disease. The child's condition was incompatible with life and he died of bronchopneumonia on the ninth day. At autopsy, further lesions were detected including arhinencephaly, polycystic kidneys, and abdominal testes. Chromosome analysis confirmed the diagnosis of trisomy 13.

## Reference

1.  Hodes ME, et al. Clinical experience with trisomies 18 and 13. J Med Genet 15:48, 1978.

**Figures 105–106  Cri du chat Syndrome (Deletion 5p-):**  Findings included craniofacial dysmorphism with microcephaly, round face, dysplastic low set ears, downward slanting palpebral fissures, hypertelorism, and micrognathia. During the first few months of life, the child had a characteristic high, shrill, cat-like cry, which led to the presumptive diagnosis of cri du chat syndrome. Analysis of chromosomes revealed a partial deletion of the short arm of chromosome 5. Psychomotor development in this child was considerably delayed.

## Reference

1.  Breg, et al. The cri-du-chat in adolescents and adults, clinical findings in 13 older patients with partial deletion of the short arm of chromosome No. 5 (5p-). J Pediatr 77:782, 1970.

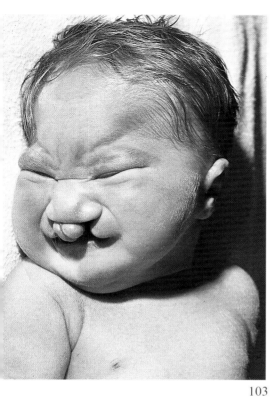

103

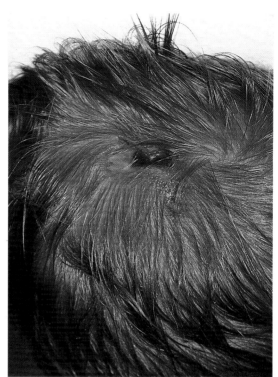

104

105

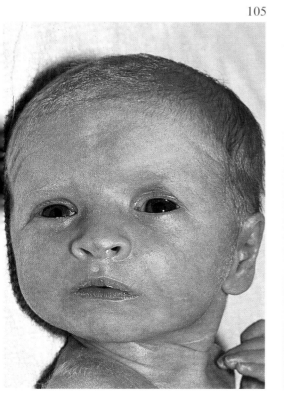

106

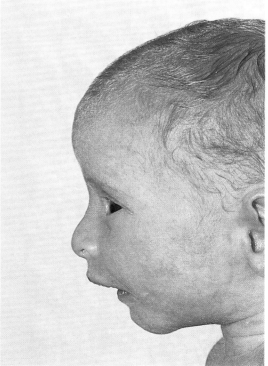

# 2. Congenital Anomalies

**Figure 107** **Polydactyly:** Polydactyly (hexadactyly) in a 6-month-old girl with multiple deformities. Radiographic examination revealed a "Y" shaped fifth metascarpal bone.

**Figure 108** **Trisomy 18 (Edwards' Syndrome):** Trisomy 18 in a 2-week-old girl. Findings in trisomy 18 include craniofacial abnormalities (dolichocephaly, prominent occiput, short palpebral fissures), short neck and sternum, clinodactyly, and rockerbottom feet.

### Reference

1. Hodes ME, et al. Clinical experience with trisomies 18 and 13. J Med Genet 15:48, 1978.

**Figure 109** **Holt-Oram Syndrome (Cardiac Limb Syndrome):** Holt-Oram syndrome in a 2-month-old boy. The syndrome is characterized by absence or dysplasia of the thumb and radial abnormalities. Cardiac defects are associated with the syndrome. In this case, the left hand lacked both the radius and the thumb, and there was phocomelia on the right (three finger rectomelia, i.e., a hand with three fingers directly connected to the shoulder). Atrial septal defect was detected on cardiac catheterization. The father, had similar deformities of the extremities (bilateral aplasia of the thumb) and an atrial septal defect.

### Reference

1. Kaufman RL, et al. Variable expression of Holt-Oram syndrome. Am J Dis Child 127:21, 1974.

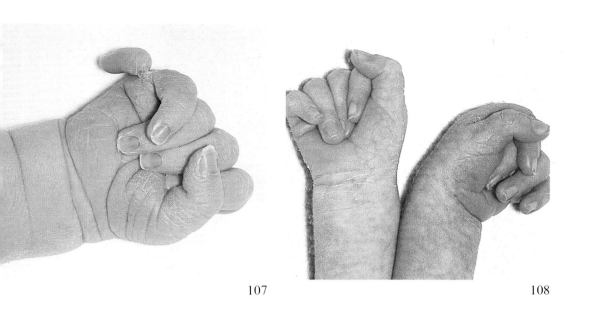

107

108

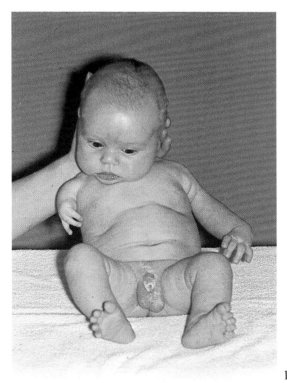

109

# 2. Congenital Anomalies

**Figures 110 and 111  Turner's Syndrome (XO Gonadal Dysgenesis):**  Turner's syndrome in a 15-year-old girl who had primary amenorrhea and lacked secondary sexual characteristics. On physical examination, a low hair line, redundant skin folds, webbing of the neck, and shield-like chest with widely spaced nipples was noted. There was no breast development and pubic hair was sparse. Analysis of chromosomes revealed X monosomy.

**Differential Diagnosis:**  Noonan's syndrome, in which there is short stature and Turner-like stigmata, must be ruled out. In Noonan's syndrome, the karyotype is normal.

### Reference

1.  Palmer CG, Reichmann A. Chromosomal and clinical findings in 110 females with Turner syndrome. Hum Genet 35:35, 1976.

**Figure 112  Turner's Syndrome:**  Turner's syndrome in a 12-year-old girl. This girl lacked breast development, had widely spaced nipples, and a shield-shaped thorax. Chromosome analysis revealed XO. Laparotomy demonstrated gonadal dysgenesis (streaks of connective tissue without follicles).

### References

1.  Weiss L. Additional evidence of gradual loss of germ cells in the pathogenesis of streak ovaries in Turner syndrome. J Med Genet 8:540, 1971.

**Figure 113  Noonan's Syndrome:**  Noonan's syndrome in a 10-year-old girl with a normal karyotype. Findings included facial abnormalities (broad forehead, downward slanting palpebral fissures, hypertelorism, micrognathia), shield shaped thorax, widely spaced nipples, pigmented nevi on the lower abdomen, microsomy, skeletal abnormalities, and developmental delay. Noonan's syndrome may also be associated with cardiovascular abnormalities including valvular pulmonic stenosis, PDA, and aortic stenosis. Typical Turner's syndrome (XO karyotype) was ruled out. However, there could be a mosaic condition for Turner's syndrome which can be detected from chromosome analysis and fibroblast culture.

### Reference

1.  Char F, et al. The Noonan syndrome—a clinical study of forty-five cases. Birth Defects 8(5):110, 1972.

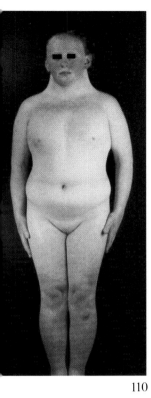

110

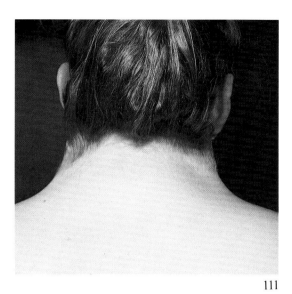

111

112

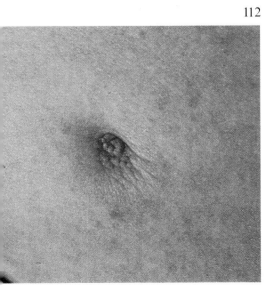

113

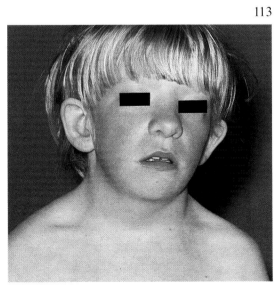

# 3. Cardiac Diseases

**Figures 114 and 115  Tetralogy of Fallot:**  Tetralogy of Fallot in a 4-year-old boy. Physical findings included generalized cyanosis, dyspnea, clubbing of the fingers, and polycythemia. In order to relieve the symptoms the child would assume the typical squatting position. The findings in tetralogy of Fallot include obstruction of right ventricular outflow, ventricular septal defect, dextroposition of the aorta, and right ventricular hypertrophy. A palliative operation was performed (aortopulmonary anastomosis) with improvement of cyanosis and dyspnea. A total correction at age 7 years was successful.

**Differential Diagnosis with Regard to Clubbed Fingers:**  Clubbing of the fingers occurs in cyanotic congenital heart disease as well as in chronic pulmonary disease (cystic fibrosis), congenital bronchiectasis and disorders of the thyroid gland. Symptoms of hereditary clubbed fingers usually develop at puberty or later in life.

**Figure 116  Tetralogy of Fallot:**  Protuberance of the sternum after operative repair of tetralogy of Fallot in a 4-year-old boy.

## Reference

1.  Stanley PH, et al. Palliative surgery in tetralogy of Fallot. Can J Surg 24:475, 1981.

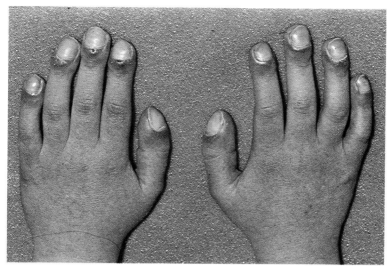

114

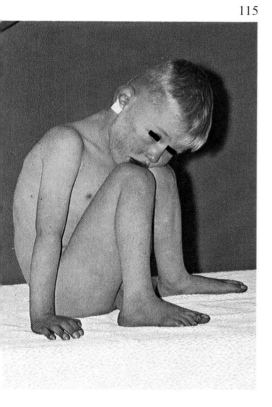

115

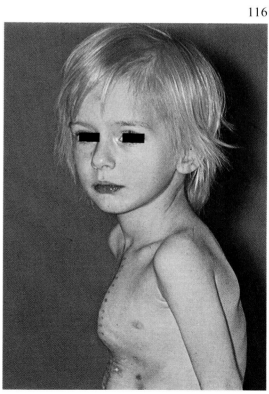

116

# 3. Cardiac Diseases

**Figure 117  Transposition of the Great Vessels:**  Transposition of the great vessels in a 6-year-old girl. Physical findings included acrocyanosis, cyanosis of the lips, and clubbing of the fingers and toes. The child had mild dyspnea at rest and considerable dyspnea with exertion. The underlying cardiac lesion was identified by means of cardiac catheterization. In transposition of the great vessels, the aorta arises from the right ventricle, the pulmonary artery from the left ventricle, and the systemic veins drain into the right atrium.

**Figure 118  Fetal Alcohol Syndrome:**  Fetal alcohol syndrome with congenital heart disease (ventricular septal defect and patent ductus arteriosus) in a 7-month-old child. The features of fetal alcohol syndrome included microcephaly, short palpebral fissures, hypoplastic midface, short nose, hypoplastic philtrum, thin vermilion border of the upper lip, micrognathia, and failure to thrive. Fetal alcohol syndrome may be associated with underlying congenital heart disease. The history of alcohol abuse during pregnancy was unclear, so other syndromes associated with congenital heart disease were ruled out. Because of a transverse palmar crease (simian crease) and mental retardation, a chromosome analysis was performed demonstrating a normal karyotype. Serologic examination ruled out intrauterine rubella infection.

**Figure 119  Pericarditis:**  Constrictive pericarditis in a 12-year-old boy. Congestive heart failure lead to protuberance of the abdomen due to ascites and hepatomegaly. Pericarditis may cause impairment of diastolic ventricular filling and compromise cardiac contractility. The child was treated with thoracotomy and pericardiectomy, with regression of symptoms afterwards. The underlying cause of the pericarditis was unknown. Possible causes of pericarditis include tuberculous pericarditis, viral pericarditis, or pericarditis secondary to irradiation or trauma.

## Reference

1.  Gersony NM, et al. Infective endocarditis and diseases of the pericardium. Pediatr Clin North Am 25:831, 1978.

**Figure 120  Marfan's Syndrome:**  Ten-year-old girl with Marfan's syndrome. Findings included tall stature (15 cm taller than average for age), long extremities, long fingers (arachnodactyly), hyperextensible joints, ectopia lentis, and flat feet. Marfan's syndrome is associated with underlying cardiac defects including aortic and mitral regurgitation and aneurysms.

**Differential Diagnosis:**  Classic homocystinuria (cystathionine synthetase deficiency) must be ruled out. In homocystinuria there may be tall stature, long extremities, arachnodactyly, and similar eye problems. Usually the homocystinine and methionine levels are elevated and the cyanide nitroprusside test in the urine is positive. Other conditions which must be ruled out include congenital contractural arachnodactyly and Ehlers-Danlos syndrome.

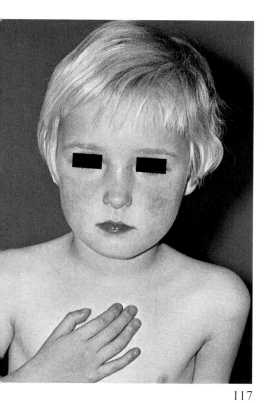

117

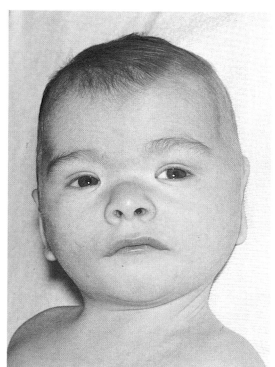

118

119

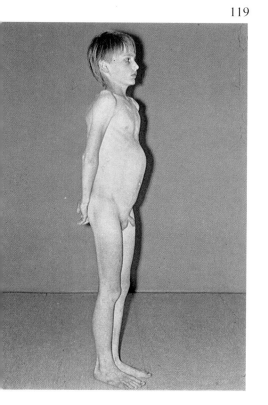

120

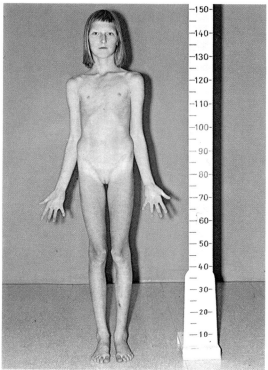

# 4.  Diseases of the Gastrointestinal Tract

**Figures 121 and 122  Imperforate Anus:**  Anal and rectal atresia with rectovaginal fistula in a 10-year old girl. Stool was passed per vagina. Radiologic examination indicated that this was a "high lesion" which the rectum does not pass through the puborectalis muscle. Usually there is an associated sacral mal formation. In females, there is usually a rectovaginal fistula. The first step in an operative repair involve forming a colostomy and closing the rectovaginal fistula. At age 8 months definitive repair was accom plished. Despite operative repair, this child remained incontinent.

**Figure 123  Imperforate Anus:**  Anal and rectal atresia without fistula in a 3-day-old boy. No re toperitoneal, rectovesicular, or rectourethral fistula could be detected. Radiographs taken with the infa held head down (Wangensteen-Rice technique) revealed the rectal fundus lying 3 cm from the perineal ski Immediate operation was performed due to symptoms of obstruction. In these "low" lesions, the operati repair may be performed using a perineal approach, with the fundus being pulled forward. Careful attentic must be paid to avoid disrupting the anal sphincter. Postoperatively, dilation must be performed to insu patency. In this case, operation led to normal stool evacuation and good sphincter tone.

**Figure 124  Gluteal Abscess:**  Gluteal abscess (after incision) as a complication of BCG injection in 4-month-old boy. Originally, the area of injection was noted to be red and swollen with purulent drainag The child was afebrile. The abscess was treated with prolonged tuberculostatic therapy.

**Figure 125  Perianal Abscess:**  Perianal abscess in a 1-year-old boy. Pictured is the completely heal perianal scar after spontaneous drainage. At the height of the illness, the child was febrile and experienc extreme pain especially when sitting or defecating. The underlying cause of the infection was anal fissure Culture of the abscess revealed a mixed infection of aerobic and anaerobic bacteria (*E. coli, Proteus, a Bacteroides fragilis*).

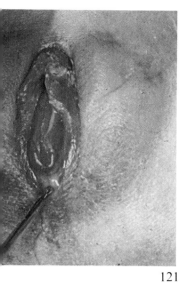

121

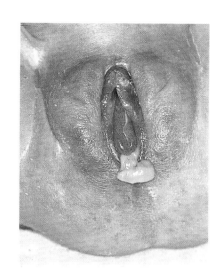

122

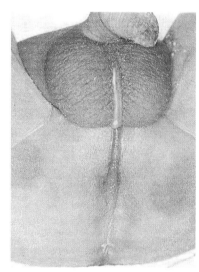

123

124

125

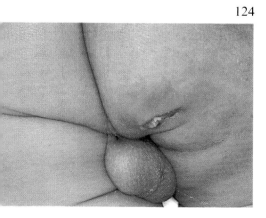

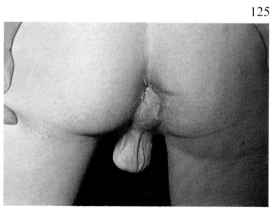

# 4. Diseases of the Gastrointestinal Tract

**Figure 126  Cystic Fibrosis:**  Cystic fibrosis in a 1-year-old child with failure to thrive and a protuberant abdomen. Cystic fibrosis involves a dysfunction of exocrine glands. A wide spectrum of problems may occur including pancreatic insufficiency, nasal polyposis, pansinusitis, metabolic dysfunction, hepatic dysfunction, failure to thrive, and chronic lung disease. Growth failure is probably on the basis of malabsorption. Children have frequent, bulky, greasy stools and protuberant abdomens. Diagnosis is confirmed through pilocarpin iontophoresis (sweat test). Treatment with pancreatic enzyme replacement leads to decreased malabsorption and weight gain. However, in this case, pulmonary problems persisted (chronic bronchitis and bronchopneumonia).

**Differential Diagnosis Regarding Failure to Thrive and Protuberant Abdomen (in the First Year of Life):**  Shwachman-Diamond syndrome (congenital pancreatic insufficiency with neutropenia and bone abnormalities), celiac disease, protein losing enteropathy, abetalipoproteinemia, cow's milk allergy, chronic intestinal infections (i.e., Giardia lamblia), and disaccharidase deficiency.

### Reference

1.  Chase HP, et al. Cystic fibrosis and malnutrition. J Pediatr 95:337, 1979.

**Figure 127  Celiac Disease:**  Celiac disease in a 21-month-old boy who had voluminous, foul-smelling stools since the age of three months. Findings included sullen facial expression, protuberant abdomen, and malnutrition. The diagnosis of celiac disease was confirmed through a perioral suction biopsy sample of the small intestine. Histologically, the biopsy specimen demonstrated villous atrophy of the epithelium of the small intestine. On a gluten-free diet, the steatorrhea ceased and the child began to gain weight.

Other causes of malabsorption (besides gluten intolerance) are chronic enteritis (especially in developing countries), short gut syndrome, cow's milk protein intolerance, protein losing enteropathy, abetalipoproteinemia, and intestinal infections such as Giardia lamblia.

### Reference

1.  Anderson CM, et al. Celiac disease - some still controversial aspects. Arch Dis Child 47:292, 1972.

**Figure 128  Cystic Fibrosis:**  Cystic fibrosis in a 5-year-old boy with meconium-ileus-equivalent. Cystic fibrosis had not been diagnosed at birth (the child had no symptoms of meconium-ileus in the newborn period). The child presented with alternating diarrhea and constipation accompanied by abdominal cramping. The abdomen was protuberant. Meconium-ileus-equivalent is caused by accumulated fecal material in the terminal portion of the ileus and cecum. Initial therapy consisted of oral N-acetylcysteine and enemas. After that, regular doses of pancreatic enzyme preparations were given at each meal.

**Differential Diagnosis:**  Protuberant abdomen with abdominal pain and symptoms of ileus may occur with intussusception or volvulus.

**Figure 129  Rectal Prolapse:**  Rectal prolapse in a 3½-year-old girl with cystic fibrosis. The rectal mucosa is prolapsed, inflamed, and swollen. The prolapse can usually be manually reduced and improves with pancreatic enzyme replacement therapy. Prolapse is due to increased intra-abdominal pressure from pulmonary disease or from malabsorption.

### Reference

1.  Stern RC, et al. Treatment and prognosis of rectal prolapse in cystic fibrosis. Gastroenterology 82:707, 1982.

**Figure 130  Cystic Fibrosis:**  Cystic fibrosis in a 10-month-old boy leading to cirrhosis of the liver. Findings included a protuberant abdomen (due to ascites) and dilatation of superficial veins. The child had biliary cirrhosis with secondary portal hypertension and esophageal varices. He presented with hematemesis which was treated with pitressin and a Sengstaken-Blakemore tube. The child died three months later due to hepatic failure.

Multilobular biliary cirrhosis of the liver occurs in about 20 percent of the cases of cystic fibrosis and frequently leads to portal hypertension, esophageal varices, and hypersplenism. The cirrhotic changes are mostly localized, leaving large parts of the liver parenchyma unaffected. Icterus is usually absent and the liver function for the most part is undisturbed.

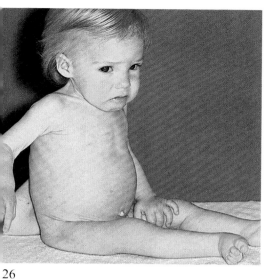

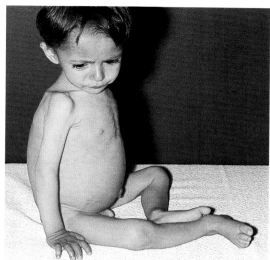

126

127

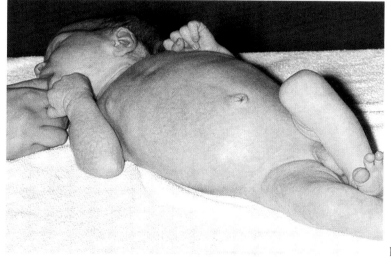

129

128

130

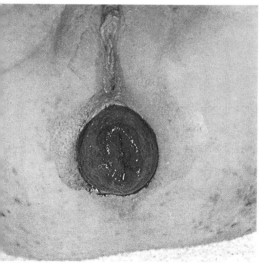

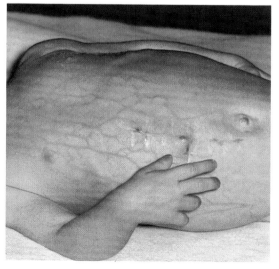

# 5. Diseases of the Urogenital Tract

**Figure 131 Phimosis:** Phimosis (narrowing of the opening of the foreskin preventing retraction) in a 3-year-old boy. The child had recently complained of pain during micturition and had a notably thin stream of urine. During micturition the foreskin would inflate like a balloon. The disorder was corrected through circumcision.

Physiologic adhesions of the foreskin to the glans (with restriction of urinary flow) in small children needs no treatment. Normal development release the adhesions, and at age 2 the foreskin can be slightly retracted. Vigorous attempts to retract the foreskin can lead to acquired phimosis because of trauma and scarring. Paraphimosis occurs in children with mild phimosis when the foreskin is forcibly retracted over the glans penis. The retracted edematous foreskin can strangle the glans and cause gangrene. Phimosis due to lichen sclerosus et atrophicus is discussed in Figure 135.

**Figure 132 Retention Cysts:** Retentions cyst of the urethra in a 2-day-old newborn. A cyst was noted at the external opening of the penis, which hindered urinary flow but regressed without therapy after a few days. No other anomalies were noted.

**Figure 133 Balanitis:** Balanitis (inflammation of the glans and foreskin) in a 4-month-old boy. Finding included diffuse erythema and swelling of the foreskin and glans with a foul-smelling, cheesy secretion (from which candida albicans was grown). A persistent diaper dermatitis was also noted.

Candidal balanitis occurs frequently in diabetics, as well as in normal adults who have had sexual intercourse with an infected partner. In the circumcised child with candidal balanitis, the glans may be inflamed and satellite lesions may be seen. Therapy involves local cleaning and topical treatment with an antifungal agent (nystatin or miconazol).

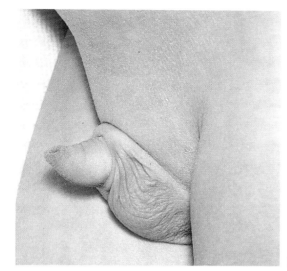

131

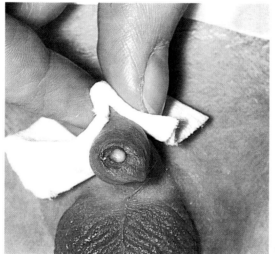

132

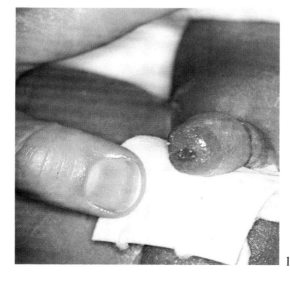

133

# 5. Diseases of the Urogenital Tract

**Figure 134   Lichen Sclerosus et Atrophicus Vulvae:**   Lichen sclerosus et atrophicus vulvae in a 7-year old girl. Findings included a white discoloration and hardening of the vulval skin with early signs of atroph of the external genitalia. Itching and burning was also noted. Symptoms improved with local applicatio of corticosteroid cream.

The prognosis for lichen sclerosus in children is usually more hopeful than it is for adults (frequentl responding without therapy). Girls have itching in 50 percent of the cases, a vaginal discharge in 20 percen In women, the skin around the anus is also involved. It can lead to considerable labial shrinkage and narrowing of the introitus. Adults may have extragenital lesions as well.

**Differential Diagnosis:**   Morphea (see p 114) and primary vulval atrophy (seen almost exclusively in adu patients).

**Figure 135   Lichen Sclerosus et Atrophicus Penis:**   Lichen sclerosus et atrophicus penis in a 6-year-ol boy. The foreskin could not be retracted over the glans (phimosis) and was noted to have a whitish discolo ration with thickening of the tissue. Symptoms have been present for a year. Histologic examination of th tissue taken at the time of circumcision revealed a superficial hyperkeratosis in the atrophic epidermis wit subepidermal sclerotic changes and lymphocytic infiltrate. The tissue gradually returned to normal afte two years (with a brief application of corticosteroid cream postoperatively).

Cases of acquired phimosis and balanitis may be caused by lichen sclerosus. In boys, the perianal are and scrotum are not affected. The diagnosis is often made only through histologic examination followin circumcision for phimosis.

## Reference

1.   Chalmers RJ, et al. Lichen sclerosus et atrophicus. A common and distinctive cause of phimosis in boys. Arch Dermat 120:1025, 1984.

**Figure 136   Priapism:**   Priapism (continual erection of the penis without sexual arousal) in a 6-year-o boy. Findings included painful penile erection that had persisted for the last 72 hours. No obstruction urinary flow was noted. Since conservative measures proved unsuccessful, a shunt operation was performe (creation of a surgical shunt between the corpora cavernosa and corpus spungeosum). Postoperative perio was free of complications. The cause in this case was not known.

During childhood, priapism has been noted in conjunction with leukemia, sickle-cell anemia, and traum to the perineal area. The treatment for priapism may be disease specific; with leukemia, chemotherap combined with radiation may be of some help; with sickle-cell disease, transfusion of packed red bloo cells may be the treatment of choice. Persistent post traumatic priapism often requires surgical correctio

## Reference

1.   Baron M, et al. The management of priapism in sickle cell anemia. J Urol 119:610, 1978.

**Figure 137   Balanitis:**   Balanitis (inflammation of the glans penis and foreskin) in a 10-year-old boy. Th penis was swollen, reddened, and partially ulcerated. Likewise, the foreskin had inflammatory changes an was very painful. Lymphadenopathy was noted in the right groin. The condition responded to antimicrobi therapy.

In uncircumcised boys, retention of smegma (due to poor hygiene) is often the cause of acute infectio with erythema, edema, and purulent drainage. Anaerobic and intestinal bacteria can frequently cause u cerations. *Trichomonas*, with or without accompanying urethritis, may also cause balanitis. Primary herpe simplex virus balanitis may be particularly painful and cause blistering edema and regional lymphadenopa thy. Herpes simplex may also cause urethritis and severe dysuria without any visible skin changes.

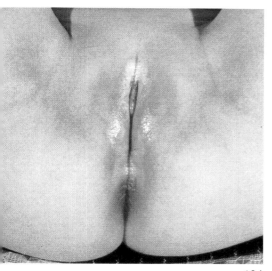

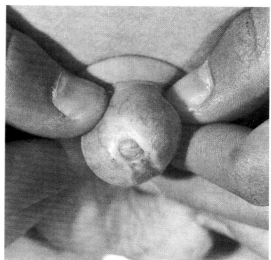

134

135

136

137

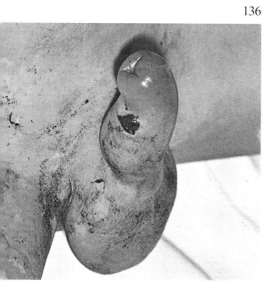

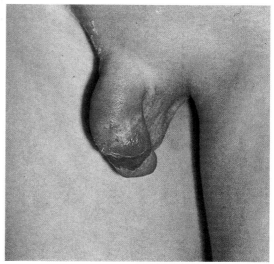

# 5. Diseases of the Urogenital Tract

**Figure 138 Vulvovaginitis:** Vulvovaginitis in a 5-year-old girl. Erythema, swelling, and purulent drainage was noted in and around the vulva. The infection was caused by *Neisseria gonorrhea* (proven microscopically and by culture). Cases of sexually transmitted diseases in the preadolescent must be approached with the diagnosis of sexual abuse in mind. The child was successfully treated with penicillin.

Vulvovaginitis in childhood must be differentiated from other forms of vulvovaginitis, which may be caused by Group A or Group B streptococci, staphylococci, *Haemophilus*, enterobacteria, *Trichomonas vaginalis*, *Candida albicans*, and herpes simplex virus. Foreign bodies, which may be introduced into the vagina, must be ruled out when dealing with children.

### Reference

1. Litt IF, et al. Gonorrhea in children and adolescents: a current review. J Pediatr 85:595, 1974.
2. Rimsza ME, Niggeman EH. Medical evaluation of sexually abused children: a review of 311 cases. Pediatrics 1982.

**Figure 139 Molluscum Contagiosum:** Molluscum contagiosum in a 4-year-old boy. The findings included several pearl-shaped papules 2 to 3 mm in diameter with central umbilication. Lesions were noted on the skin of the penis. A caseous material could be expressed from these lesions. This viral cutaneous infection was apparently caused by autoinoculation from lesions originally found on the face of the child.

Skins lesions in molluscum contagiosum can vary widely in size, from the size of a pinhead to pea sized lesions. Central dimpling or umbilication is usually noted. Microscopic analysis of the caseous material reveals many intracellular inclusion bodies. Eczematous or impetiginous changes are frequent. Molluscum contagiosum has a predilection for the axillae or the anogenital area, but may also be seen on the face, the head, and in the mouth. Opinion on treatment varies. Without treatment, molluscum contagiosum may heal within six to nine months, but some cases may take years to resolve. Some advocate mechanical extraction of the central plug.

**Differential Diagnosis:** Similar discrete pearly papular lesions may be seen with warts or milia (see p 146).

**Figure 140 Condylomata Acuminata:** Condylomata acuminata (genital or venereal warts) in a 7-year-old girl. In the area of the labia minora and the perineum there were white, moist papillomatous growth of warty tissue (identified histologically as genital warts). This is an example of papovavirus infection which may be transmitted either by sexual intercourse or direct contact. In girls, condylomata acuminata are usually located in the introitus, the labia minora, the labia majora, the perineum, the anus, the clitoris, or the urethra. Typical venereal warts are soft, red papules which sometimes may be pedunculated.

Differential diagnosis includes condylomata lata (secondary syphilis) and, in adults, carcinoma.

### Reference

1. Stringel G, et al. Condyloma acuminata in children. J Pediatr Surg 20:499, 1985.

**Figure 141 Condyloma Acuminata:** Condyloma acuminata (venereal warts) in a 4-year-old boy. Cauliflower-like, hyperplastic warts were noted on the penis and glans. Venereal warts may be skin colored or reddened papules with a raw appearing surface. They are frequently found on the foreskin, the meatus, the shaft of the penis, the anus, and the scrotum. They can last for a few weeks or up to a year. Differential diagnosis should consider molluscum contagiosum, milia, and condyloma lata.

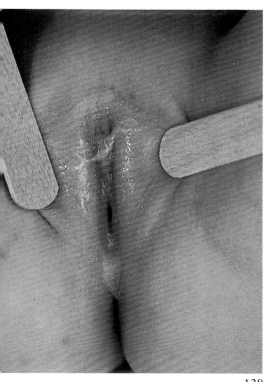

138

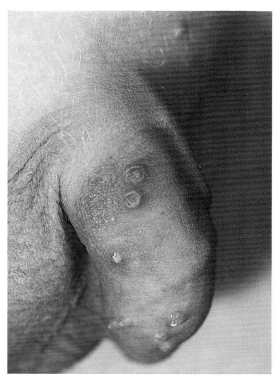

139

140

141

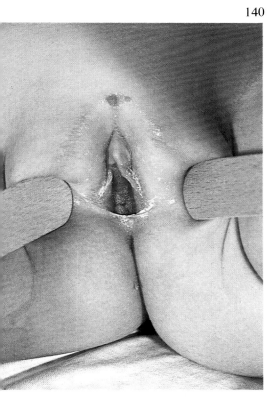

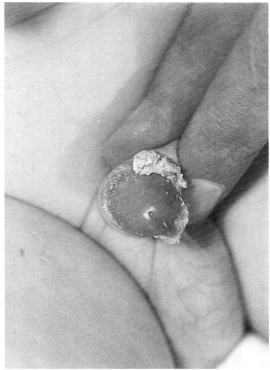

# 5. Diseases of the Urogenital Tract

**Figure 142  Indirect Hernia:**  Indirect hernia in a 3-month-old boy. Of note was the swelling of the right groin near the pubic symphysis. The swelling extended into the scrotum. When the child cried, the swelling increased. The hernia was easily reducible.

**Differential Diagnosis:**  Hydrocele of the spermatic cord or testes must be differentiated from an indirect hernia. A hydrocele will transilluminate unlike an indirect hernia.

**Figure 143  Hydrocele:**  Bilateral hydrocele of the testes and spermatic cord in a 5-month-old boy. Hydrocele is due to the failure of obliteration of the tunica vaginalis. Due to the abnormal collection of fluid inside the tunica vaginalis, both the left and right scrotum were taught and painfully swollen. Since there was also hydrocele of the spermatic cord, the swelling was also noted in the groin. The fluid collection could be easily transilluminated. In cases of an indirect hernia, transillumination is negative. Presence of a hydrocele was confirmed at the time of surgical repair. Hydrocele of the testes or the spermatic cord is usually associated with an indirect hernia.

**Figure 144  Hypospadias:**  Hypospadias in a 2-year-old boy. The narrowed urethral opening was on the ventral surface of the penis close to where the penis joins the scrotum. The penis was bent ventrally due to a fibrous band or chordee, and urine was passed in a very thin stream. Intravenous pyelogram and voiding cystourethrogram demonstrated no distention of the bladder, ureter, or renal pelvis. Both testes were descended and no hernia was detected. Surgical repair is recommended prior to school age.

## References

1. Belman AB and Kass EJ. Hypospadias repair in children less than 1 year old. J Urol 128:1273, 1982.
2. Nobel MJ, Wacksman J. Screening excretory urography in patients with cryptorchidism or hypospadias: a survey and review of the literature. J Urol 124:98, 1980.

**Figure 145  Exstrophy of the Bladder:**  Exstrophy of the bladder with epispadias in a 1-day-old newborn. Extrophy of the bladder is a developmental defect in which there is abnormal midline fusion of endoderm and ectoderm. The defect may involve the anterior abdominal wall, the bladder, and the urethra. In this case, the bladder was everted and the opening to the ureter could be seen on the posterior wall of the bladder. The ureter and renal pelvis were not distended. The urethra opened on the dorsal side of an abnormally short penis (epispadias). The child was treated with antimicrobial agents to prevent infection. At 1 year of age rectal prolapse developed, which required operative correction. Corrective surgery for exstrophy of the bladder (cystectomy and ureteral diversion into a sigmoid conduit) was planned at a later date.

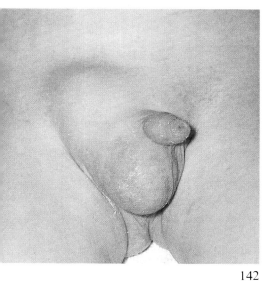

142

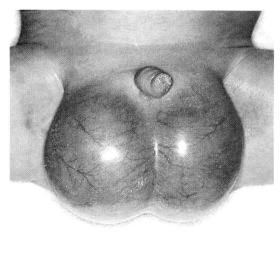

143

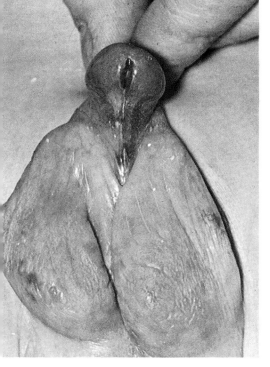

144

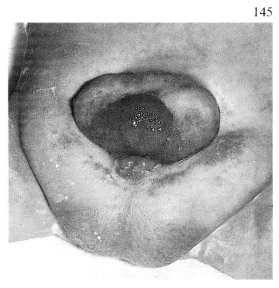

145

# 6. Diseases of the Nervous System

**Figure 146   Asymmetric Tonic Neck Reflex (ATNR):**   Asymmetric tonic neck reflex is elicited by rapidly turning the head of the supine infant to one side. This maneuver will lead to extension of the arm and leg on the side the face is turned to. The opposite side will adopt a flexion posture; the so-called "fencing-"position. The reflex may be normal during the first two to four months of life.

**Figure 147   Galant Reflex:**   Stroking the back along the paravertebral spine causes sideward bending of the spinal column, with the concave side toward the side being stimulated.

**Figure 148   Foot-Grasp Reflex:**   Light pressing on the soles of the feet causes the toes to curl (like claws).

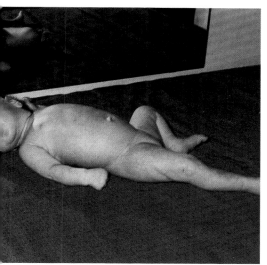

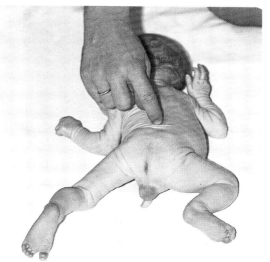

146

147

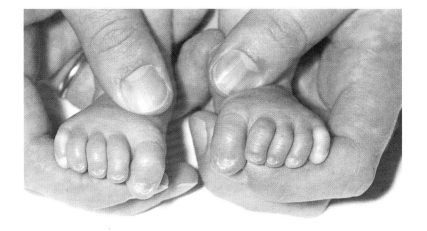

148

# 6. Diseases of the Nervous System

**Figure 149  Palmar Grasp:**  Palmar grasp reflex in a 2-week-old healthy child. This primitive reflex involves the grasping of a finger laid on the inner surface of the child's hand.

**Figure 150  Rooting Reflex:**  This healthy 2-week-old child demonstrates the rooting reflex. The mouth is open and the head turns towards the finger, which gently strokes the mouth.

**Figure 151  Stepping Reflex:**  The stepping reflex (automatic walking) in a healthy 2-week-old child. The child will stimulate the movements of walking when the infant is held upright, inclined forward, and the soles are gently touched to a flat surface.

**Figure 152  Placing Reflex (Climb Reflex):**  Placing reflex (climb reflex) in a healthy 2-week-old child. After touching the edge of the table with the dorsum of the foot, the child lifts his or her leg and sets the foot flatly on the table.

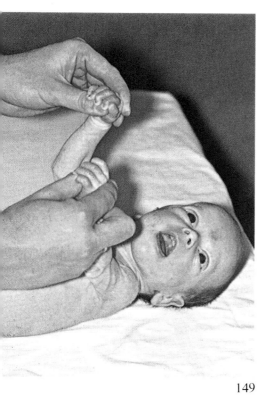

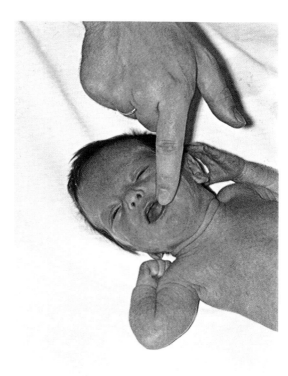

149

150

151

152

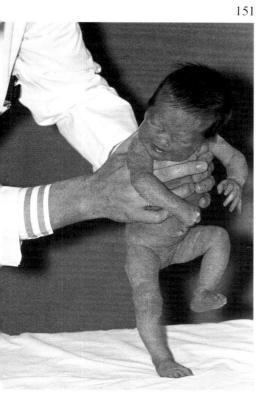

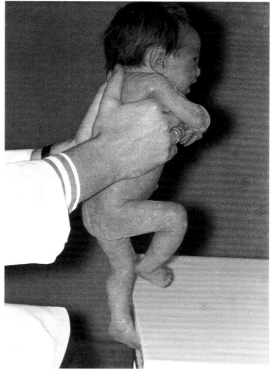

# 6. Diseases of the Nervous System

**Figure 153 Moro Reflex:** Moro reflex in a healthy 2-week-old child. The Moro relex is elicited when the child is placed supine and the infant is either gently shaken or support is suddenly withdrawn. The reflex has two phases. The infant will first demonstrate extension and abduction of the arms, followed by flexion and adduction of the arms and splaying of the fingers. The Moro reflex is a primitive reflex which usually disappears by three months of age.

**Figure 154 Asymmetric Moro Reflex:** Asymmetric response to an attempt at eliciting the Moro reflex in a 3-week-old child. The left arm extended and abducted appropriately, but the right arm did not change position. The cause of this asymmetric response was severe birth trauma that led to right-sided hemiplegia.

**Figure 155 Parachute Reflex:** Forward parachute reflex, triggered by the sudden bending forward of a 7-month-old child who had previously been held in an upright position. The child protects himself or herself by extending the arms and splaying the fingers.

**Figure 156 Parachute Reflex:** Attempts to elicit forward parachute reflex in a 1-year-old boy with cerebral palsy. When the child is held upright and bent forward, the arms and fingers remain flexed (pathological response). The child had cerebral palsy due to intrauterine asphyxia. After birth, there was still evidence of asphyxia and the child had to be supported with mechanical ventilation for several days. The long-term effects of this intrauterine asphyxia included cerebral palsy, seizure disorder and developmental delay.

Cerebral palsy may present with:
1. Persistence of primitive reflexes (such as atonic neck reflex).
2. Absence of complex reflexes (such as the parachute reflex, support reflex, placement reflex and balance reactions).
3. The occurrence of pathological reflexes (such as extension reflexes).
4. Changes in muscle tone (such as spastic dyplegia).
5. The inability to learn motor skills such as grasping, sitting, standing, walking, and crawling.
6. Asymmetric posture and disturbances of spontaneous movements.

## Reference

1. Nelson KB, Ellenberg JH. Antecedents of cerebral palsy: multivariate analysis of risk. N Engl J Med 315:81, 1986.

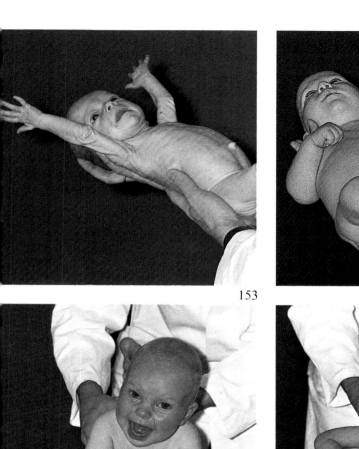

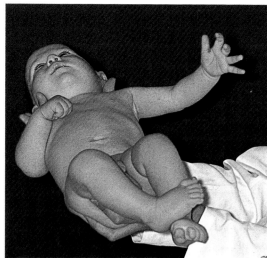

153

154

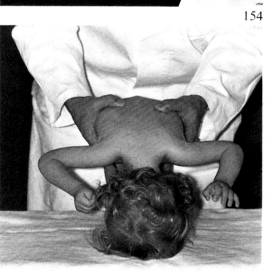

155

156

**Figure 157   Sidewards Parachute Reflex (Support Reaction):**   When pushed to one side, positive place ment reaction of the torso and head occurs, along with shortening of the unweighted left side of the torso and support from the open hand of the outstretched right arm (demonstrated in a healthy 8-month-old boy). A positive sideways parachuete reflex (support reaction) usually begins at age 7 months.

**Figure 158   Sideways Parachute Reflex (Support Reaction):**   When pushed to one side, negative place ment reaction of the head and torso occurs, with no support from the right hand. The hands remain rolled in a fist. This is demonstrated in an 8-month-old boy with cerebral palsy.

**Figure 159   Positive Standing with Support (Readiness to Stand):**   Standing with support (readines to stand) is demonstrated in this healthy 8-month-old boy. The posture is symmetric, the trunk is held slightly forward, the hips are extended, and the legs rotated slightly outwards and abducted. At 10 months of age a normal child will begin to stand while holding on to something for support, and lift himself up to stand.

**Figure 160   Negative Standing with Support (Readiness to Stand):**   Negative standing with suppor (readiness to stand) is demonstrated in a 1-year-old girl with cerebral palsy. The arms are in a jughandl position. The hands are closed in a fist, the thumbs are tucked in, the hips slightly bent, and the legs rotated inward and crossed.

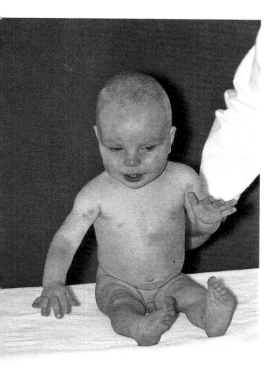

157

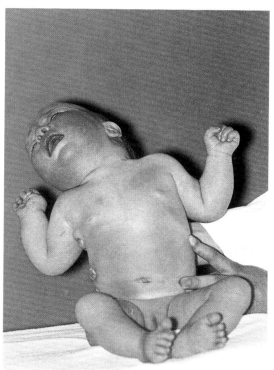

158

159

160

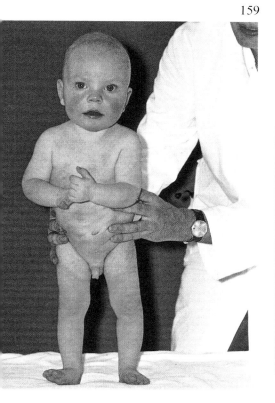

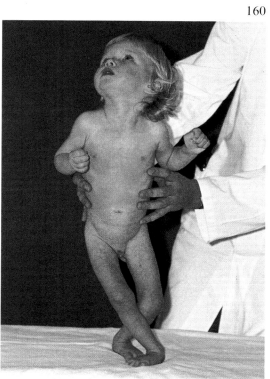

# 6. Diseases of the Nervous System

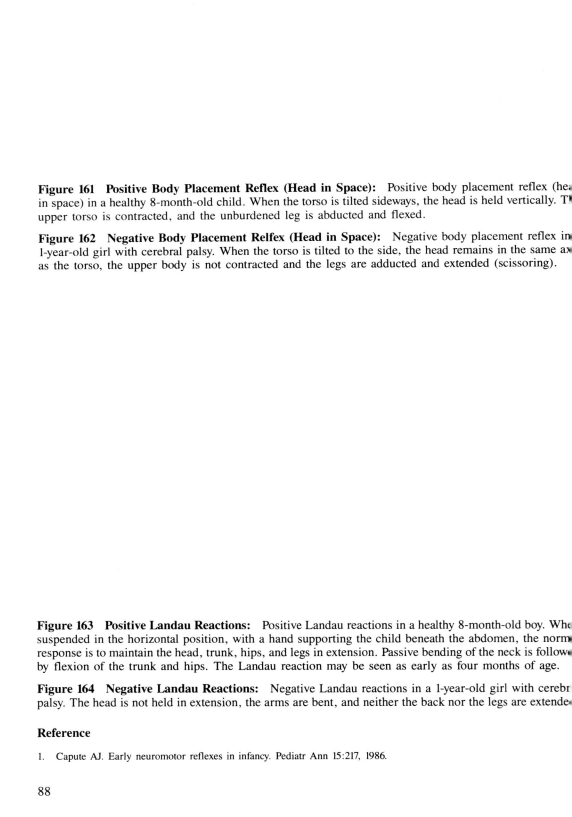

**Figure 161  Positive Body Placement Reflex (Head in Space):**  Positive body placement reflex (head in space) in a healthy 8-month-old child. When the torso is tilted sideways, the head is held vertically. The upper torso is contracted, and the unburdened leg is abducted and flexed.

**Figure 162  Negative Body Placement Relfex (Head in Space):**  Negative body placement reflex in a 1-year-old girl with cerebral palsy. When the torso is tilted to the side, the head remains in the same axis as the torso, the upper body is not contracted and the legs are adducted and extended (scissoring).

**Figure 163  Positive Landau Reactions:**  Positive Landau reactions in a healthy 8-month-old boy. When suspended in the horizontal position, with a hand supporting the child beneath the abdomen, the normal response is to maintain the head, trunk, hips, and legs in extension. Passive bending of the neck is followed by flexion of the trunk and hips. The Landau reaction may be seen as early as four months of age.

**Figure 164  Negative Landau Reactions:**  Negative Landau reactions in a 1-year-old girl with cerebral palsy. The head is not held in extension, the arms are bent, and neither the back nor the legs are extended.

### Reference

1.  Capute AJ. Early neuromotor reflexes in infancy. Pediatr Ann 15:217, 1986.

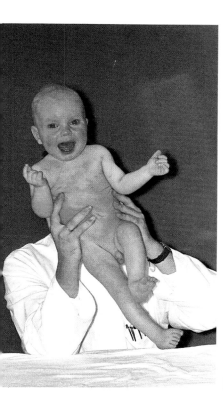

161

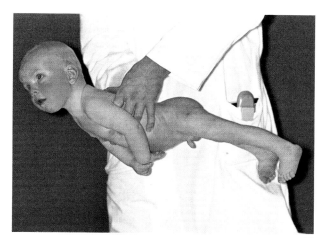

163

162

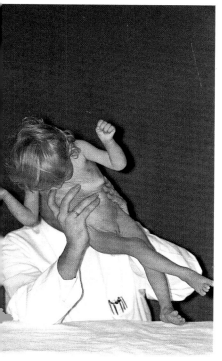

164

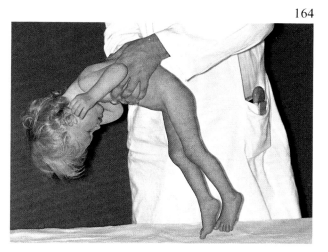

**Figure 165 Traction Attempt (Pull to Sitting Position):** Attempts to pull to a sitting position in a 3-month old boy. The arms remain slightly bent and the head is brought up in the process of sitting.

**Figure 166 Traction Attempt (Pull to Sitting Position) in a Child with Cerebral Palsy:** Attempts to pull to a sitting position in a 4-month-old girl with cerebral palsy. The arms were extended during the maneuver and the head was noted to fall back.

**Figure 167 Obligatory Neck Reflex:** Obligatory neck reflex in a 4-year-old boy with cerebral palsy. Obligatory extension and turning of the head was noted. Other signs of abnormal neurological development in this child include hyperextension of the legs (scissoring), plantar flexion of the feet, extension and pronation of the arms, and arching of the back.

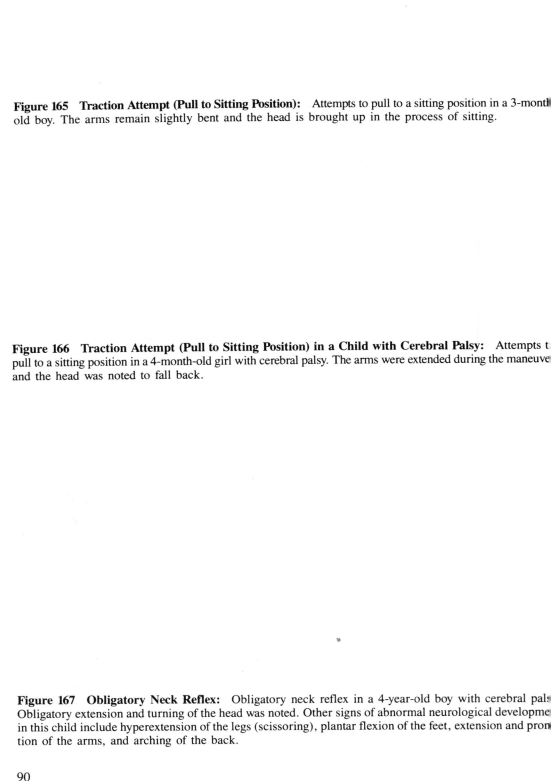

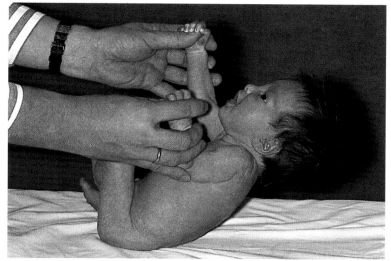

165

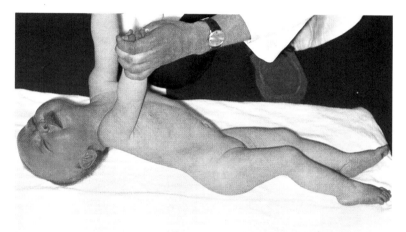

166

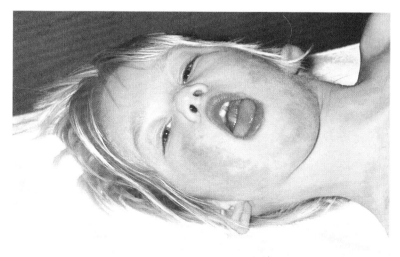

167

# 6. Diseases of the Nervous System

**Figure 168  Spastic Hemiplegia:**  Spastic hemiplegia of the right side in a 3-month-old boy with cerebral palsy. The right arm is always flexed, adducted, and pronated. The fist is closed with the thumb tucked in. The right leg is rotated inward and adducted; the left leg is rotated outwards. The right foot is maintained in a slightly equinovarus position. Muscle tone of the right arm and leg is increased, Achilles tendon reflexes are greater on the right and the grasp reflex on the right is strongly positive. A left convex scoliosis of the spine was also noted. The cause of the hemiplegia was uncertain. The child became involved in intensive physical therapy with some improvement.

**Figure 169  Decorticate Posture:**  Decorticate posture noted after drowning in a 4-year-old boy. The arms are flexed, the hands tightly fisted, and the legs extended. Bilateral contractures were noted. The child maintained an opisthotonic posture. The child remained in a comatose state, apparently awake, but with no response to external stimuli (coma vigile).

## Reference

1.  Peterson B. Mortality of childhood near drowning. Pediatrics 59:364, 1977.

**Figures 170 and 171  Infantile Spinal Muscular Atrophy (Werdnig-Hoffmann Disease):**  Werdnig-Hoffmann disease in an 11-year-old boy. Findings included widespread muscular atrophy leading to weakness, hypotonia, and areflexia. The child was unable to sit or stand and had contractures of the hands and feet. Other findings included paradoxical respirations (due to weakness of the intercostal muscles with otherwise normal diaphragmatic function) as well as vesiculation of the tongue. The disease became manifest at 1 year of age presenting with muscle weakness. The child had normal intelligence.

Werdnig-Hoffmann disease is caused by atrophy of the anterior horn cells of the spinal cord, as well as atrophy of the motor nuclei in the brain stem. Nerve atrophy leads to secondary muscular atrophy. The disease is complicated by frequent bronchopneumonia. The diagnosis may be confirmed through electromyography (demonstrating denervation) and muscle biopsy (demonstrating degeneration).

**Figure 172  Friedreich's Ataxia:**  Hereditary Friedreich's ataxia in an 11-year-old boy. Since the age of 1 year, pes cavus (high arched feet) and muscular atrophy of the lower extremities had been noted. This neurological disorder may present with ataxic gait, muscle weakness (due to peripheral neuropathy), sensory loss, (especially in the feet), intention tremor, dysarthria, and loss of reflexes. Friedreich's ataxia is a progressive cerebellar and spinal cord dysfunction due to the degeneration of the spinocerebellar and corticospinal tract. Nerve conduction studies will demonstrate decreased velocity.

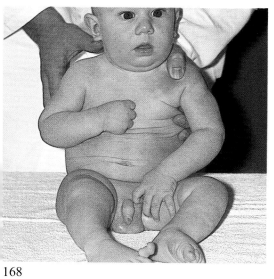

168

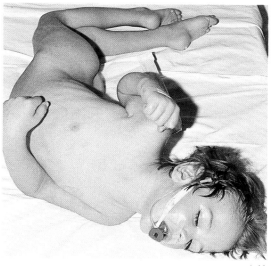

169

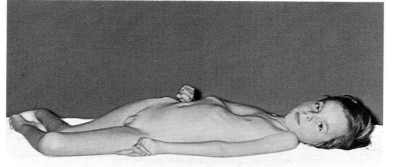

170

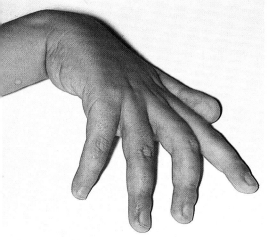

171

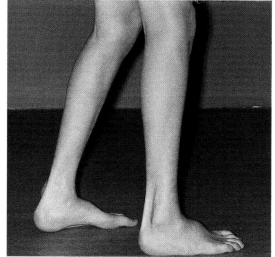

172

# 6. Diseases of the Nervous System

**Figure 173 Hydrocephalus:** Hydrocephalus in a 14-month-old girl as a result of intrauterine toxoplasmosis. Enlargement of the head had been noted since birth, along with thinning of the cranial bones, dilation of the scalp veins, and downward deviation of the eyes ("sunset phenomenon"). Funduscopic examination of the eyes revealed chorioretinitis, findings typically seen in toxoplasmosis. Protein content of the cerebrospinal fluid was elevated. On skull radiographs, intracranial calcifications could be detected. Serum IgM specific for toxoplasmosis was detected using indirect fluorescent antibody technique.

## Reference

1.  Desmonts G, Couvreurj J. Congenital toxoplasmosis: a prospective study of 378 pregnancies. N Engl J Med 290:110, 1974.

**Figure 174 Hydrocephalus:** Progressive hydrocephalus in a 4-week-old boy. The findings included increasing head circumference, large bulging anterior fontanel, and "sunset" phenomenon of the eyes (downward displacement of the eyes with retraction of the upper eyelid). The diagnosis of communicating hydrocephalus was made through ventriculography; the cause remains uncertain. In order to control the symptoms of progressive hydrocephalus, a shunt procedure was performed (ventriculoatrial shunt).

**Differential Diagnosis:** Abnormal enlargement of the head within the first year of life may be due to chronic subdural effusion. In this case, the parietal region protrudes more than the frontal area (the opposite of hydrocephalus). In cases of familial macrocephaly (see Figure 176), no symptoms of illness appear. Enlargement of the head due to excessive brain growth (megalocephaly) appears in storage diseases such as Hurler's disease, Tay-Sachs disease, and metachromatic leukodystrophy. With hydranencephaly (absence of cerebral hemispheres) only the cerebellum and brain stem are present; the cerebrum is replaced by a fluid-filled cavity. The head circumference is normal or only slightly enlarged and the shape of the head may be normal. When transilluminated, the skull will light up brightly. There is a striking absence of voluntary motor movements in these hydranencephalic children.

## Reference

1.  Ignelize RJ, Kirsch WM. Follow-up analysis of ventriculoperitoneal and ventriculoatrial shunts for hydrocephalus. J Neurosurg 42:679, 1975.

**Figure 175 Hydrocephalus:** Congenital hydrocephalus in a 1-day-old premature infant. The infant was born four weeks before the expected due date and weighted 4,800 g. The child had a greatly enlarged head (OFC 54 cm) with widely open cranial sutures, large bulging fontanels, low set ears, large forehead, and a relatively small face. Prenatal infection was not suspected due to the lack of other deformities or symptoms. Death resulted from respiratory failure after five weeks. The autopsy identified the cause of hydrocephalus as congenital aqueductal stenosis. Congenital aqueductal stenosis may lead to obstructive hydrocephalus with extreme enlargement of the lateral and third ventricles.

**Figure 176 Macrocephaly:** Familial macrocephaly in a 4-month-old boy. At birth, the head circumference was 37.5 cm. As can be seen in Figure 176, the head is enlarged (OFC 44 cm), but of normal configuration. The fontanel is of normal size, the cranial sutures are not widened, and the face appears relatively normal. Psychomotor development is commensurate with age. Computerized tomography revealed no signs of hydrocephalus, subdural effusion, or brain tumor. Both the father and 5-year-old brother are macrocephalic as well.

## Reference

1.  Lorber J, Priestly BL. Children with large heads: a practical approach to diagnosis in 557 children, with special reference to 109 children with megalocephaly. Develop Med Clin Neurol 23:494, 1981.

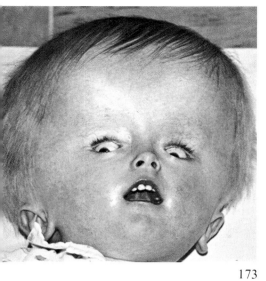

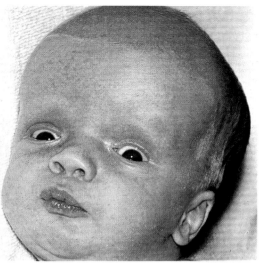

173

174

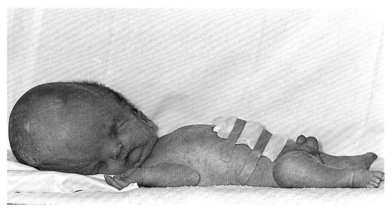

175

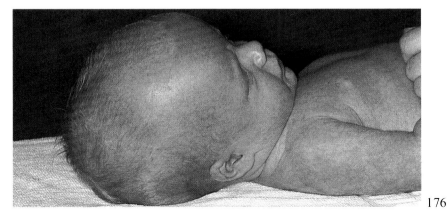

176

# 6. Diseases of the Nervous System

**Figures 177 and 178  Hydrocephalus:**  The figure demonstrates the findings in a 3½-month-old girl after ventriculoatrial shunt for hydrocephalus. The child was born prematurely at 30 weeks gestation and developed progressive hydrocephalus. After the operation, the head circumference decreased from 42 cm to 39.5 cm. The large fontanel and widely spread cranial sutures were no longer noted. After the operation the parietal and occipital bones overlap. The cause of the hydrocephalus was uncertain, but was probably related to intraventricular hemorrhage and posthemorrhagic hydrocephalus.

**Figure 179  Dandy-Walker Syndrome:**  Dandy-Walker syndrome in a 1-day-old girl. Dolichocephaly, bulging anterior and posterior fontanels, and widely spread cranial sutures were noted. Occipital transillumination of the cranium revealed enlargement of the fourth ventricle. Computerized tomography demonstrated not only enlargement of the ventricles (due to congenital obstruction of the foramen of Luschka and foramen of Magendie), but also shifting of the cerebellar hemispheres.

### Reference

1.  Hart MN, et al. The Dandy-Walker syndrome: a clinical-pathological study of 28 cases. Neurology 22:771, 1972.

**Figure 180  Oxycephaly:**  Oxycephaly in a 2-week-old boy. The "tower like" cranium is caused by craniosynostoses involving the coronal sutures. The high forehead and exophthalmos are a result of the depression of the roof of the orbits. Later, there may be papilledema and optic atrophy.

Other malformations occur with oxycephaly such as syndactyly, cardiac defects, or choanal atresia. Oxycephaly is one of the main symptoms of Apert's syndrome, Carpenter's syndrome, and Crouzon's syndrome (see p 28).

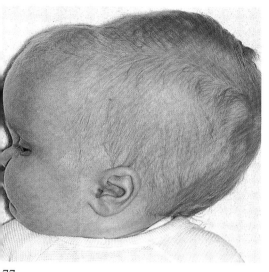

77

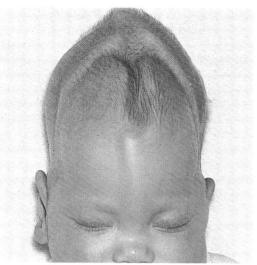

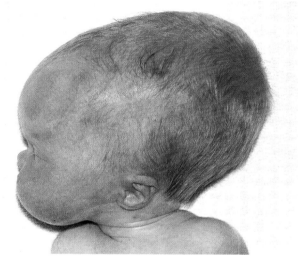

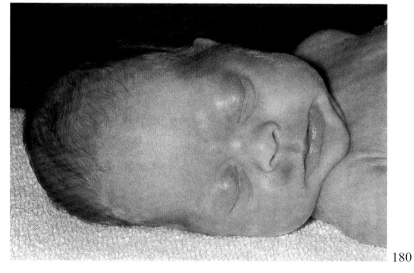

# 6. Diseases of the Nervous System

**Figure 181 Meningocele:** An apple-sized sacral meningocele in a 4-day-old newborn. The infant wa without symptoms of hydrocephalus or other neurological disease. The diagnosis of meningocele with spin bifida was confirmed radiologically and at the time of operative repair.

Spina bifida with meningocele (or meningomyelocele) may present as a midline defect usually in th lumbosacral area. The defect is covered by a thin membrane of meninges. Spina bifida is associated witl Arnold-Chiari malformation and aqueductal stenosis.

## Reference

1. Gross RH. Newborns with myelodysplasia-the rest of the story. N Engl J Med 312:1632, 1985.
2. McLaughlin JF, et al. Influence of prognosis on decisions regarding the care of newborns with myelodysplasia. N Eng J Med 312:1589, 1985.

**Figure 182 Meningomyelocele:** Closed lumbosacral meningomyelocele which caused partial paralys: of the legs and incontinence of urine and stool. The lesion was repaired on the first day of life. The infa did not develop hydrocephalus.

**Figure 183 Meningomyelocele:** Open thoracolumbar meningomyelocele in a newborn infant. The chi was completely paralyzed below the level of the lesion. Surgery to close the spinal defect was performe on the second day of life. A ventriculoatrial shunt was performed during the fourth week of life due t progressive hydrocephalus.

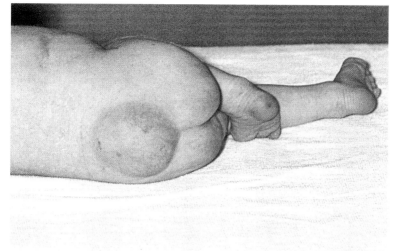

181

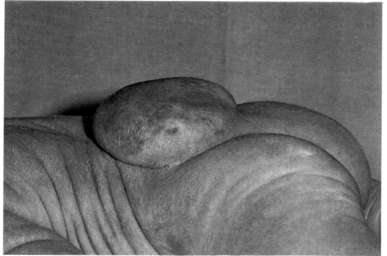

182

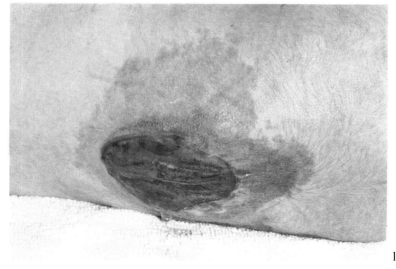

183

# 6. Diseases of the Nervous System

**Figure 184  Cranial Meningocele:**  Cranial meningocele in a 3-day-old newborn. In cranial meningocele there is herniation of meninges through a skull defect. The fluid filled mass transilluminated in a uniform fashion. Surgical correction was undertaken and there were no neurological sequelae.

Cranial meningocele (and meningoencephaloceles) associated with cranial defects usually occur in the occipital area. They are frequently associated with underlying problems of the ventricular system such as hydrocephalus.

**Figure 185  Meningoencephalocele:**  Occipital meningoencephalocele in a newborn infant. The infant had a large cranial defect in the occipital area and multiple other anomalies (ventriculoseptal defect, coarctation of the aorta, hydronephrosis). No operation was attempted and the child died on the 24th day of life due to increasing intracerebral pressure. At autopsy, the brain showed a large meningoencephalocele, obstructive hydrocephalus, cerebellar aplasia, microgyria of the right cerebral hemisphere, and gliosis.

An encephalocele involves herniation of the brain through a skull defect and may be accompanied by other cerebral malformations or hydrocephalus.

**Figure 186  Teratocarcinoma:**  Malignant teratocarcinoma in a 6-month-old girl. Since birth, a plum sized doughy tumor at the upper end of the anal cleft was noted. There were no neurological symptoms. On palpation of the abdomen, no masses were appreciated. At surgery, a cystic teratocarcinoma which extended to the spinal column and into the abdominal cavity was removed. Although there were no immediate post operative complications, one month after the operation, a grapefruit sized tumor was discovered in the child's pelvis. The mass could be palpated in the lower abdomen. It displaced both ureters laterally and shifted the rectosigmoid colon forward. Laparotomy revealed that this was part of the original teratocarcinoma which had penetrated the pelvis. After the second operation, radiation and chemotherapy were given.

Germ cell tumors such as teratocarcinoma can occur in the gonads, in the central nervous system, in the sacrococcygeal area, in the retroperitoneum, and in the mediastinum. The mass may cause obstruction of either the genitourinary or the gastrointestinal system, as seen in this case.

**Differential Diagnosis:**  A similar sacrococcygeal mass may occur in cases of lipoma or meningomyelocele. Hemangiomas and neurogenic tumors must also be considered.

## Reference

1.  Noseworthy J, et al. Sacroccocygeal germ cell tumors in childhood: an updated experience with 118 patients. J Pediatr Surg 16:358, 1981.

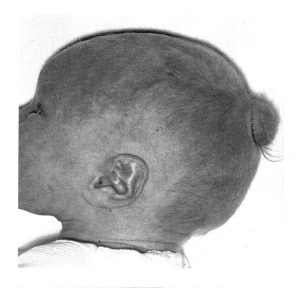

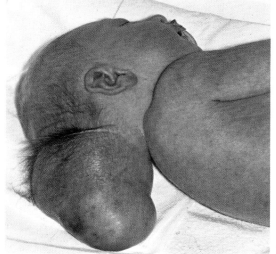

185

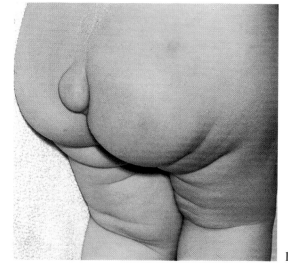

186

# 6. Diseases of the Nervous System

**Figure 187  Gingival Hypertrophy:**  Twelve-year-old girl with gingival hypertrophy caused by takin diphenylhydantoin for a seizure disorder. Hypertrophy may be so severe as to cover the crowns of the teeth Because of gingival hypertrophy, the mouth is more prone to trauma, and poor oral hygiene may lead t increased inflammation.

**Differential Diagnosis:**  Idiopathic gingival hyperplasia may occur and can lead to thickening of the lip and anomalies of tooth placement. Patients with idiopathic gingival hyperplasia may also suffer from men tal deficiency and hypertrichosis.

**Figure 188  Acrodynia:**  Acrodynia (Feer's disease) in a 3-year-old girl. Findings included redness an swelling of the gums with increased salivation. Characteristic of acrodynia is the red color of the tips c the fingers and toes, and extreme pruritus and pain in the hands and feet. Detailed medical history reveale the presence of chronic mercury poisoning.

**Figure 189  Hypertrichosis:**  Hypertrichosis in a 12-year-old boy who had been treated with dipheny hydantoin for a seizure disorder. An excess of body hair was first noted on the extensor surface of the arn and later noted on the torso and face. Therapy with diphenylhydantoin is also associated with gingival hype trophy.

Hypertrichosis is caused by many medications including prolonged therapy with corticosteroids, d azoxides, androgens, and other anabolic agents. While hypertrichosis caused by many medications may di appear 6 to 12 months after cessation of therapy, the hirsutism seen with androgens or anabolic steroic is usually irreversible. Specific syndromes may also be associated with hypertrichosis including Brachmar de Lange syndrome, craniofacial dysostosis, trisomy 18, and Bloom's syndrome.

**Figure 190  Cushingoid Syndrome:**  Cushingoid syndrome in a 1½-year-old boy who had been treate with dexamethasone for infantile myoclonic seizures. Findings included "full moon" face, obesity, and hype trichosis. Glucose intolerance also occurred due to the steroid treatment. Later, use of clonazepa (clonopin) for control of the seizures proved effective, and the Cushingoid syndrome disappeared with th cessation of the dexamethasone therapy.

## Reference

1.  Riikonen R, Donner M. ACTH therapy in infantile spasms: side effects. Arch Dis Child 55:664, 1980.
2.  Singer WD, et al. The effect of ACTH therapy upon infantile spasms. J Pediatr 96:485, 1980.

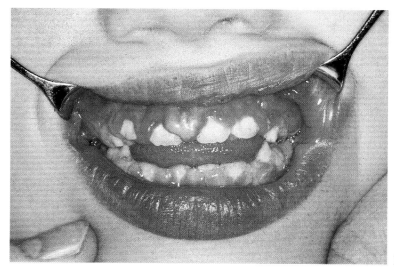

187

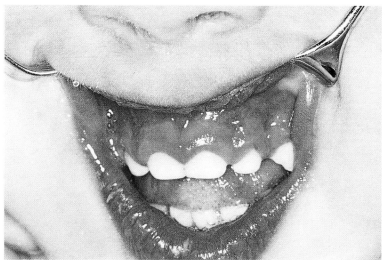

188

190

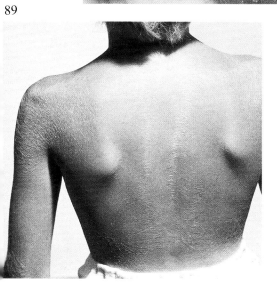

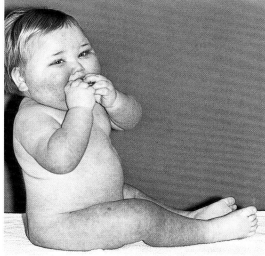

# 7. Diseases of the Musculoskeletal System

**Figures 191 and 192  Pseudohypertrophic Muscular Dystrophy:**  Progressive muscle weakness with pseudohypertrophy of the calf muscles in an 8-year-old boy with Duchenne muscular dystrophy. Since the age of 1 year, the child has suffered with increasing muscle weakness of the legs. Findings included slow motor development, waddling gait, difficulties in climbing stairs, and difficulty in getting up from a reclining posture (Gower's sign). Hyperreflexia of the lower extremities was noted. Serum creatine kinase (CK) was raised tenfold. Electromyography was typical for primary muscle disease (decreased amplitude and duration).

**Figure 193  Charcot-Marie-Tooth Disease:**  Charcot-Marie-Tooth disease (peroneal muscular atrophy) in a 7-year-old girl. Findings included bilateral pes cavus (high arched feet), and symmetrical atrophy of the muscles enervated by the peroneal nerve. Muscle atrophy of the lower extremity leads to a "stork leg" appearance. Gait abnormalities are noted including foot drop and "steppage" gait. Tendon reflexes may be decreased and a sensory deficit may be noted as well. Diagnosis was made by demonstrating decreased nerve conduction along with the typical findings on muscle biopsy and electromyography.

**Differential Diagnosis:**  Pes cavus (high arched foot) may occur with other neurological disorders:
1. Déjerine-Sottas disease (hypertrophic interstitial neuritis) a slowly progressive neuropathy associated with peripheral nerve enlargement and an increase in cerebrospinal fluid protein.
2. Hereditary Friedreich's ataxia (progressive cerebellar and spinal cord dysfunction) with signs of ataxia, decreased tendon reflexes, and positive Babinski's sign. Pes cavus, hammertoe, and scoliosis are commonly
   seen in this disorder.
3. Roussy-Lévy syndrome. The symptoms are similar to Friedreich's ataxia, but the disease may show little or no progression. Pes cavus and hammertoe may appear before ataxia and muscular atrophy.
4. Cerebral palsy.
5. Lumbosacral meningomyelocele (with spina bifida).

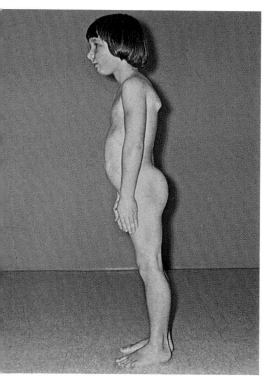

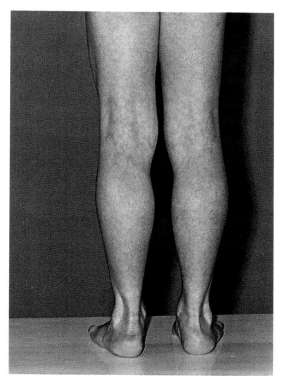

191

192

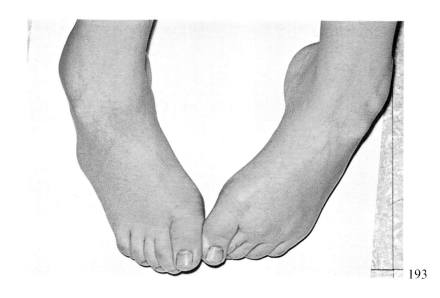

193

# 7. Diseases of the Musculoskeletal System

**Figures 194 and 196  Dermatomyositis:**  A 9-year-old girl with dermatomyositis. Symptoms included skin findings and muscular pain and weakness. The face had a butterfly-shaped erythema over the malar area and a lilac coloring of the upper eyelids. Gingival and nasal mucous membranes were also reddened. Over the arms and legs there was thickening of the skin resembling scleroderma, nonpitting edema, and a maculopapular rash. Scaly erythematous areas with atrophy were noted over the extensor surfaces of the knee, elbow, and finger joints; later, these areas were noted to be hyperpigmented. Extension at both elbow joints was restricted. Evidence of myositis was seen in the painful response to palpation of the muscles, diminished strength (making standing impossible), areflexia, and typical findings on electromyography. Laboratory investigation revealed elevated serum levels of creatine kinase, transaminase, and aldolase. A dermal muscle biopsy confirmed the diagnosis of dermatomyositis. The child rapidly improved after being started on prednisone therapy, but recovery (disappearance of muscle weakness and skin changes) occurred only after several months of treatment.

**Differential Diagnosis:**  During the chronic stage, with the absence of any visible skin findings, dermatomyositis may be difficult to distinguish from other muscular diseases (poliomyelitis, viral myositis, muscular dystrophy, myasthenia gravis). Differentiation can be made through electromyography, through enzyme analysis, through muscle biopsy, or through the presence or absence of specific neurological symptoms.

Since arthritis or arthralgia may be associated with dermatomyositis, dermatomyositis must be differentiated from juvenile rheumatoid arthritis and mixed connective tissue disease. Butterfly-shaped erythema of the face is also seen in systemic lupus erythematosus. Hardening of the skin and structures under the skin may occur in scleroderma.

## Reference

1.  Pachman LM. Juvenile dermatomyositis. Pediatr Clin North Am 33:1097, 1986.

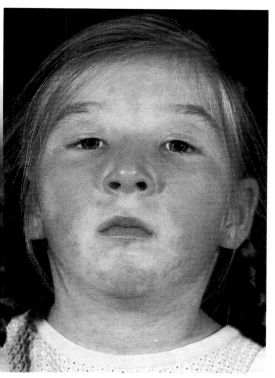

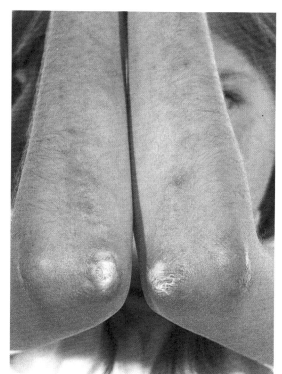

194

195

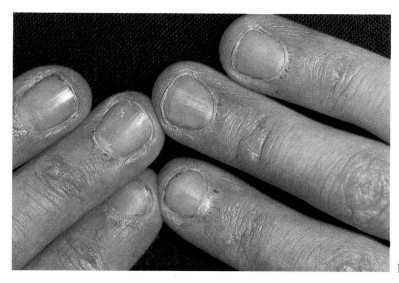

196

# 7. Diseases of the Musculoskeletal System

**Figures 197 and 198   Juvenile Rheumatoid Arthritis:**   Juvenile rheumatoid arthritis in a 9-year-old girl. Findings included painful swelling (with restricted movement) of the metacarpal phalangeal joints and the metatarsal phalangeal joints. The right knee joint was also involved. Despite treatment with acetylsalicylic acid (aspirin), there was chronic progression of disease, with bouts of fever, leukocytosis, and worsening arthritis. Temporary treatment with indomethacin, prednisone, and chloroquine was required. Aggressive treatment was able to control the symptoms. There was no other organ involvement (as there is in Still' disease) and no iridocyclitis was noted. There are several clinical subgroups of juvenile rheumatoid arthritis. This girl apparently suffered from polyarticular disease, in which there is multiple joint involvement. The onset of polyarticular JRA is frequently late in childhood. Serum rheumatoid factor and antinuclear antibodies are frequently positive. Polyarticular JRA is associated with HLA type DR4. The long term outcome of children with polyarticular disease is poor (severe arthritic disease).

**Differential Diagnosis:**   The early stages of rheumatoid arthritis must be distinguished from other causes of acute arthritis including osteomyelitis, viral infections, sepsis, and gonorrhea. Tuberculous joint disease, gout, leukemia, trauma, and aseptic necrosis must all be considered. In rheumatic fever, the arthralgia and arthritis may be migratory and endocarditis can occur. Systemic lupus erythematosus may exhibit very similar arthritic symptoms and must be differentiated by means of other clinical findings. Ankylosing spondylitis is rare in childhood, but can follow juvenile rheumatoid arthritis of the pauciarticular type. Patients with ankylosing spondylitis are more commonly HLA type B 27 (which is noted in 90 percent of patients with ankylosing spondylitis, but in only 5 to 7 percent of the remainder of the population).

### References

1.   Brewerton DA, et al. Ankylosing spondylitis and HLA-27. Lancet 1:904, 1973.
2.   Shaller J, Wedgewood RJ. Is juvenile arthritis a single disease? A review. Pediatrics 50:940, 1972.

**Figures 199 and 200   Osteomyelitis:**   Acute hematogenic osteomyelitis in a 6-week-old infant. Findings included swelling and restricted movement in the area of the left shoulder joint and both knee joints. The left leg was maintained in an adducted position. The infant was febrile and had hepatosplenomegaly. Culture from both the blood and joint aspirate revealed *Staphylococcus aureus*. Characteristic radiographic findings of osteomyelitis (periosteal elevation in the metaphyseal area) were seen in the left proximal femur, in both distal femurs, and in the left proximal humerus. The child was successfully treated with antibiotics.

**Differential Diagnosis:**   In older children, the differential diagnosis of joint swelling includes rheumatic fever (pain and swelling in several joints, carditis), leukemia, Ewing sarcoma, metastatic tumors (such as neuroblastoma), and scurvy. With chronic osteomyelitis of uncertain etiology, tuberculosis, syphilis, brucellosis, actinomycosis, and other systemic mycoses must be considered.

### Reference

1.   Weissberg ED, et al. Clinical features of neonatal osteomyelitis. Pediatrics 53:505, 1974.

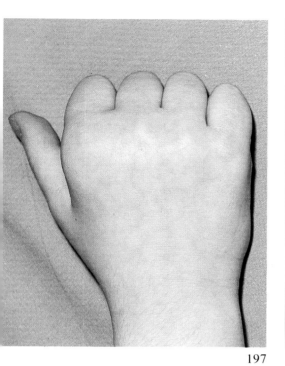

197

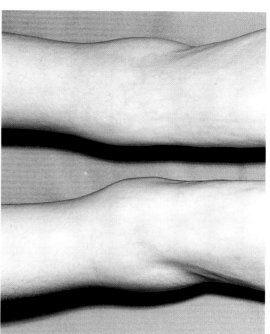

198

199

200

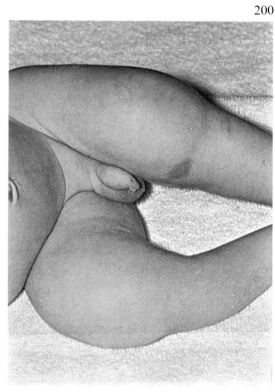

# 7. Diseases of the Musculoskeletal System

**Figure 201   Juvenile Rheumatoid Arthritis:**   Arthritic involvement of the right knee in a 10-year-old girl. Of note was the painful, nonerythematous swelling of the right knee, with restricted movement. Initially a high fever was noted, lasting for one week. The probable diagnosis was juvenile rheumatoid arthritis (pauciarticular form). Pauciarticular juvenile rheumatoid arthritis usually affects one or more of the large joints. Antinuclear antibodies are positive in the majority of these cases. Rheumatoid factor is usually negative. The diagnosis was confirmed by aspiration of joint fluid and synovial biopsy during an acute episode.

**Differential Diagnosis:**   Acute septic monarthritis must be considered. Causative agents include *Haemophilus influenzae, Neisseria gonorrhea, Salmonella*, or *Brucella*. Other causes of more persistent monarthritis of infectious etiology may include tuberculosis and congenital syphilis. Noninfectious causes for swelling of the knee include synovial chondromatosis and pigmented villonodular synovitis. Characteristic of pigmented villonodular synovitis is proliferation of the synovial membrane and hemosiderin impregnation. Joint aspirate usually reveals pigmented or serosanguineous fluid. Other causes of joint swelling may include fibroma, hemangioma, xanthoma, and sarcoma which emanate from the synovial membrane, and under certain circumstances may cause swelling of the joint.

**Figure 202   Juvenile Rheumatoid Arthritis:**   Juvenile rheumatoid arthritis (systemic onset or Still's disease) in a 5-year-old boy. Systemic JRA may have prominent extraarticular manifestations. The findings included a red evanescent macular rash on the face, torso, and extremities. The child had frequent bouts of fever and arthralgia (especially of the hands, fingers, and knee joints) without arthritis or lymphadenopathy. The child had pleuritis, but had no symptoms of pericarditis. The acute febrile episodes responded well to prednisone therapy, but, due to several relapses over a 12-year period, the child was also treated with D-penicillamine.

**Figure 203   Erythema Marginatum:**   A 12-year-old boy with rheumatic fever (presenting with chorea and rheumatic carditis). Erythema marginatum, the characteristic skin rash of rheumatic fever, was noted in this case. The typical numerous bright red macules (rings or stripes) were seen over the back and abdomen. The appearance of the rash varied day by day, and after two days the rash was no longer detectable. Gradual improvement of the chorea and carditis followed treatment with acetylsalicylic acid (aspirin) and prednisone.

Erythema marginatum may occur in 5-10 percent of children with rheumatic fever (especially when there are cardiac findings), but is not pathognomonic. The rash is evanescent and may come and go during the several weeks the child is affected.

**Differential Diagnosis:**   Erythema annulare centrifigum (see p 118, 196).

## Reference

1.   DiSciascio G, Tarant A. Rheumatic fever in children. A review. Am Heart J 99:635, 1980.

**Figure 204   Arthrogryposis:**   A 3-month-old boy with arthrogryposis. Congenital joint contractures were noted at birth (both of the large and small joints). Other findings included muscular hypoplasia, generalized thickening of the skin with dimpling, hip subluxation, bilateral talipes equinovarus, opisthotonic posture, and scoliosis of the lumbar spine. Treatment included physical therapy, casting, and surgical correction.

## Reference

1.   Hall JG. An approach to congenital contractures (arthrogyrposis). Pediatr Ann 10:249, 1981.

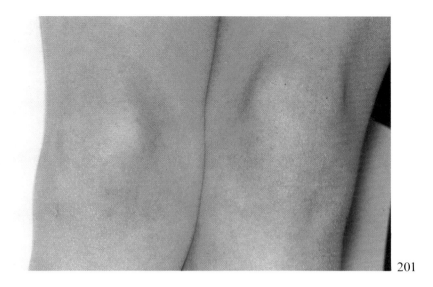

201

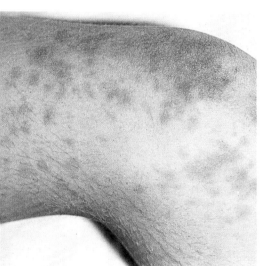

02

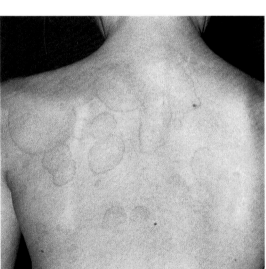

203

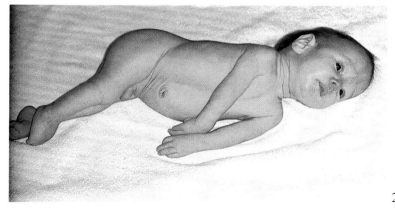

204

# 7. Diseases of the Musculoskeletal System

**Figure 205  Systemic Lupus Erythematosus:**  Systemic lupus erythematosus in a 6-year-old boy. Of note was a butterfly-shaped, nonpruritic, scaly, erythematous rash involving the malar area and the bridge of the nose. In approximately one-third of the cases, there is hypersensitivity to sunlight which can lead to blistering. Cutaneous facial symptoms of systemic lupus erythematosus include discoid lupus, nonpruritic urticaria, and changes similar to erythema multiforme.

**Differential Diagnosis:**  See pages 106, 120 and 200.

### References

1.  Fish AJ, et al. Systemic lupus erythematosus within the first two decades of life. Am J Med 62:99, 1977.
2.  King KK, et al. The clinical spectrum of systemic lupus erythematosus in childhood. Arthritis Rheum 20(S):287, 1977.
3.  Wallace DJ, et al. Systemic lupus erythematosus - survival patterns. Experience with 609 patients. JAMA 245:934, 1981.

**Figure 206  Systemic Lupus Erythematosus:**  Systemic lupus erythematosus in a 7-year-old girl. Findings included several irregular ulcerations of the mucous membranes that were covered with a white pseudomembrane. Other cutaneous symptoms and evidence of systemic disease lead to the diagnosis. Twenty-five percent of all patients with systemic lupus erythematosus experience changes of the mucous membrane (especially the palate, inner cheek, or gums). In the early stages, one finds erythematous hemorrhagic lesions that may evolve into painful ulcers.

**Differential Diagnosis:**  Similar findings may be seen in ulcerative stomatitis (see p 176).

**Figure 207  Erythema Nodosum:**  Erythema nodosum in a 10-year-old boy. Physical findings included painful, indurated nodules over both legs, and arthritis of the knees. Over the shins of both legs were found numerous round and elliptical nodules of varying sizes, which were raised above the skin surface and felt hot and painful when touched. The overlying skin was taught and glistening. At first, the skin overlying the nodules was a bright red color which later developed a bluish red discoloration. The underlying cause of erythema nodosum was apparently an infection with *Yersinia pseudotuberculosis* (serum antibody titer 1:5,000). Within three weeks of appropriate antibiotic therapy, the lesions healed without scar formation, leaving behind a brown discoloration. Erythema nodosum may be associated with an underlying infection of tuberculosis, *Yersinia*, or various fungal infections. Erythema nodosum may also be seen in rheumatoid arthritis, sarcoidosis, ulcerative colitis, systemic lupus erythematosus, and secondary to drug allergy.

**Differential Diagnosis:**  Erythema nodosum must be differentiated from erythema induratum, polyarteritis nodosa, Weber-Christian syndrome (nodular panniculitis), subcutaneous fat necrosis, thrombophlebitis, and fungal infection.

### Reference

1.  Biomgren SE. Erythema nodosum. Semin Arth Rheum 4:1, 1974.

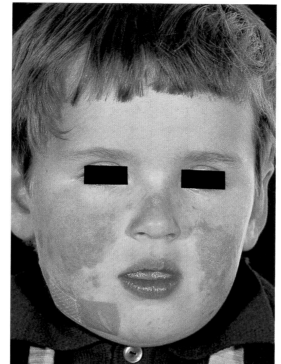

205

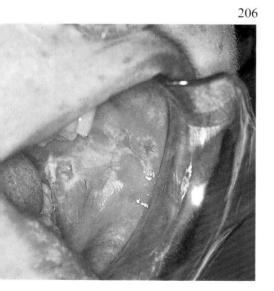

206

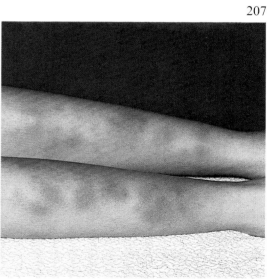

207

# 8. Diseases of the Skin

**Figure 208 Scleroderma:** Morphea (localized scleroderma) in an 8-year-old girl. The skin finding began as indurated, erythematous lesions on the flexor surface of the right leg and on the back. These foci later faded centrally and appeared violet in color at the margins. After several weeks the lesions became indurated and waxy in appearance. Scaring and fibrosis occurred, causing the lesions to be firmly adhered to the underlying tissue. The lesions gradually resolved, without therapy, over eight months.

Scleroderma is a chronic inflammatory disturbance of connective tissue. Isolated cutaneous involvement, as seen in this case, is referred to as morphea.

**Differential Diagnosis:** Skin changes resembling scleroderma frequently occur after bone marrow transplant (chronic graft-versus-host disease). Atrophic plaques resembling morphea can also beeen seen following injections of corticosteroids. In cases of scleredema adultorum, which rarely occurs in children localized, nonerythematous, nonpitting, induration of the skins occurs, which may limit mobility. Scleredema adultorum develops suddenly, 1 to 6 weeks after an acute streptococcal infection. The lesions appear on the face, neck, back, and later on the arms and thorax. The condition is self limited and resolves within months or years. Effective treatment is not known.

## Reference

1.  Cassidy JT, et al. Scleroderma in children. Arthritis Rheum 20:351, 1977.
2.  Winkelmann RK. Symposium on scleroderma. Mayo Clinc Proc 46:77, 1971.

**Figure 209 Scleroderma:** Morphea (frontoparietal scleroderma, "en coup de sabre") on the left side of the forehead of a 17-year-old girl. The lesion was an elongated, indurated, hyperpigmented area of skin 1 to 2 cm wide, which extended from the forehead to the parietal area. Where the lesion extended into the scalp there was alopecia. There were no other lesions. Hemiatrophy of the face, which frequently occurs, was absent in the case. The ESR was normal. In other cases of morphea, similar frontoparietal lesions with an ivory colored, hardened plaque, with hyperpigmented borders may occur. Usually there are no other lesions. Treatment is difficult; however, spontaneous regression of scleroderma is possible.

## Reference

1.  Singsen BH. Scleroderma in childhood. Pediatr Clin North Am 33:1119, 1986.

**Figure 210 Scleroderma:** Progressive scleroderma in a 16-year-old girl. For 3 years she had experienced increasing pain and swelling of the fingers. When her hand was closed in a fist, the skin over the swollen fingers was taught and shiny. In addition, the skin over the hand and the knees was hardened causing restricted movement. A 2 cm long hardened area of skin was noted on the left side of the neck. The girl also complained of coldness, paresthesia, and acrocyanosis of the hands (Raynaud's phenomenon). Involvement of the gastrointestinal tract, the heart, the lungs, or the kidneys, was not noted. As is typical in scleroderma the ESR was only slightly elevated and the serum rheumatoid factor was positive. No antinuclear antibodies could be detected.

**Differential Diagnosis:** Scleroderma must be differentiated from disseminated morphea (which does not affect the internal organs). Scleroderma may be differentiated from dermatomyositis by the lack of muscle involvement.

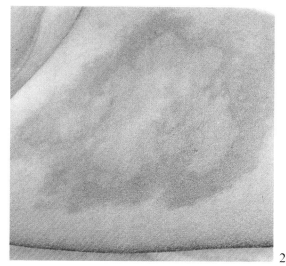

208

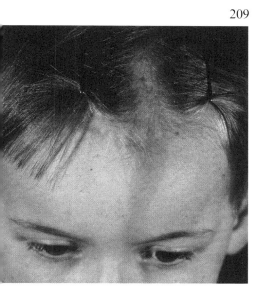

209

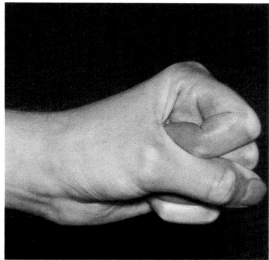

210

# 8. Diseases of the Skin

**Figure 211  Erythema Multiforme Exsudativum:**  Erythema multiforme (Stevens-Johnson syndrom in a 12-year-old boy. After treatment of bronchopneumonia with antibiotics, the child developed a nonpruri generalized exanthem. The rash was characterized by circular lesions, 1 to 2 cms in diameter on the a and legs; the lesions had a sunken, blue, discolored center, with a bright red raised border. Some of lesions developed central vesiculation. The rash rapidly responded to 4 days of prednisone treatment. cause of the rash was unknown. In only half the cases of erythema multiforme, the underlying caus determined. Erythema multiforme is associated with viral infections (herpes simplex), bacterial infecti (micoplasma) and certain medications (sulfonamide, anticonvulsants, penicillin, barbiturates). In appro mately 40 percent of the cases, the oral mucous membranes are affected (Stevens-Johnson syndrome, p 120). The characteristic skin rash usually presents no difficulty with regard to differential diagnos

## References

1. Ginsburg CM. Stevens-Johnson syndrome in children. Pediatr Infec Dis 1:155, 1982.
2. Marvin JA, et al. Improved treatment of Stevens-Johnson syndrome. Arch Surg 119:601, 1984.
3. Yetiv JZ, et al. Etiologic factors of the Stevens-Johnson syndrome. South Med J 73:599, 1980.

**Figure 212  Scarlatiniform Exanthem:**  Scarlatiniform exanthem in a 12-year-old boy. The child was trea with carbamazepine (Tegretol) for a seizure disorder. Three weeks after therapy was initiated, the ch became febrile and a generalized skin rash was noted. The rash was slightly pruritic and consisted of den red papules the size of a pinhead. The mucous membranes were not affected. There was no arthrit lymphadenopathy, or hepatosplenomegaly. After discontinuing the anticonvulsant medication, the exanthe disappeared after 2 days and the child's fever abated.

Other known allergic side affects of carbamazepine include maculopapular and urticarial exanthe edema, and agranulocytosis.

**Figure 213  Urticaria:**  Urticaria in a 3-year-old boy. The rash is characterized by pruritic, erythemato raised skin lesions (approximately the size of a penny) that appear suddenly over the entire body. The r may be accompanied by facial edema. Fever is not associated with the rash. The cause of urticaria is f quently unknown. Individual lesions may be resolved quickly (within 2 days), but new lesions may app later. The diagnosis of urticaria is generally simple. However, sometimes it is difficult to differenti urticarial lesions from erythema multiforme or anaphylactoid purpura.

**Figures 214 and 215  Urticaria:**  Generalized urticaria in a 5-year-old boy. The rash appeared every ti the child ate fish. The rash was characterized by pruritic wheals with a white edematous center surround by an erythematous base. Lesions were found on the face and over the body. Some of the lesions form ring- and garland-like patterns. Along with the urticarial rash, the child developed subglottic edema whi rapidly responded to intravenous corticosteroids.

There are many forms of urticaria in childhood. Papular urticaria occur in small children at the s of insect bites. The lesions have a papular center on an urticarial base, often with a small blister in t center. These pruritic lesions are arranged in groups and are usually located on the exposed parts of t extremities. Other forms of urticaria include cholinergic urticaria. Cholinergic urticaria are brought on exertion, heat, and emotional stress. The rash is characterized by small wheals or papules, 2 to 3 mm diameter, surrounded by a 2 to 3 mm wide erythematous base. The lesions are nonpruritic and devel on the torso, upper arms, and upper legs. They may disappear in minutes or after 1 to 2 hours. Seve outbreaks of cholinergic urticaria may be accompanied by systemic cholinergic sympto (sweating, salivation, abdominal pain, diarrhea).

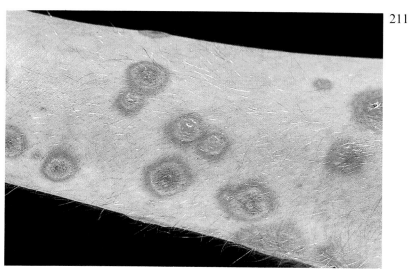

211

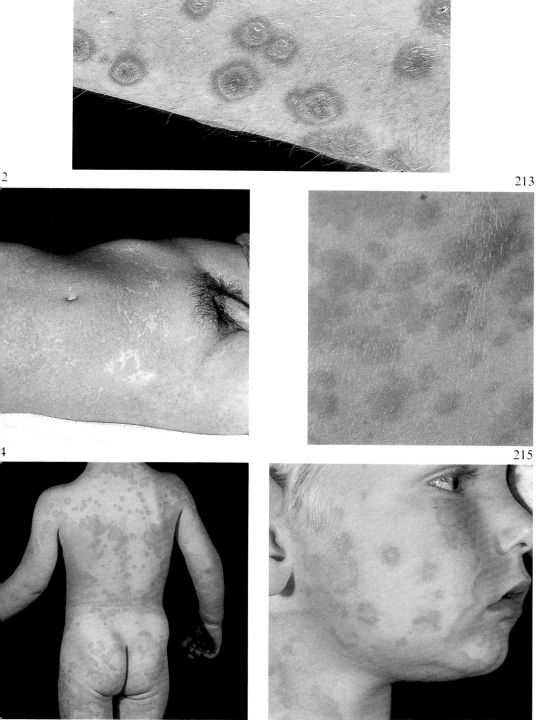

213

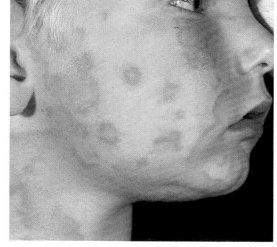

215

# 8. Diseases of the Skin

**Figures 216 and 217   Erythema Muliforme Exudativum:**   Erythema multiforme in an 8-year-old b▮ The typical lesions are dark erythematous, nonpruritic macules on the face and torso, which may becom▮ partially confluent. There may be characteristic central clearing, the so-called iris or target lesions. Mucos▮ involvement is common.

The term "multiforme" is applied to this skin disease because the rash may manifest in various wa▮ (either as erythematous macules or papules, or as vesiculobullous lesions). In contrast to urticaria, the▮ is no itching, the course of the disease is longer, and relapses occur more frequently.

## Reference

1.   Edmond BJ, et al. Erythema multiforme. Pediatr Clin North Am 30:631, 1983.

**Figure 218   Erythema Annulare Centrifugum (Darier):**   Erythema annulare centrifugum on the che▮ of a 1-year-old boy. The rash consists of nonpruritic, erythematous, edematous lesions which may take ▮ an annular- or garland-shaped form. The center may be pale red, with an erythematous border. The ra▮ is found on the torso and extremities; it may spread centrifugally and remain for several weeks. The exa▮ cause is uncertain.

Characteristic of erythema annulare centrifugum is the chronic, progressive nature of the rash, a▮ the development of ring-shaped lesions from the small, red papules. The edge may be flat or slightly rais▮ and may be slightly scaly.

**Differential Diagnosis:**   Differential diagnosis of erythema annulare centrifugum includes tineal infe▮ tions, granuloma annulare, and systemic lupus erythematosus.

**Figure 219   Erythema Multiforme Exudativum:**   Erythema multiforme on the arm of a 6-year-old b▮ Due to the confluence of the erythematous lesions, the rash took on a garland-shaped appearance. Chara▮ teristic target lesions were seen on the arms and legs (sunken livid centers with bright red borders). T▮ rash was symmetrically arranged in a garland-shaped pattern on the extensor surfaces of the extremiti▮ At the time the rash appeared, the child was febrile. Pneumonia was detected by chest radiograph. T▮ rash appeared in bursts over several days, and disappeared after 2 weeks.

**Differential Diagnosis:**   Erythema multiforme must be differentiated from other erythematous rash▮ including the rashes associated porphyria, systemic lupus erythematosus, and Kawasaki disease (see p 12▮

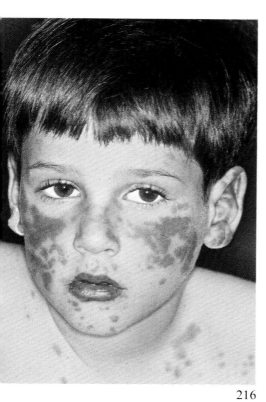

216

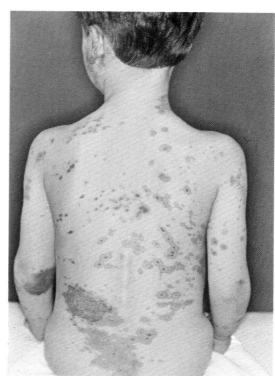

217

218

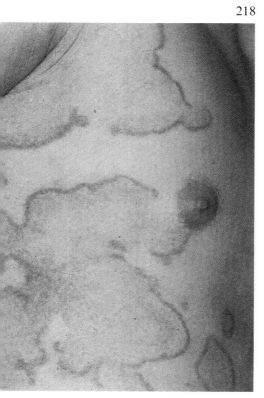

219

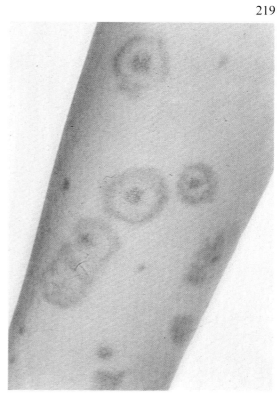

# 8. Diseases of the Skin

**Figure 220  Stevens-Johnson Syndrome:**  Butterfly-shaped erythematous facial rash with hemorrhag exudative, vesicular inflammation of the oral mucosa, nasal mucosa, and conjunctiva in a 9-year-old bc Stomatitis was present and led to an inability to tolerate feeding. A generalized maculopapular and bullo rash was noted over the body. Due to the stomatitis, the child had to be parenterally fed. Systemic cc ticosteroid treatment and local treatment of the mucous membrane lesions were successful in treating th illness. The rash resolved after 1 week, with no scarring.

**Figure 221  Stevens-Johnson Syndrome:**  Stevens-Johnson syndrome in a 3-year-old boy. Of note v inflammation of the urethra and the foreskin, with swelling and purulent drainage. The child had pain urination. In addition, the child had a high fever and developed a rash compatible with erythema multifor exudativum (maculopapular lesions with partial vesiculation and hemorrhage). A bullous eruption was n ed over the mouth, the anus, and the eyes. Stevens-Johnson syndrome was secondary to the administrati of barbiturates 10 days previously. After 2 weeks of illness, the symptoms were brought under contro

**Figure 222  Stevens-Johnson Syndrome:**  Stevens-Johnson syndrome in a 3½-year-old. The findin included redness and swelling of the skin surrounding the anus without vesicle formation. There were la blisters of the mouth which ulcerated and were covered with hemorrhagic crusts. Other mucous membra and skin changes were characteristic of Stevens-Johnson syndrome. The patient responded to oral prednis and symptomatic therapy.

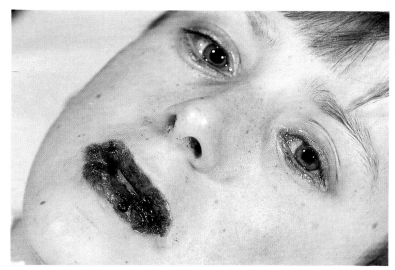

220

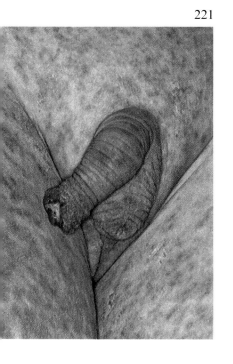

221

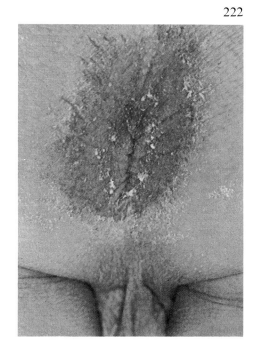

222

# 8. Diseases of the Skin

**Figure 223** **Acrodynia:** Acrodynia (Feer's disease) in a 3½-year-old girl. The child had absorb abnormally high levels of mercury because of exposure to a topical treatment containing mercury. Symptoi included redness and swelling of the hands (pink disease), and scaling of the fingers associated with acu pain (acrodynia) and itching. Similar skin changes were noted on the feet. Other findings included musc lar hypotonia (with diminished Achilles and patellar tendon reflexes), tachycardia, elevated blood pressui increased perspiration, anorexia, behavior changes (irritability), and insomnia. After the exclusion of oth causes, mercury intoxication was diagnosed. The child was removed from the source of mercury poisoni and gradually improved with symptomatic treatment.

**Figures 224 and 225** **Kawasaki Disease:** Kawasaki disease (mucocutaneous lymph node syndrome) a 9-year-old boy who suddenly developed high fever and systemic illness. Symptoms included nonpurule conjunctivitis, stomatitis (strawberry tongue), cherry red lips, and painful cervical lymphadenopathy. T hands were erythematous and swollen, and the fingers tips had a bluish discoloration. Subsequently t rash began to desquamate (as is typical of Kawasaki disease). Kawasaki disease may sometimes cause my carditis, pericarditis, arthritis, arthralgia, aseptic meningitis, and hepatitis. Kawasaki disease is also associat with coronary artery vasculitis, especially in the younger male patients. Corticosteroid therapy is not indicate

**Differential Diagnosis:** Scarlet fever may be confused with Kawasaki disease. Both have a "strawber tongue" and desquamation of the skin of the finger tips. The cutaneous findings and stomatitis are al characteristic of erythema multiforme exudativum and Stevens-Johnson syndrome.

## References

1. Kawasaki T, et al. A new infantile acute febrile mucocutaneous lymph node syndrome (MLNS) prevailing in Japan. Pe atrics 54:271, 1974.
2. Melish ME, et al. Mucocutaneous lymph node syndrome in the United States. Am J Dis Child 130:599, 1976.

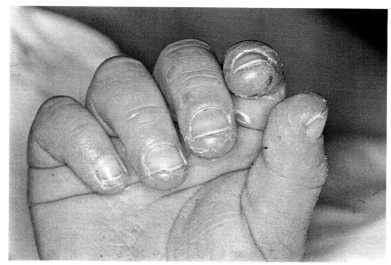

223

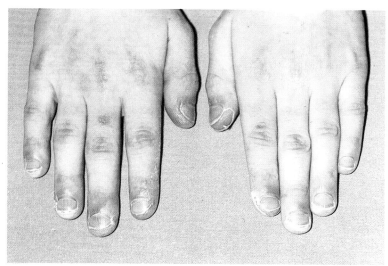

224

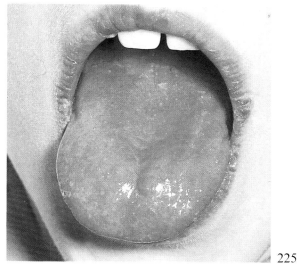

225

**Figure 226  Granuloma Annulare:**   Granuloma annulare in a 16-year-old boy. Of note was an erythematous firm, painless nodule, 1 × 2 cm in size, at the base of a finger on the right hand. The characteristic feature of granuloma annulare were demonstrated histologically (granuloma with central necrosis, mucin deposition and peripheral infiltration of lymphocytes, histiocytes, and giant cells). In granuloma annulare, there is typically a ring of dense, small, firm, skin colored or light red colored papules found primarily on the extensor surface of the fingers, hands, arms, legs, and feet.

**Differential Diagnosis:**   Granuloma annulare must be differentiated from necrobiosis lipoidica diabeticorum

## Reference

1.   Muhlbauer JE. Granuloma annulare. J Am Acad Dermatol 3:217, 1980.

**Figure 227  Granuloma Annulare:**   Granuloma annulare in a 15-year-old boy. The rash takes on a ring like appearance with a raised reddened border. In contrast to tinea corporis, there is no desquamation After persistence for several months, the rash healed following local and systemic corticosteroid treatment

**Figure 228  Granuloma Annulare:**   Granuloma annulare in a 14-year-old girl. A large erythematous area of skin with a slightly atrophic center is noted on the dorsum of the foot. More typical of this lesion is a ring of erythematous papules around a sunken center. The cause of granuloma annulare is uncertain Granuloma annulare is relatively frequent and occurs primarily in children. Generally, it does not bring about discomfort and can disappear after months or years without scarring.

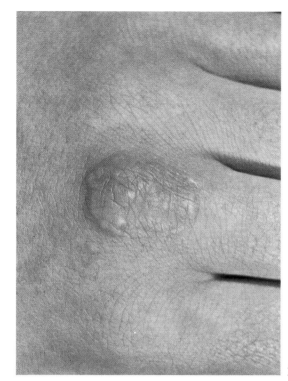

226

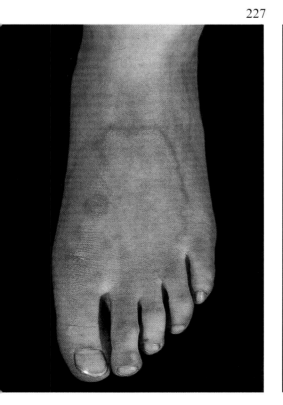

227

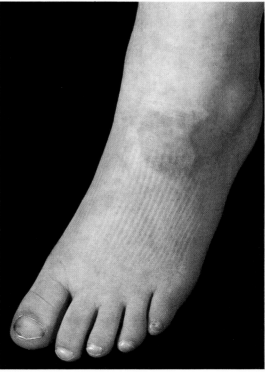

228

# 8. Diseases of the Skin

**Figures 229 and 230  Seborrheic Dermatitis:**   Seborrheic dermatitis in a 3-month-old boy. Generalized scaling and yellow crusting of the scalp was noted. Round erythematous lesions converged to form larger honeycomb-like areas over the torso and extremities. The lesions on the trunk and extremities were scaly and erythematous. Seborrheic dermatitis is frequently found in the scalp, in the flexor surface of the joints, and in the anogenital area. The rash was nonpruritic. The dermatitis began in the child's sixth week of life and resolved in the seventh month of life after various trials of symptomatic therapy.

**Differential Diagnosis:**   Seborrheic dermatitis must be differentiated from a variety of other dermatological conditions including atopic dermatitis (see p 132), contact dermatitis, diaper dermatitis (see p 128), psoriasis (see p 154), tinea versicolor (see p 184), tinea capitis (see p 184), tinea corporis (see p 182), and pityriasis rosea.

**Figures 231 and 232  Leiner's Disease:**   Leiner's disease in a 3-month-old boy. Of note is the generalized erythema and scaling of the skin. Children with Leiner's disease may have a disorder of the compliment system. Complications include anemia, hypoproteinemia, protracted diarrhea, failure to thrive, and secondary bacterial infection. The dermatitis improved after 4 weeks of treatment.

**Differential Diagnosis:**   The differential diagnosis includes other scaling dermatoses (seborrhea, ichthyosiform erythroderma, and candida dermatitis).

126

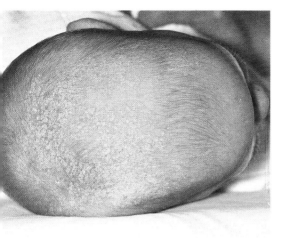

229

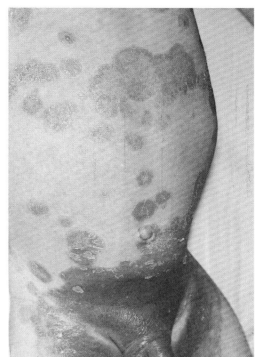

230

232

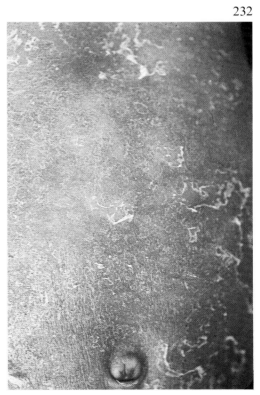

231

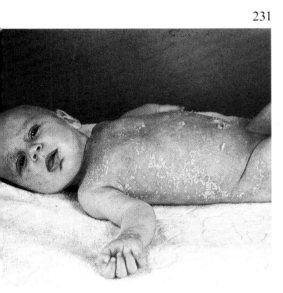

# 8. Diseases of the Skin

**Figure 233  Candida Dermatitis:**  *Candida* dermatitis in a 8-month-old girl. The skin around the anogenital area (including the labia majora) was reddened, swollen, and slightly scaly. KOH preparation revealed numerous microscopic *Candida* hyphae. Fungal cultures were also positive for *Candida albicans*. *Candida* dermatitis has a predilection for the folds of the skin, the diaper area, the areas near orifices, and the fingers (due to contact with saliva). The lesions have bright erythematous centers and irregular scaling edges. Satellite lesions may be found nearby.

**Differential Diagnosis:**  The differential diagnosis includes many other forms of dermatitis.

**Figure 234  Candida Dermatitis:**  *Candida* dermatitis in a 4-month-old boy. The skin of the anogenital area (including the foreskin) was erythematous and scaly, with a sharply defined erythematous border. *Candida albicans* was detected in culture. The child originally had a seborrheic dermatitis that became infected with *Candida*. The child rapidly improved with the use of a topical nystatin preparation, although several relapses occurred. The rash completed resolved by 11 months of age. During relapses, vesiculopustular lesions on an erythematous base were noted, which were also caused by *Candida albicans*.

**Figure 235**  Crusted areas on both sides of the groin in a 3-month-old girl.

**Figure 236  Diaper Dermatitis:**  Diaper dermatitis in a 4-month-old boy. Of note was a sharply outlined deeply erythematous, fine scaling rash over the entire diaper area. Papules and small blisters on erythematous bases were also noted. The rash was chronic and progressive in nature. The cause of the dermatitis was maceration of the skin due to contact with urine and feces in the diaper. The rash responded well to topical treatment.

Seborrheic or atopic dermatitis may predispose to contact diaper dermatitis. Frequently candida or bacterial infections may complicate this rash.

## Reference

1.  Rasmussen JE. Diaper dermatitis. Pediatr Rev 6:77, 1984.

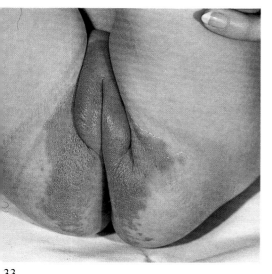

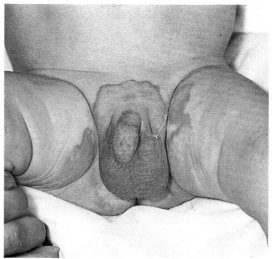

33

234

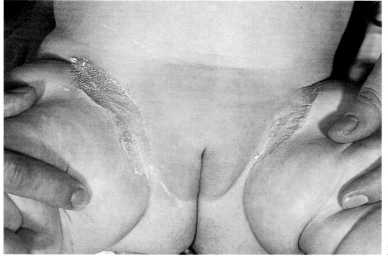

235

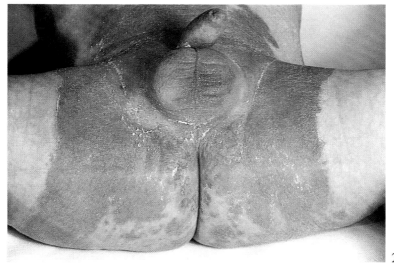

236

# 8. Diseases of the Skin

**Figure 237  Atopic Dermatitis:**  Atopic dermatitis in a 12-year-old boy. Findings included lichenified dried skin wth excoriations over the hands and arms, (evidence of long standing disease). During the firs year, the skin changes were localized to the face and the extensor surface of the extremities, and consistec of raised, confluent, pruritic, edematous papules that later formed crusted blisters. The course of the condi tion was chronic and progressive in nature, with intermittent spontaneous remissions. The lichenified area were treated with topical corticosteroid cream.

Atopic dermatitis during the first year of life (infantile atopic dermatitis) frequently appears on the face, but may involve the extensor surfaces of the extremities and the hands. Later in childhood, atopic dermatitis typically involves the flexural surfaces of the extremities. During the first year, edematous erythematous papules which may be single or confluent predominate; later in childhood, thickening and lichenification is more common.

## References

1.  Krafchik BR. Atopic dermatitis. Pediatr Clin North Am 30:669, 1983.

**Figures 238 and 239  Atopic Dermatitis:**  Atopic dermatitis in a 10-year-old boy. Findings include lichenifi cation of skin and excoriation due to scratching. The prognosis for atopic dermatitis is relatively good. At age 14 years, half of the patients will usually show marked improvement. Rarely does the disease extene beyond the age of 30 years. A familial history is positive in 70 percent of the cases.

## Reference

1.  Hanifin JM. Atopic dermatitis. J Allergy Clin Immunol 73:211, 1984.

**Figure 240  Atopic Dermatitis:**  Impetiginized atopic dermatitis in a 6-month-old boy. Findings include pruritic papules and blisters on the dorsal side of the hands and fingers, which were excoriated and became infected with staphylococci. Erythematous pruritic lesions with partial scaling and vesicle formation were also found on the arms, the scalp, and the torso. The child had other allergic manifestations, including hay fever and bronchial asthma (seen in 30 to 50 percent of all cases).

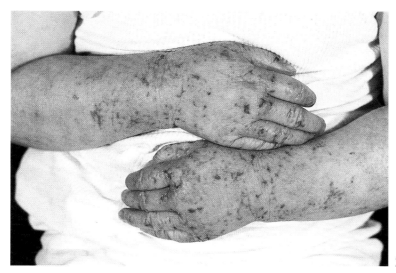

237

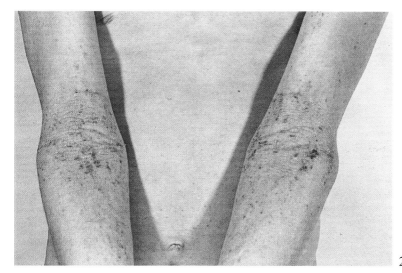

238

240

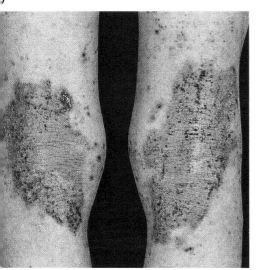

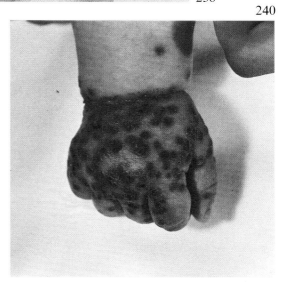

# 8. Diseases of the Skin

**Figure 241  Infantile Atopic Dermatitis:**  Infantile atopic dermatitis (infantile eczema) in an 8-mont old girl. Raw, scaly, excoriated lesions were found over the entire body (including flexor surfaces); crust lesions were also found in the scalp. The cause of infantile eczema is unknown. The child responded topical treatment with corticosteroid cream and tar containing preparations. Serum IgE levels were n increased, but this does not rule out the possibility of atopic dermatitis. Increased serum IgE occurs mo frequently in patients suffering from bronchial asthma. Delayed hypersensitivity may be compromised these cases (decreased T-lymphocytes and decreased reactivity of T-lymphocytes in vitro towards mitoge and specific antigens).

## Reference

1.  Yates VM, et al. Early diagnosis of infantile seborrhoic dermatitis and atopic dermatitis—clinical features. Br J Derma 108:633, 1983.

**Figure 242  Atopic Dermatitis.**  Atopic dermatitis (infantile eczema) in a 3-month-old boy. There we scaly, erythematous lesions over the body, and scaling, crusting lesions in the scalp. Later (at 4 years age), the child was also noted to have bronchial asthma. The family history was positive for allergic manifes tions. The only way to distinguish infantile atopic dermatitis from seborrheic dermatitis is to observe t course of the condition (seborrheic dermatitis will disappear after several weeks or months and will not recu

**Figure 243  Atopic Dermatitis:**  Atopic dermatitis in a 3-year-old boy. Generalized erythema and eder of the skin was noted. The lesions on the face were extremely scaly and the lesions on the neck we exudative and secondarily infected (impetiginization). The pinnas of the ears and the external auditory can: were also inflamed. In addition to secondary bacterial infection, complications may include eczema he peticum (p 172), conjunctivitis, and cataract. The child died suddenly, due to an anaphylactic reactio

**Figure 244  Photoallergic Dermatitis:**  Photoallergic reaction in an 8-year-old boy after treatment w: tetracycline. The parts of the body exposed to light (especially the cheeks and nose) were red and swolle Some areas were blistered and excoriated. The lesions were extremely pruritic. In susceptib individuals, exposure to light may lead to a delayed hypersensitivity reaction. Preventive treatment involv either the use of sunscreens or avoidance of specific medications which may cause photoallergic respons

**Differential Diagnosis:**  The differential diagnosis, when the immediate cause of photosensitivity is unknow includes several photodermatoses:
1.  summer prurigo (pruritic papules with secondary excoriation)
2.  immune disorders including polymorphous light eruptions (papulovesicular lesions) or urticaria sola: (urticarial lesions)
3.  genetic disorders associated with photosensitivity including xeroderma pigmentosum (presenting w: a wide variety of skin lesions) and Bloom's syndrome (photosensitivity and dwarfism)
4.  inborn errors of metabolism including porphyria (associated with erythematous wheals and bliste: and Hartnup disease
5.  hydroa vacciniform (vesiculobullous eruption with scarring)
6.  infectious disease including recurrent herpes simplex infection.

## Reference

1.  Ramsay CA. Photosensitivity in children. Pediatr Clin North Am 30:687, 1983.

132

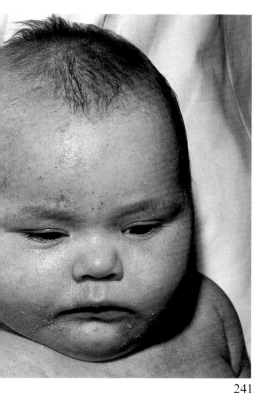

241

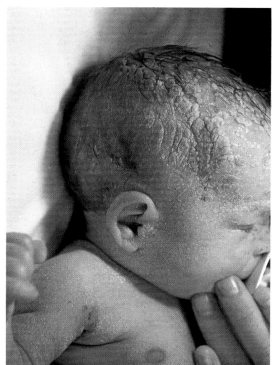

242

243

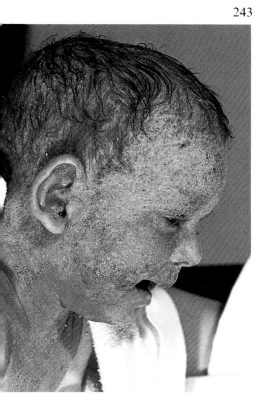

244

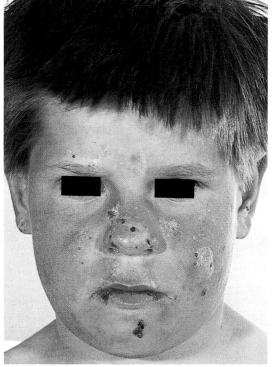

# 8. Diseases of the Skin

**Figures 245 and 246 Staphylococcal Scalded Skin Syndrome:** Staphylococcal scalded skin syndrom (Ritter's disease) in a 6-day-old boy. The skin was erythematous with vesicle formation and widespre wrinkling and loosening of the epidermis. Signs of systemic illness included high fever, irritability, a leukocytosis. Nasopharyngeal cultures grew *Staphylococcus aureus* (Group II Phage type). Systemic antib otic treatment lead to gradual healing, without scar formation.

Staphylococcal scalded skin syndrome may be a specific form of toxic epidermal necrolysis (Lyel disease) in the young infant. Both conditions may be caused by a *Staphylococcus* which produces exfoliative toxic substance.

## Reference

1.  Elias PM, et al. Staphylococcal scalded skin syndrome. Arch Dermatol 113:207, 1977.

**Figure 247 Toxic Epidermal Necrolysis:** Toxic epidermal necrolysis (Lyell disease) in a 4-year-old b A painful erythematous rash was noted on the face and chest. Some areas of skin formed flaccid bulla wh were filled with a clear liquid. When the skin was lightly rubbed, bulla would form or skin would exfoli (Nikolsky's sign). There were signs of systemic ilness (high fever, malaise). The cause in this case w sulfonamide medication. The child was successfully treated with systemic corticosteroid therapy and loc antibacterial treatment (to prevent secondary bacterial infection).

The changes of toxic epidermal necrolysis are often first noted in the axilla and groin. Toxic epiderm necrolysis may more often be fatal than staphylococcal scalded skin syndrome. Toxic epidermal necroly is a hypersensitivity phenomenon usually caused as a reaction to medication (sulfonamide, barbiturat infection, or neoplasm.

## Reference

1.  Manzella JP. Toxic epidermal necrolysis in childhood: differentiation from staphylococcal scalded skin syndrome. Pe atrics 66:291, 1980.

**Figure 248 Toxic Epidermal Necrolysis:** Toxic epidermal necrolysis (Lyell's disease) in a 2-year-c girl. An erythematous rash was noted over the hand, with vesicle formation on the palms and finger ti The cause in this case was unknown. Fluid loss across the denuded skin may lead to dehydration. In ad tion to the usual skin lesions, conjunctivitis and stomatitis were noted.

**Differential Diagnosis:** The differential diagnosis for toxic epidermal necrolysis should include staphy coccal scalded skin syndrome (Ritter's disease), burns (either secondary to heat or chemical skin damag and Stevens-Johnson syndrome. In adults, pemphigus vulgaris (flat blisters on nonerythematous skin) sho be considered.

**Figure 249 Photoallergic Reaction:** Photoallergic reaction in a 10-year-old girl. Rapid appearance vesicles and bulla (partially covered with crusting areas) on the back of the hands after exposure to su light. The lesions were nonpruritic. These lesions healed leaving hyperpigmented areas. The cause in th case was exposure to cologne. (see Figure 244).

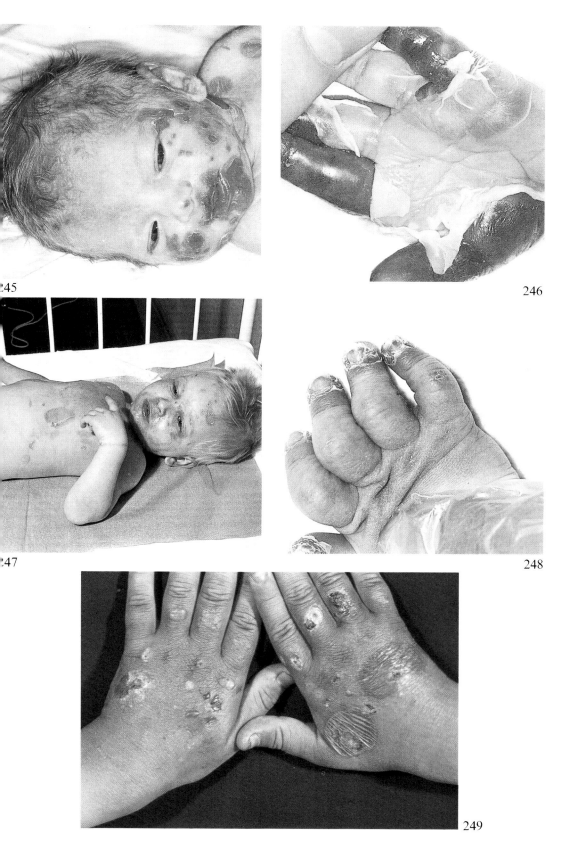

245

246

247

248

249

# 8. Diseases of the Skin

**Figure 250 Infantile Acne:** Infantile acne in a 1-year-old boy. Typical skin lesions (comedones) were noted on the face. These lesions were noted during the first year of life. Infantile acne may be progressive. The lesions resolved after regular local treatment with soap and water and application of a mild keratolytic lotion (benzoyl peroxide).

Infantile acne may be seen in precocious puberty and adrenogenital syndrome. Exposure to halogenated compounds may lead to acne during the first year of life. In this case, the rash is more progressive (with pustules or granulomas). *Candida* dermatitis can resemble infantile acne.

**Figure 251 Acne Vulgaris:** Acne vulgaris in a 1-year-old boy. Of note was a papular/pustular rash on the face which developed from closed (white) comedones. Acne vulgaris is an inflammatory process of sebaceous follicles. In this case, the probable cause was phenobarbital treatment. Acne may be brought on by a variety of medications including ACTH, corticosteroids, phenobarbital, isoniazid, certain vitamin or mineral preparations, and iodine or bromide.

**Figure 252 Photodermatitis:** Summer prurigo in a 6-year-old boy after exposure to sunlight. The findings included pruritic papules on the face, which eventually became excoriated and crusted, leaving small superfical scars. The skin changes were restricted to the face, but they may also occur on clothed parts of the body. Lesions may persist for a lengthy period of time.

**Figure 253 Xeroderma Pigmentosum:** Xeroderma pigmentosum in a 7-year-old girl. Pigmented macules resembling freckles of various sizes were located on the face, the lips, and the conjunctiva. White atrophic spots were also noted. The child had extreme hypersensitivity to sunlight and required regular application of sunscreen as a protective measure. Later in the course of the disease, the child developed characteristic telangiectasia and small angiomas. Xeroderma pigmentosa is a rare genetic disorder thought to be caused by a hereditary endonuclease defect causing cellular DNA damaged by ultraviolet light to be left unrepaired.

**Differential Diagnosis:** Milder cases of xeroderma pigmentosum must be differentiated from simple freckles. Other entities to be considered include Peutz-Jeghers syndrome (see p 164), and other photodermatoses.

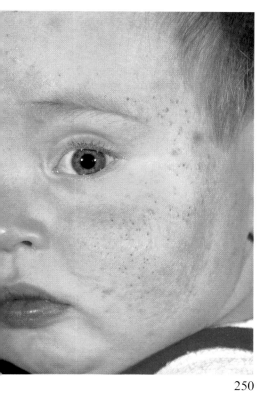

250

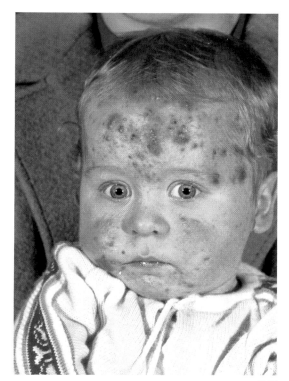

251

252

253

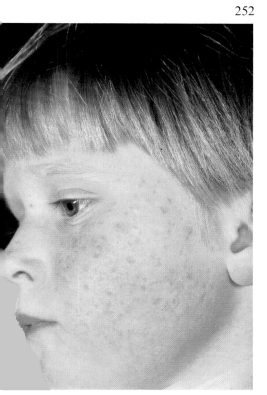

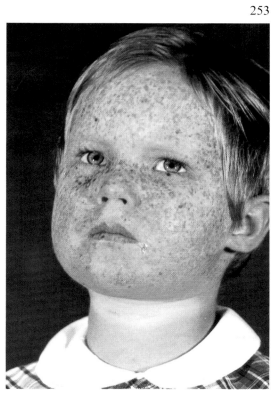

# 8. Diseases of the Skin

**Figure 254  Calcinosis:**  Localized calcinosis (calcium deposition in connective tissue) in a 10-year-o
girl. The findings included small, hard irregular papules which occurred on the arms, the legs, and th
torso. Deposition of calcium in the skin and subcutaneous tissue were confirmed by biopsy. Serum calciu
and phosphorous levels were normal. The cause in this case was uncertain (idiopathic form).

Inflammatory processes, as well as disorders of calcium and phosphorous metabolism, may lead
calcinosis cutis. Calcinosis cutis may be the symptom of the following diseases: hyperparathyroidism, ren
disease, vitamin D intoxication (due to hypercalcemia), dermatomyositis (due to chronic inflammation
and scleroderma. Calcinosis cutis may also be caused by ruptured epidermal cysts (epithelioma of Malherb
or local trauma (foreign bodies, hematoma, fat tissue necrosis). Hereditary diseases, such as fibrodysplas
ossificans, and pseudohypoparathyroidism, may also lead to localized dermal calcinosis. In calcinosis unive
salis, calcium deposition occurs symmetrically in the skin and musculature of the torso and extremitie
without previous trauma or metabolic illness. In later stages, erythema of the overlying skin and ulceratic
may occur.

**Figure 255  Branchial Cleft Sinus:**  External branchial cleft sinus on the anterior aspect of the neck
a 14-year-old girl. Since birth, there were two cutaneous openings located at the anterior aspect of the ste
nocleidomastoid muscle. They appeared as slightly erythematous papules which secreted no mucou
Branchial cleft cysts or sinuses are the result of incomplete closure of the first and second branchi
arches during embryonic development. The defects are usually unilateral. Mucous secretion sometim
occurs. The external branchial sinus can open into the pharynx and secrete saliva while the patient is eatin
The external opening lies at the anterior edge of the sternocleidomastoid muscle (usually at the lower third
Unlike external sinuses, the internal branchial sinuses may have no connection to the skin. Complicatio
related to the external branchial cleft sinus include secondary bacterial infection and cyst formation. Branch
cysts usually lie higher along the sternocleidomastoid muscle (upper third of the neck) and become manife
later in childhood. They may be confused with tuberculous lymphadenitis. Thyroglossal fistulas and cys
lie in the midline of the neck and may be attached to the base of the tongue. In addition to mucous, thyrogloss
duct cysts may contain thyroid tissue.

**Figure 256  Nevus Araneus:**  Nevus araneus (spider nevus) on the cheek of a 12-year-old boy. Arour
the red point in the middle of the lesion (the central artery), there is a radial mesh of vessels. If one pu
pressure on the central artery, the nevus becomes pale. These nevi are frequently solitary and vary
diameter from a few millimeters to several centimeters. They are commonly found on the face, the ea
the dorsum of the hand, and under the arms. These lesions are found in 15 percent of preschool aged chi
dren and up to 45 percent of healthy school aged children. Multiple spider nevi may be seen with pregnan
and in hepatic cirrhosis (due to elevated estrogen levels). Spider-like telangiectasia are noted in Osler-Webe
Rendu disease (hereditary hemorrhagic telangiectasia). In Osler-Weber-Rendu disease, telangiectasia usua
ly develop during puberty and appear primarily on the face, the palms, the nail beds, the tongue, and m
cous membranes of the lips. These lesions may involve internal organs and may lead to severe hemorrha
and anemia.

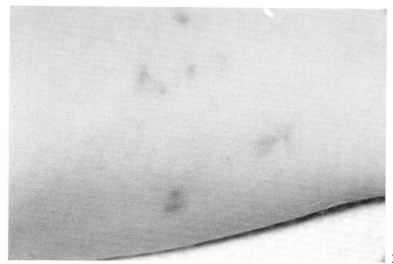

254

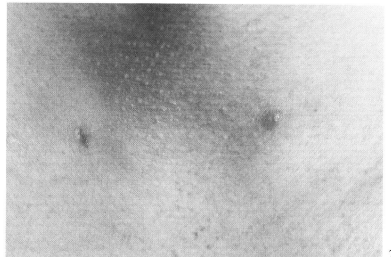

255

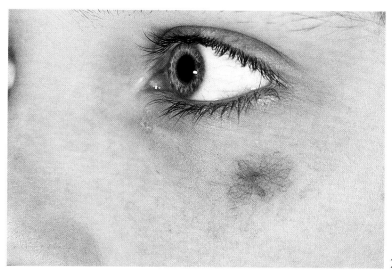

256

# 8.  Diseases of the Skin

**Figure 257  Nevus Flammeus:**  Nevus flammeus (port wine nevus, or flat hemangioma) on the right cheek and chin of a 1-year-old girl. The lesion is a sharply outlined, erythematous, macular lesion of irregular shape. The lesion had been present since birth and demonstrated no tendency toward regression.

Nevus flammeus occur frequently on the face, but may occur on other sites as well. If the neck is involved, it is known as Unna nevus. Color may be varying shades of red. The lesion may involve the mucous membranes. Over time, nevus flammeus may become slightly raised or fade considerably. Nevus flammeus may be associated with several syndromes including:

1.  Sturge-Weber syndrome (see p 38)
2.  Klippel-Trenaunay-Weber syndrome (see p 42)
3.  Rubinstein's syndrome
4.  Cobb's syndrome (arteriovenous malformation of the spinal cord)
5.  Beckwith-Wiedemann syndrome (see p 202)
6.  Trisomy 13 (Patau's syndrome, see p 58).

In contrast to nevus flammeus, macular hemangioma (salmon patch) is usually present at birth and is localized to the base of the nose, the upper eyelid, or the upper lip. Salmon patches are poorly defined, bright red in color, and, usually, disappear during the first year of life.

**Figure 258  Pigmented Nevus:**  Pigmented nevus (junctional nevus) in a 4-year-old boy. The findings include a superficial, discrete, brown, hyperpigmented lesion on the left cheek. The lesion is not raised. As a rule, pigmented nevi are benign; very seldom do malignant melanoma develop.

**Figure 259  Nevus Sebaceous:**  Nevus sebaceous (Jadassohn) in a 2-year-old girl. The findings include an elongated, sharply demarcated, hairless, orange-yellow, elevated area of skin over the scalp. These findings had persisted since birth. Typical findings on biopsy included hyperkeratosis, hyperplasia of the epidermis, deformed hair follicles, and an abundance of sebaceous glands. Since malignant degeneration during adolescence may occur, the nevus was fully resected.

Nevus sebaceous may develop later in children and appear on the face, the ears, or the neck. Nevus sebaceous must be differentiated from epidermal nevus (nevus verrucosus) which appear in various forms. Nevus sebaceous must also be differentiated from ichthyosis hystrix. In ichthyosis hystrix, one finds brown verrucose papules arranged in a linear fashion; histologically, one sees epidermolytic hyperkeratosis, papillomatosis, and acanthosis.

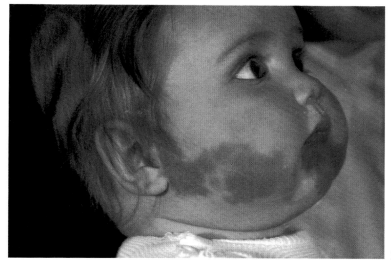

257

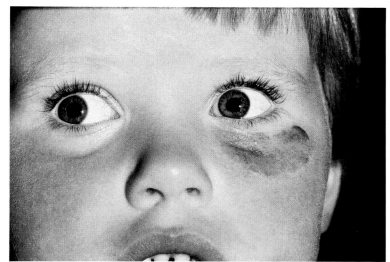

258

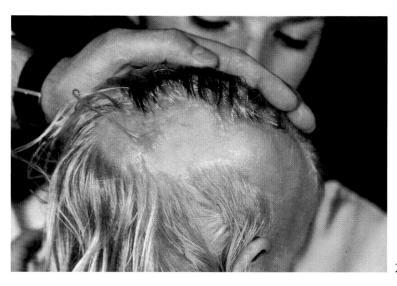

259

# 8. Diseases of the Skin

**Figure 260  Congenital Giant Pigmented Nevus:**  Congenital giant pigmented nevus (giant hairy nevus) in a 7-month-old girl. This extensive lesion is dark brown in color with thickened partially hairy skin that extended from the waist down to the knees. Several small pigmented macules on the back, hands, and arms were noted. There were no other malformations. Because of the extent of the lesion, surgical removal was not possible. As the child grew older, the thickness and hairiness of the nevus increased.

**Figure 261  Congenital Giant Pigmented Nevus:**  Congenital giant pigmented nevus (giant hairy nevus) in a 1½-year-old girl. The findings included extensive, sharply outlined, hairy, hyperpigmented lesions on the back and several smaller pigmented lesions over the body. Histologically, this would be classified as a compound nevus (both epidermal and intradermal).

Congenital giant pigmented nevi may be epidermal (junctional type) or intradermal. In about 10 per cent of the cases, malignant change may occur (malignant melanoma). Further complications include leptomeningeal melanocytosis that can lead to hydrocephalus, seizures, and developmental delay. In these cases, cells containing melanin may be detected in the cerebrospinal fluid.

**Figure 262  Intradermal Pigmented Nevus:**  Intradermal pigmented nevus in a 2-month-old infant. Several sharply outlined, raised, dark brown, pigmented growths were noted at the base of the nose and below the left eye. The lesions were noted since birth and grew considerably. Histological examination identified them as being benign intradermal pigmented nevus.

**Figure 263  Pigmented Nevus:**  Pigmented nevus (compound nevus) in a 3-day-old newborn. The lesion was a palm sized, slightly raised, dark brown area of skin on the anterior chest and abdomen. Histologically, the nevus was found to be a compound nevus (located in both the epidermis and the dermis). In contrast to a compound nevus, a junctional nevus lies only on the epidermal surface and is flat, smooth, and relatively small. Junctional nevi vary in color from light to dark brown, and over time may become compound nevi. Pigmented nevi can occur in 1 to 2 percent of all children. Junctional nevi are the most common. Intradermal nevi stand out more prominently from the body surface than do compound nevi. Generally, these pigmented nevi get larger during adolescence, but remain stable thereafter, and may diminish in size after 60 years of age. Nevi may undergo malignant transformation. Lesions which demonstrate a rapid change in growth, or become otherwise symptomatic, should be removed because of the possibility of malignant degeneration.

142

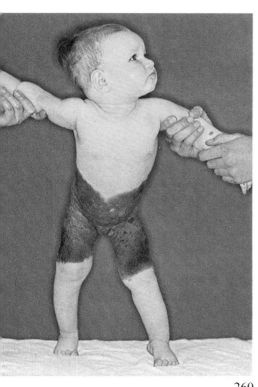

260

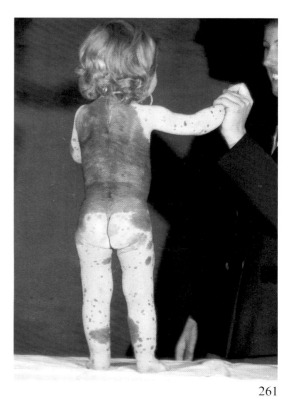

261

262

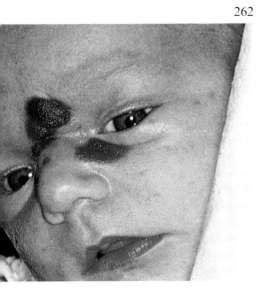

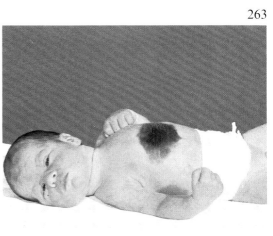

263

# 8. Diseases of the Skin

**Figure 264  Nevus Sebaceous:**  Nevus sebaceous (Jadassohn) in a 10-month-old boy. The lesion, whic was present since birth, consisted of several densely grouped, small, yellow nodules in front of the le ear. After surgical removal, the diagnosis was confirmed histologically. Histologically, these lesions demo strate hyperkeratosis, abnormal hair follicles, and an abundance of sebaceous glands. For differential dia nosis see p 140.

**Figure 265  Nevus Sebaceous:**  Nevus sebaceous (Jadassohn) in an 8-year-old boy. The lesion was a extensive, irregularly outlined, hardened, nonhairy area of the scalp above the parietal bone. The nev was surgically removed (because of the risk of malignant degeneration) and the skin defect was cover by skin transplant.

**Figure 266  Blue Nevus:**  Blue nevus in a 12-year-old girl. Of note was a pea-sized, dark blue, smoot nodule arising from the skin next to the right eye. The lesion had developed during the first year of li and then ceased to grow. Despite the benign nature of the blue nevus, the lesion was surgically remove for cosmetic reasons. On histologic examination, there were groups of deeply pigmented, spindle-shape melanocytes.

Blue nevi are usually solitary and found primarily on the face, neck, arms, upper legs, hands, an feet. They must be differentiated from the cellular blue nevi, which are larger than 1 cm and found primaril on the thigh or sacrum. Since these lesions can become malignant, they must be surgically removed.

**Figure 267  Congenital Pigmented Nevus:**  Congenital pigmented nevus in a 3-year-old boy. The lesio was a 3 × 7 cm, hyperpigmented area of the skin over the forehead. The lesion had abundant hair. Afte surgical removal, the skin defect was covered by grafting.

**Figure 268  Leukoderma Acquisitum Centrifugum:**  Leukoderma acquisitum centrifugum (halo nevus in a 13-year-old girl. The lesion is unique in appearance; a central pigmented nevus is surrounded peripherall by a depigmented area of skin (halo). The pigmented nevus has been noted since birth, whereas the depig mented base first appeared at puberty. After 4 to 5 months, the pigmented nevus became pale, smalle and disappeared. Although repigmentation may occur, it did not in this case.

Halo nevi may appear as solitary or multiple lesions. Generally, the depigmented base is not large than 5 mm in diameter. In the early stages, histologic examination may reveal a junctional or intraderma nevus; in later stages, a dense infiltrate of lymphocytes or histiocytes may be seen. Melanocytes are lackin in the depigmented base. Therapy is usually not necessary, since halo nevi tend to resolve on their ow Malignant melanoma may look similar to halo nevi (including depigmented base); in case of doubt, a com plete removal and histological examination must take place.

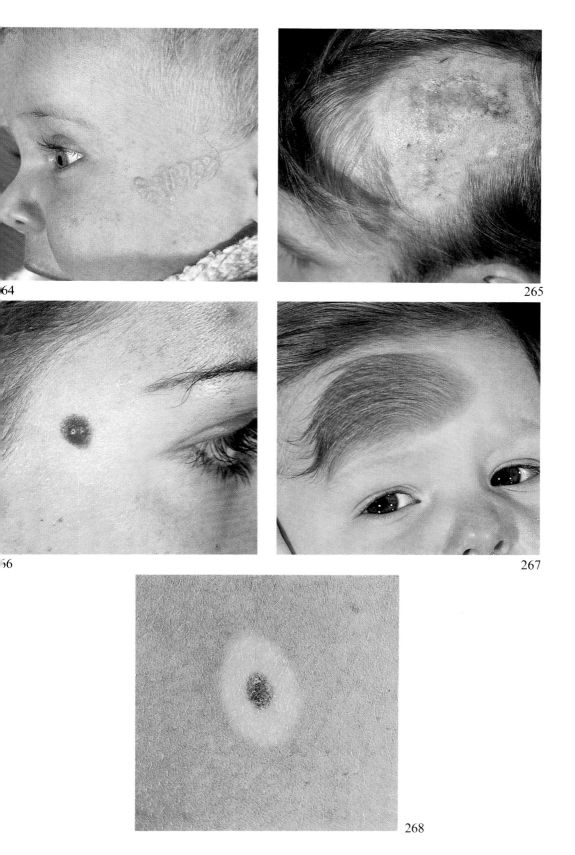

264

265

56

267

268

# 8. Diseases of the Skin

**Figure 269 Shagreen Patches:** Shagreen patches, in association with tuberous sclerosis, in a 14-year old girl. Raised indurated areas of skin were noted on the lower back (the most frequent location). These shagreen patches are typical findings in tuberous sclerosis. In addition the girl had adenoma sebaceum on the face.

**Figure 270 Granuloma Telangiectaticum:** Granuloma telangiectaticum (pyogenic granuloma) in a 2-year old boy. Findings included a red, pea-sized, sometimes bleeding nodule with a crusted surface on the right cheek. The lesion had persisted for several months without healing.

Granuloma telangiectaticum is frequent in children and is usually an isolated lesion found on the face, arms, or hands. The lesion probably stems from an unobserved episode of trauma. Secondary infection leads to exuberant granulation tissue. Pyogenic granulomas grow rapidly at first, but then remain stationary in size. It may be difficult to differentiate these lesions from small hemangiomas.

**Figure 271 Granuloma Telangiectaticum:** Pyogenic granuloma on the underarm of a 10-year-old girl. The lesion was a bean–sized, broad based, elevated, red nodule with an irregular surface. The nodule was moist on the surface and at its base had a narrow epithelial collar. The granuloma was excised because it was persistent and had a tendency to bleed. Microscopically, in the dense, capillary rich connective tissue, one could see numerous granulocytes. After surgical excision, histologic examination should always be performed because granuloma telangiectaticum may vary greatly in size and can be confused with neoplastic disorders (melanoma, Kaposi's sarcoma, metastatic carcinoma).

**Figure 272 Milia:** Milia on the eyelids of a 16-year-old girl. Of note were numerous 1 mm large, firm pearly white papules. Histologically, these are inclusion cysts of the pilosebaceous follicles, which contain keratin. They occur on the cheek, forehead, nose, and nasolabial cleft of newborn infants. They disappear within the first weeks of life without treatment. In the case of older children and adults, they can persist for longer periods of time; lesions may be removed by making a small incision with a fine needle and expressing the keratin.

146

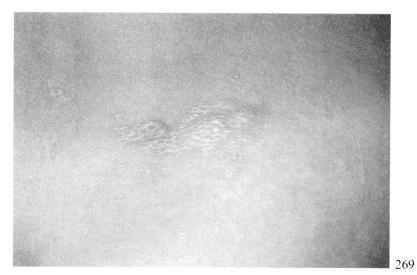

269

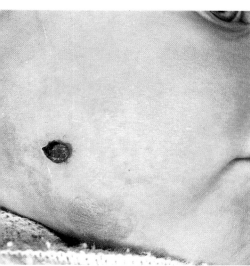

0

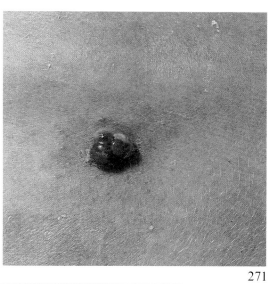

271

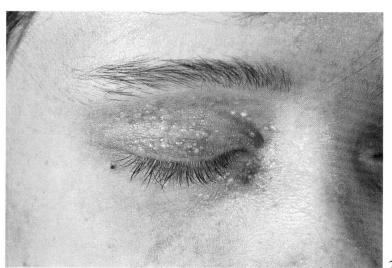

272

# 8. Diseases of the Skin

**Figure 273  Histiocytoma:**  Histiocytoma (dermatofibroma) of the thigh of a 15-year-old girl. The lesion is a flat, round, hyperpigmented, firm nodule, 1 cm in diameter, which contains histiocytes, fibroblasts and capillaries. Histiocytoma is a benign tumor. In this case, the lesion was firm, but in other cases the lesions may be soft and pedunculated. They are usually solitary and primarily develop on the arms or legs (possibly as the result of trauma).

Differential diagnosis should consider hemangiomas, epidermal cysts, juvenile xanthogranulomas, and neurofibromas.

**Figure 274  Lymphocytoma:**  Lymphocytoma (lymphadenosis cutis benigna) of the underarm of a 4-year-old boy. The lesions were round, coarse, red brown nodes, 2 cm in diameter, which had developed within the past several months. The etiology is uncertain. Many of these lesions regress spontaneously. Lymphocytoma may occur at any age, may be solitary or multiple, and occur primarily on the face, the earlobes, the scrotum and on the breast.

**Figure 275  Spitz Nevus:**  Spitz nevus (spindle and epithelioid cell nevus, or juvenile melanoma) under the left eye of a 4-year-old boy. Of note was a ½ cm slightly raised, firm nodule that was red–brown color and appeared suddenly under the child's left eye. Spitz nevi are usually solitary and are frequently located on the face, shoulders, and arms. Children ages 3 to 13 years are most commonly affected. A Spitz nevus may grow rapidly and attain a diameter of 1.5 cm. The Spitz nevus is considered a variant of the compound nevus (see p 142). After excision there is no danger of spreading. The Spitz nevus must be differentiated from pyogenic granuloma (see p 142), hemangioma, other pigmented nevi, and basal cell carcinoma.

**Figure 276  Spitz Nevus:**  Spitz nevus (juvenile melanoma) in a 5-year-old girl.

**Figure 277  Leiomyoma:**  Benign leiomyoma of the upper arm in a 7-year-old boy. Of note were multiple rough, bright red nodules of varying size. The lesions contain muscle tissue. Characteristically, there are paroxysmal bouts of pain. The pain, caused by muscle contractions, can be relieved through massage or cold compresses. Solitary lesions occur and may be treated with surgical excision.

**Figure 278  Pigmented Nevus:**  Pigmented nevus of the lower arm of a 2-year-old boy.

148

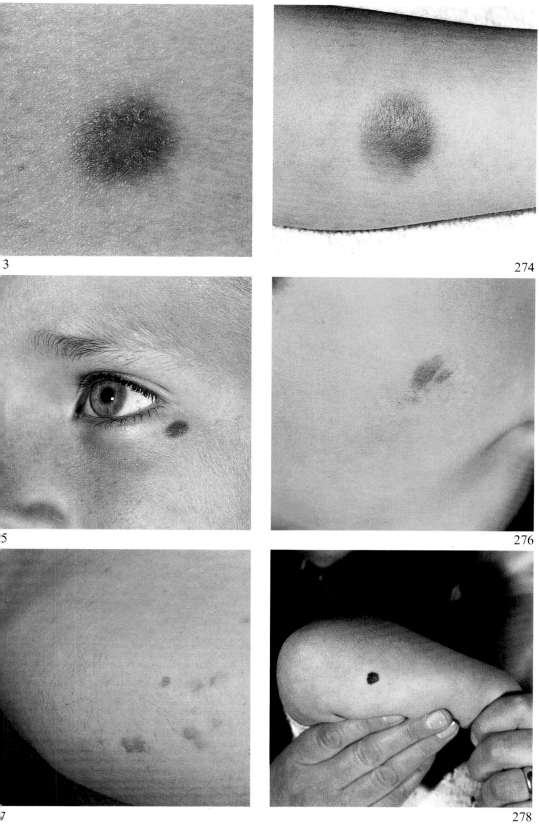

273

274

275

276

277

278

# 8. Diseases of the Skin

**Figure 279 Ichthyosis Vulgaris:** Ichthyosis vulgaris (X-linked ichthyosis) in an 8-year-old boy. Finding included large, brown, firmly attached scales on the neck, forehead, and body including the flexor surface of the extremities, but sparing the palms and the soles. The condition first became manifest at 2 month of age. There was a poor response to therapy.

**Differential Diagnosis:** X-linked ichthyosis must be differentiated from autosomal dominant heredita ichthyosis vulgaris. In the autosomal dominant form, one finds scaling over the back and extensor surface of the extremities. The flexor surfaces of the extremities and the face are apparently spared. The palm and soles are thickened and partially chapped. The first manifestations of disease occur after the first ye of life, but sometimes do not present until late childhood or adulthood. In contrast to hereditary x-linke ichthyosis, symptoms may improve with increasing age. In addition to hereditary autosomal ichthysosis vu garis, there is also a rare acquired form of ichthyosis vulgaris. The acquired form can appear at any ag and has been observed in patients with malignant disease (Hodgkin's disease). The skin changes do n differ from those seen in the inherited form.

**Figure 280 Lamellar Ichthyosis:** Lamellar ichthyosis (congenital ichthyosiform erythroderma) in 6-month-old girl. Since birth there had been diffuse erythema and scaling (without vesicle formation) ov the torso, the flexor surfaces of the extremities, the palms, and the soles. The skin condition improved ter porarily with symptomatic treatment.

**Differential Diagnosis:** The differential diagnosis of Lamellar ichthyosis includes other forms of ichthyos and certain syndromes with ichthyosiform skin changes:
1. Sjögren-Larsson syndrome (ichthyosis, spastic diplegia, and developmental delay)
2. Netherton's syndrome (ichthyosis, abnormal breakage of the hair, urticaria or angioneurotic edem
3. Conradi-Hunermann syndrome (autosomal dominant syndrome with chondrodysplasia punctata "stipple epiphyses, shortening of the long bones, joint contractures, and ichthyosis)
4. Refsum's syndrome (disturbance of the metabolism of phytic acid caused by alpha-decarboxyla deficiency leading to mild ichthyosis in the first or second decade of life, chronic polyneuritis, progre sive paralysis, and ataxia).

**Figures 281 and 282 Lamellar Ichthyosis:** Lamellar ichthyosis (congenital ichthyosiform erythrode ma) in a 3-week-old boy. Skin changes included generalized erythema and scaling (including the flexor s faces, palms, and soles) with numerous dermal fissures. Bilateral eversion of the lid margin (ectropiu was noted.

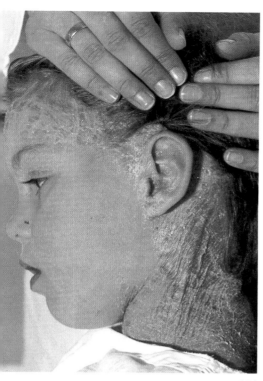

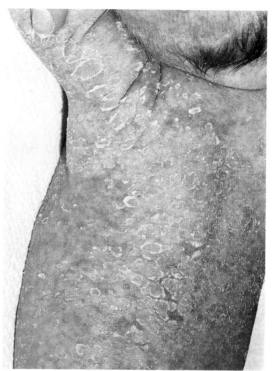

279

280

281

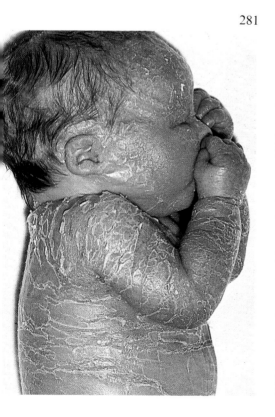

282

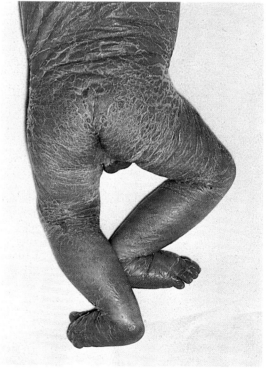

# 8.   Diseases of the Skin

**Figure 283   Ichythosis:**   Congenital ichythosis in a 1-day-old child ("Harlequin fetus"), who died at 8 days of age. The skin over the entire body was thickened and fissured causing extreme disfigurement. The mouth was constantly held open and the lips everted. There was also severe ectropium and chemosis. The hair was sparse and the nails were absent. Movement at the joints was severely limited. This severe form of ichthyosis (autosomal recessive inheritance) almost always leads to death after a few days or weeks. This child died due to an aortic thrombus.

**Figure 284   Ichthyosis Congenita:**   Ichthyosis congenita (ichthyosiform erythroderma) with unilateral cataract in a 4-week-old girl. The "white pupil" (due to cataract) of the left eye had been noted since birth. Ophthalmologic examination was performed to detect complications such as glaucoma and amblyopia e anopsia.

      The differential diagnosis of congenital or infantile cataracts includes:
1. cataracts associated with hereditary dermatoses such as intercontinentia pigmenti, Rothmund's syndrome (atrophic telangiectatic dermatosis) and other ectodermal dysplasia syndromes
2. cataracts associated with other malformations such as various trisomy and deletion syndromes, chondrodysplasia punctata, and Torsten-Sjögren syndrome
3. inborn errors of metabolism including galactosemia, homocystinuria, Lowe's syndrome
4. intrauterine infection including rubella embryopathy or toxoplasmosis
5. diseases of the eye that can secondarily lead to cataract (retrolental fibroplasia)
6. hereditary form (isolated malformation).

**Figure 285   Lamellar Ichthyosis:**   Lamellar ichthyosis (congenital ichthyosiform erythroderma) in a 11-month-old girl. Since the age of 1 month, a generalized, scaly erythroderma, without vesicle formation was noted. The facial skin showed diffuse erythema with patches of fine scaling. The flexor surfaces, the palms, and the soles were also affected. Because of the skin loss through dermal scaling, the child has a constant loss of protein and was considerably underweight. Improvement followed symptomatic treatment with keratolytic lotions, bath oil, and emollients.

**Figure 286   Ichthyosis Vulgaris:**   Ichthyosis vulgaris (autosomal dominant form) in an 8-year-old girl. Characteristic lamellar scaling of the extensor surfaces of the legs was noted. The flexor surfaces were not affected. The palms and soles were thickened and partially chapped. The father was likewise affected. The prognosis of ichthyosis vulgaris is relatively favorable, with improvement in adulthood.

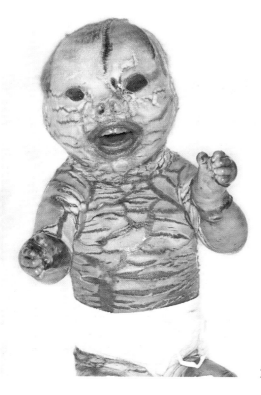

283

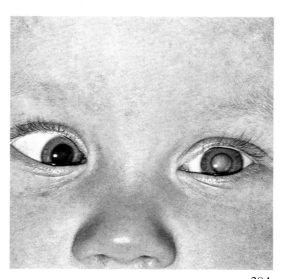

284

285

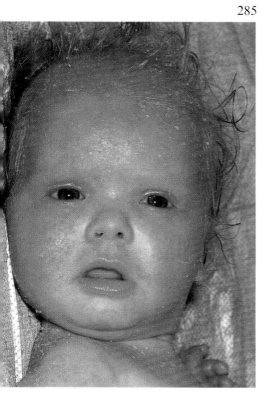

286

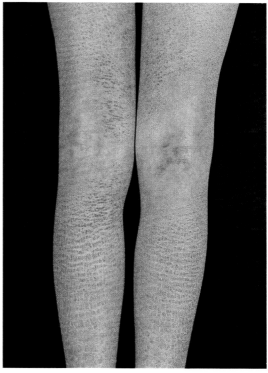

# 8. Diseases of the Skin

**Figures 287–289 Psoriasis:** Psoriasis in a 10-year-old boy. Shown is the generalized rash (Figure 287), an individual psoriatic lesion with the slightly raised, reddish plaque covered with thick, shiny, silvery scales (Figure 288), and discoloration of the nail plate with early onycholysis (Figure 289). In this case, the lesions were nonpruritic. Characteristic of psoriasis were the following:
1. candle-spot phenomenon (with light scratching, the lesions attain the color of candle wax)
2. the phenomenon of "last membrane" (with more vigorous scratching, the whole lesion can be lifted off)
3. dew-drop phenomenon or Auspitz sign (on the remaining skin surface, now free from scales, dot shaped hemorrhages appear)
4. Koebner's phenomenon (loosening of the typical skin lesions by scratching with the fingernail).

In this case, psoriasis was first noted at age 5. It was chronic and progressive in nature, with periods of spontaneous remission. Many family members were similarly affected.

**Differential Diagnosis:** The differential diagnosis of psoriasis varies depending on the morphology and location of the lesions, as well as the age of the patient. In cases where there is doubt, a skin biopsy should be performed. Typical findings of psoriasis include thickening of the stratum corneum with parakeratosis, hyperplasia of the epidermis with elongation of the rete ridges, micro-abcesses, vascularization of the dermis and infiltration of inflammatory cells. In cases in which psoriasis affects the scalp, fungal infection (tinea capitis) and seborrheic dermatitis must be ruled out. In cases of nail involvement, mycotic infection of the nails and lichen ruber planus must be considered. Chronic forms of psoriasis with extreme scaling must be differentiated from tinea corporis. Acute forms of psoriasis (with numerous, disseminated, small erythematous papules) must be distinguished from pityriasis rosea and secondary syphilis. Other forms of dermatitis associated with scaling must be considered. When psoriasis is localized to the anogenital area, *Candida* dermatitis (so called diaper dermatitis), seborrheic dermatitis and intertrigo must be considered. Guttate psoriasis, which occurs more frequently in children, can be confused with pityriasis rosea, secondary syphilis, and certain drug rashes.

## References

1. Nyfors A, Lemholt K. Psoriasis in childhood. Br J Dermatol 92:437, 1975.
2. Watson W, Farber EM. Psoriasis in childhood. Pediatr Clin North Am 18:875, 1971.

**Figure 290 Erythema Elevatum Diutinum:** Erythema elevatum diutinum on the legs of a 10-year-old boy. Of note are red–blue, scaling, nodular lesions of varying size with partial central indentation, ulceration, and crusting. The primary location is the extensor and flexor surfaces of the extremities, and the hand. The cause is unknown.

**Differential Diagnosis:** Erythema elevatum diutinum may be differentiated from facial granuloma because of its location. Granuloma annulare, histiocytoma, and sarcoidosis can be differentiated by histologic examination. Lichen ruber planus (light red, shiny papules) and xanthoma (yellow–brown papules or nodules) are usually distinguished without difficulty.

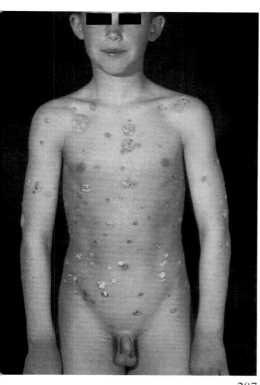

287

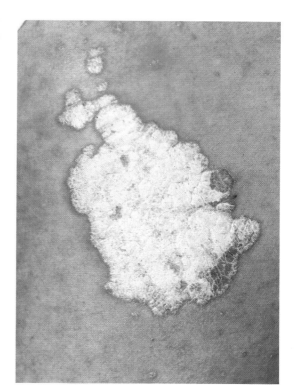

288

289

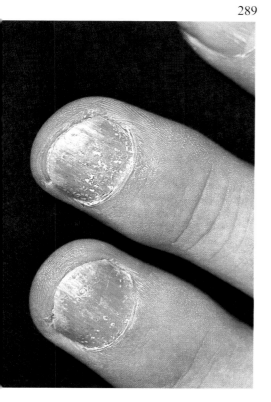

290

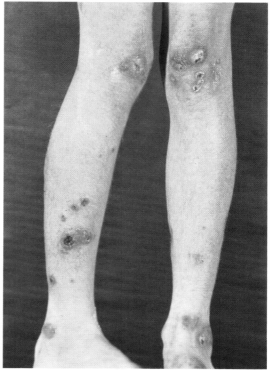

# 8. Diseases of the Skin

**Figures 291 and 292  Pityriasis Lichenoides et Varioliformis Acuta:**  Pityriasis lichenoides et varioliform acuta (Mucha-Habermann disease) in a 6-year-old boy. Varicella-like lesions (small, grouped, red, prurit papules and vesicles with red brown crusts) were noted over the entire body. The child was febrile for short period of time. The lesions healed leaving pigmented, sunken scars. The areas primarily affected in cluded the trunk, the upper arms, and the thighs. As a rule, the mucous membranes are spared. Mucha Habermann disease is currently considered to be vasculitis, which may occur at any age.

**Differential Diagnosis:**  Processes that must be differentiated from Mucha-Habermann disease includ varicella and other viral exanthems, papular urticaria (strophulus), and drug rashes.

**Figures 293 and 294  Pityriasis Lichenoides Chronica:**  Pityriasis lichenoides chronica (parapsorias guttate) in a 7-year-old boy. Of note were erythematous partially scaling macules and papules of varyin sizes over the body and face. The rash was nonpruritic. Characteristic of the condition is that scratchin the overlying scales will uncover a red brown papule. Parapsoriasis guttate may have a prolonged cours lasting for months or years. The cause is unknown. In early stages, or when lesions are not dense, th condition may be confused with viral exanthems or insect bites. More persistent cases must be distinguishe from guttate psoriasis (bright red centers with silvery, shiny scales) and lichen ruber planus (sharply ou lined, reddish blue, flat papules with white oval striations noted on the flexor surfaces and often affectin the mucous membranes).

**Figure 295  Parapsoriasis:**  Parapsoriasis in an 8-year-old girl. The findings included numerous roun elongated, poorly defined, yellow–red macules of different sizes. The rash was pruritic and scaly. It w noted on the torso and, on the extremities. The center of the lesions were slightly raised. The rash w chronic and progressive in nature and was difficult to treat.

**Differential Diagnosis:**  In the early stages one must consider mycosis fungoides or poikiloderma (derm atrophy). In addition, nummular eczema (coin shaped atopic dermatitis) must be considered.

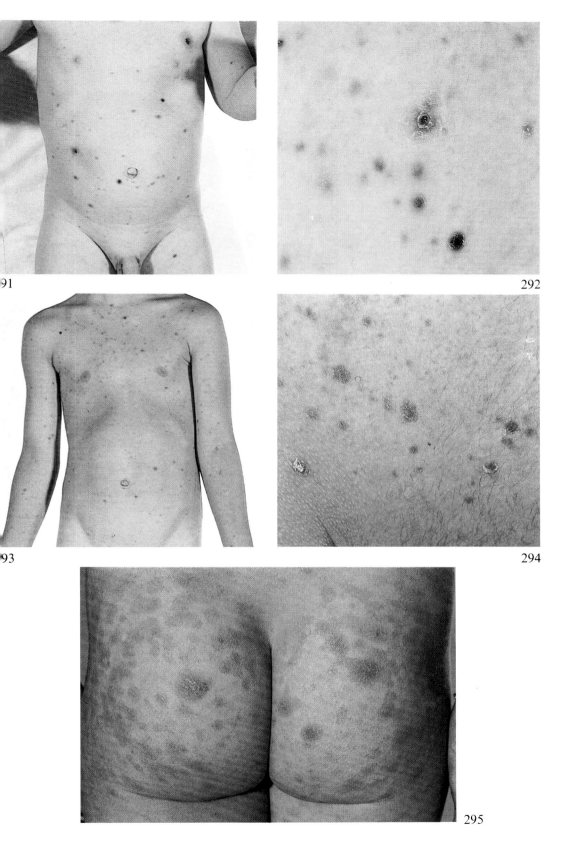

291

292

293

294

295

# 8.  Diseases of the Skin

**Figures 296–298  Papillon-Lefèvre Syndrome:**  Papillon-Lefèvre syndrome (keratoderma of palms an soles associated with periodontitis) in a 4-year-old boy. Of note is erythematous hyperkeratosis of the kne (Figure 297), the soles of the feet (Figure 298), and the palms. Anomalies of the nails and teeth, as we as gingivitis and severe periodontitis occur (Figure 296). As a rule, this syndrome includes palmar an plantar hyperhydrosis, which can result in calcification.

This autosomal recessive hereditary syndrome must be distinguished from other syndromes that occ with keratoderma (excessive accumulation of stratum corneum):

1. keratosis palmaris et plantaris simplex
2. mal de Meleda (hyperkeratosis of the extensor surfaces of the extremities associated with developmen delay)
3. Vohwinkel's syndrome (keratoma hereditaria mutilans associated with hyperkeratosis, autoamputatic of the fingers, alopecia, and deafness)
4. Nockemann's syndrome (keratoma hereditaria mutilans associated with deafness)
5. classic ectodermal dysplasia.

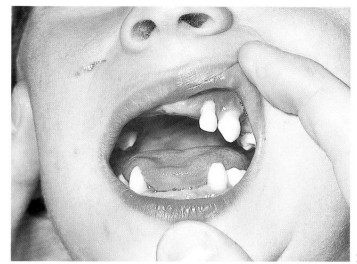

296

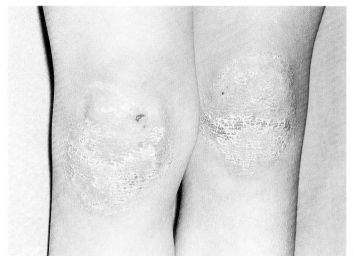

297

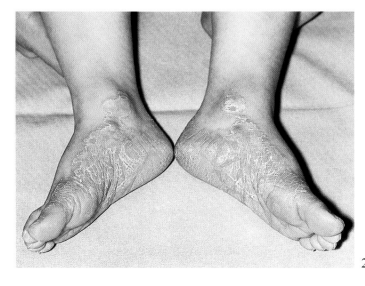

298

# 8.  Diseases of the Skin

**Figures 299 and 300  Urticaria Pigmentosa:**  Numerous tan or brown pigmented spots of varying size were noted over the skin and scalp. The lesions were pruritic and, in this case, were without vesicular change. Rubbing the skin causes the formation of urticaria (Darier's sign). In cases of doubt, the diagnosis can be confirmed through skin biopsy (revealing mast cell infiltration). Spontaneous remission usually occurs in adolescence.

**Figure 301  Urticaria Pigmentosa:**  Urticaria pigmentosa in a 13-month-old girl. Red–brown macules and papules were noted over the entire body, especially the torso. When rubbed, these lesions became urticaria. When brought to the clinic at 12 years of age, only a few pigmented areas (without urticaria) remained.

**Differential Diagnosis:**  Urticaria pigmentosa must be differentiated from papular urticaria (strophulus). In papular urticaria, the lesions on the extremities are more numerous than those on the torso, and are rarely pigmented. Central facial lentiginines (elevated dark brown macules not to be confused with epithelides) are easily ruled out, as is healing lichen ruber planus. The nodular forms of urticaria pigmentosa must be differentiated from xanthomas and juvenile xanthogranulomas.

**Figure 302  Urticaria Pigmentosa:**  Urticaria pigmentosa in a 4½-year-old boy. Numerous, indistinctly outlined, irregular brown spots of varying sizes were noted. The child had no systemic complaints. The prognosis is good, as long as there are no signs of systemic mastocytosis (bone involvement, gastrointestinal involvement, or hepatosplenomegaly). Flushing and tachycardia occur more frequently in systemic mastocytosis (10 percent of the cases) than in cases with isolated skin findings.

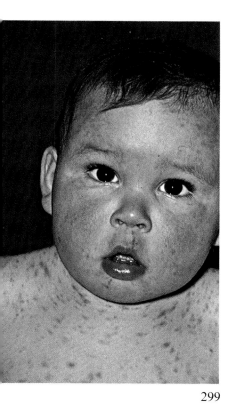

299

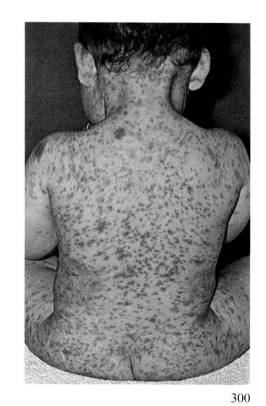

300

301

302

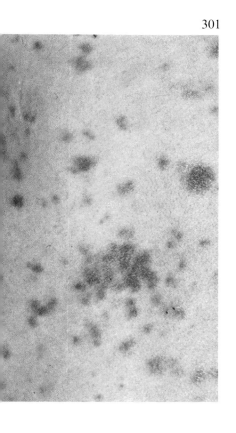

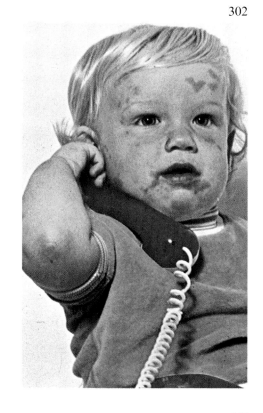

# 8. Diseases of the Skin

**Figure 303 Urticaria Pigmentosa:** Urticaria pigmentosa (bullous mastocytosis) in a 2-month-old infant. Vesicular skin lesions were noted over the entire body since birth. Later, these lesions became hyperpigmented. At first, this was thought to be pyoderma, but the skin biopsy demonstrated that it was urticaria pigmentosa. The father had also been affected with urticaria pigmentosa. A familial predisposition is known, but the specifics of inheritance are uncertain. Vesicles that may change to urticaria are frequently an expression of urticaria pigmentosa in younger children (up until 3 years of age). The lesions are localized primarily to the feet and the legs and are often accompanied by flushing of the skin.

**Differential Diagnosis:** Differential diagnosis for bullous urticaria pigmentosa includes juvenile pemphigoid, bullous impetigo, epidermolysis bullosa, intercontinentia pigmenti, and the bullous form of ichthyosiform erythroderma (ichthyosis congenita).

**Figure 304 Urticaria Pigmentosa:** Urticaria pigmentosa in a 3-month-old boy. Several pruritic, maculopapular, and vesicular lesions of varying size were noted on the extensor surface of the left thigh. There was no involvement of the internal organs or systemic symptoms (diarrhea, tachycardia, flushing). Skin biopsy demonstrated infiltration of mast cells with intracellular metachromatic pigmentation.

Localized mastocytomas occur in about 5 percent of all cases of mastocytosis. The lesions may be solitary or in groups of vesicles. The lesions may be present at birth or may develop during the first few weeks of life. Seldom does a generalized skin rash follow.

**Figure 305 Intercontinentia Pigmenti Syndrome:** Intercontinentia pigmenti syndrome (Block-Sulzberger disease) in a 2-month-old girl. Linearly arranged vesicles and red nodules appeared on the flexor surface of both legs during the first month of life and remained for several months. The contents of the vesicles were predominantly eosinophilic granulocytes. Between 6 and 12 months of age, red-brown, hyperpigmented lesions appeared in a symmetrical distribution on the arms and legs. These lesions persisted. Fortunately, the child did not develop the associated occular or central nervous system abnormalities which have been observed in 30 percent of all patients. Therapy was not required.

**Differential Diagnosis:** In the early vesicular stage, intercontinentia pigmenti syndrome is difficult to differentiate from pemphigoid; in cases of intercontinenti pigmenti one characteristically finds eosinophilia and, on biopsy of the lesion, eosinophilic infiltrate. Other vesicular or bullous rashes must be ruled out, including epidermolysis bullosa and bullous impetigo. If only pigmentation is present, post inflammatory hypermelanosis (seen in papular urticaria, herpes zoster, lichen ruber planus, and certain allergic rashes) as well as inherited pigment disturbances must be differentiated.

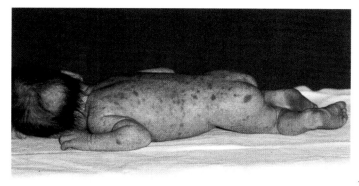

303

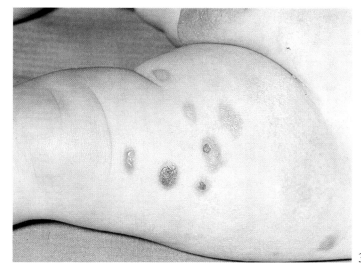

304

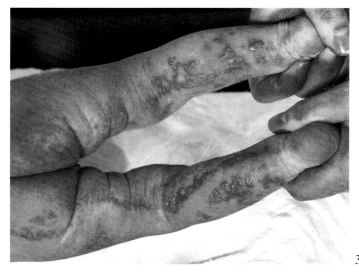

305

# 8. Diseases of the Skin

**Figures 306 and 307   Peutz-Jeghers Syndrome:**   Peutz-Jeghers syndrome in a 9-year-old boy. Numerou brown, melanin-containing macules of varying sizes were found in the areas surrounding the mouth an oral mucous membranes. The condition persisted for years, but the diagnosis was made only after the child father died of the same disease (due to intestinal problems). The boy suddenly developed an ileus due an intussusception (the lead point being a large intestinal polyp). Further radiologic studies detected mor polyps in the small intestine and the stomach.

**Differential Diagnosis:**   In cases of Addison's disease, the skin on various parts of the body (not onl the mucous membranes), is hyperpigmented. Freckles, which occur in fair skined people exposed to sur light, are never located in the oral cavity. In the case of multiple lentigines syndrome, the mucosa is als spared, and polyposis of the gastrointestinal tract is absent. In Capute-Rimoin-Konigsmark syndrome (gene alized lentigines with deafness), there are no pigmented lesions of the oral mucosa, an almost constant findir in Peutz-Jeghers syndrome. Cronkheit-Canada syndrome (polyposis associated with ectodermal defects ir cluding alopecia and nail atrophy) becomes manifest in the fifth or sixth decade of life while the pigmente lesions of Peutz-Jeghers syndrome are either present at birth or develop in early childhood (seldom appea ing later in life).

**Figure 308   Turner's Syndrome:**   Turner's syndrome in a 12-year-old girl. The skin findings include multiple pigmented nevi on the legs. At an earlier age, the findings of pterygium colli, low hairline, shiel shaped thorax, and widely spaced nipples were noted, which led to the presumptive diagnosis of Turner syndrome. Chromosome studies detected X-monosomy.

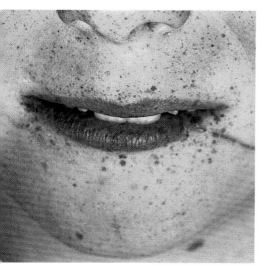

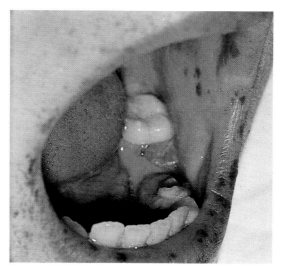

306

307

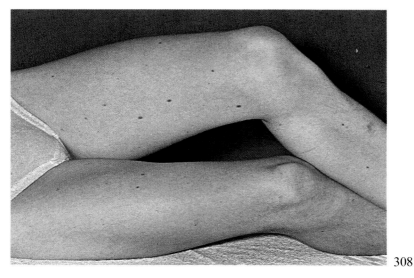

308

# 8.  Diseases of the Skin

**Figures 309–311  Ehlers-Danlos Syndrome:**  Ehlers-Danlos syndrome (cutis hyperelastica) in a 16-year old boy. Findings included hyperelastic skin, (Figure 309) and joints which were hypermobile (which le to subluxation and gait problems—Figure 310). Flat scars with paper thin scar tissue (Figure 311) were see over the knees, as were characteristic subcutaneous hematomas. The hematomas appeared after mild traum and calicified on resolution.

Ehlers-Danlos syndrome (which stems from a collagen defect) has at least seven different forms tha differ in regards to pattern of inheritance, degree of severity, and enzyme defect.

**Differential Diagnosis:**  Milder forms of Ehlers-Danlos syndrome could be confused with inherited cuti laxa (diminished elastic tissue). In cases of cutis laxa, the skin hangs down in loose folds; upon being picke up, the skin does not return as quickly to its previous position as does the skin in Ehlers-Danlos syndrome Hypermobile joints occur in Marfan's syndrome (p 66) and with hydroxylysine-deficient collagen. Easil damaged skin with poor wound healing is characteristic of osteogenesis imperfecta.

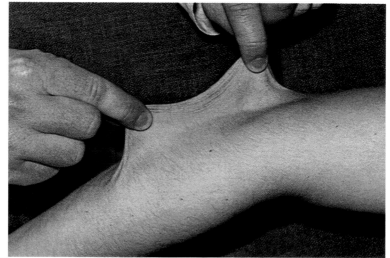

309

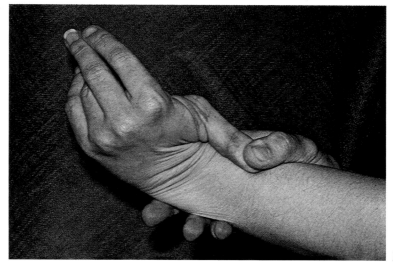

310

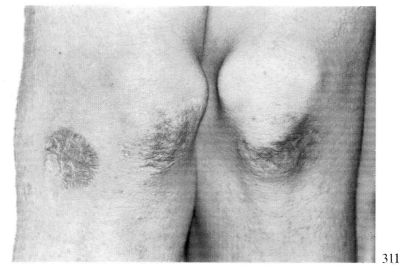

311

# 8. Diseases of the Skin

**Figure 312   Epidermolysis Bullosa Simplex:**   Epidermolysis bullosa simplex in a 6-year-old girl. Finding included ulcerated vesicles and bullae grouped closely together over the back. The child was treated witl antibiotics and the lesions resolved without scar formation. The mucous membranes and the nails wer not affected. The autosomal dominant inherited form of epidermolysis bullosa becomes manifest shortl after birth with vesicle formation. After only minimal trauma (rubbing of the skin), vesicles and bulla appeared that were fluid filled and broke easily. Biopsy of skin lesions revealed disintegration of the cytoplasn of the cells in the basal layer of the epidermis.

**Figures 313 and 314   Dystrophic Epidermolysis Bullosa:**   Dystrophic epidermolysis bullosa (recessiv inherited form) in a 2-month-old boy. Findings included vesicle and bullous formation and extensive erc sions (after rupture of the vesicles). These areas gradually healed leaving behind atrophic scars, keloid and contractures. The heavily involved areas included the skin of the back and the extremities (especiall over bony structures). Nikolski's phenomenon was positive (vesicle formation when the skin is rubbed) Dystrophy of the nails was noted, leading to loss of some nails. Feeding was complicated by vesicles i the oral cavity. The child had a prolonged hospital course, requiring hospitalization until age 2 years. Fre quent secondary bacterial infections required treatment with antibiotics.

**Figures 315 and 316   Dermatitis herpetiformis:**   Dermatitis herpetiformis in an 11-year-old girl. Grour of vesicles and papules on an erythematous base were symmetrically distributed on the extensor surface of the extemities, the buttocks, and the neck. These lesions were pruritic, partially excoriated, and cruste over. Other affected areas included the knees, the elbows, the shoulders, and the scalp. As is typical c dermatitis herpetiformis, the mucous membranes were not affected.

In small children, one finds larger vesicles often in the anogenital area. Excoriation can give rise t large, oozing surfaces. Dermatitis herpetiformis is chronic and progressive in nature and is frequently con plicated by secondary bacterial infection. The etiology is probably related to an immune complex diseasr

**Differential Diagnosis:**   Dermatitis herpetiformis must be differentiated from scabies, papular urticari (strophulus), erythema multiforme (with vesicle formation), and certain forms of atopic dermatitis.

168

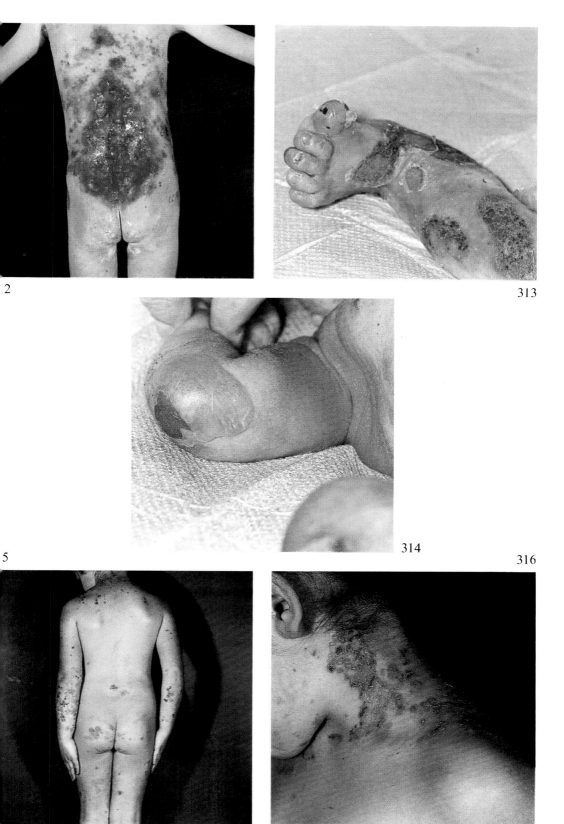

2

313

314

5

316

# 8. Diseases of the Skin

**Figure 317  Ecthyma:**  Ecthyma in a 10-year-old boy. Crusted pea-sized pustules on an indurated, erythema-tous base were found on both knees. After removal of the firmly attached crusts, an irregularly outline purulent ulcer was noted. Culture of these lesions isolated beta hemolytic Group A streptococci. After pe sisting for several weeks, the lesions healed leaving a scarred area.

Ecthyma is frequently located on the legs. Autoinnoculation can cause new lesions to appear. Seconda infection with coagulase positive staphylococci is possible. In cases of ecthyma gangrenosum, *Pseudom nas aeruginosa* can be detected in the ulcers (during *Pseudomonas* septicemia).

**Figure 318  Bullous Impetigo:**  Bullous impetigo on the abdomen of a 4-year-old boy. Of note were broke loose, large blisters of skin associated with a staphylococcal skin infection. The bullous lesions may res in scar formation. Bullous impetigo is most frequent in the newborn.

**Figure 319  Bullous Impetigo:**  Bullous impetigo on the knee of a 14-year-old girl. Pictured are la ruptured bullae, previously filled with cloudy fluid, on a narrow erythematous base with slight crusti This form of impetigo contagiosa is usually caused by *Staphylococcus aureus.*

**Differential Diagnosis:**  In older children, the differential diagnosis of bullous impetigo includes eryt ma multiforme exuditivum, toxic epidermal necrolysis (Lyell's syndrome), and other chronic bullous d matoses. In the newborn period, the following should be considered: epidermolysis bullosa, urtica pigmentosa (bullous mastocytosis), and dermatitis exfoliativa (Ritter's disease).

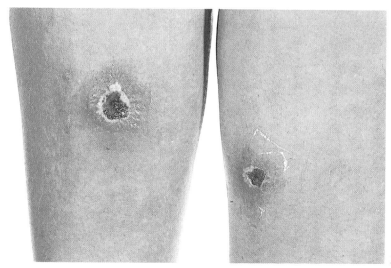

317

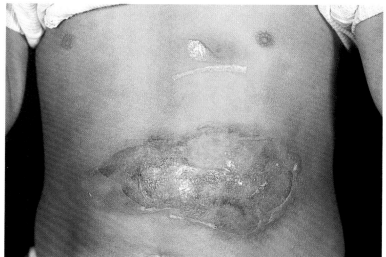

318

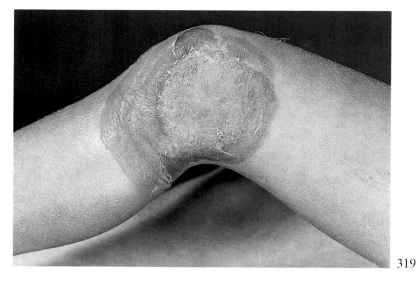

319

# 8. Diseases of the Skin

**Figure 320   Impetigo Contagiosa:**   Impetigo contagiosa on the face of a 4-year-old boy. Findings include numerous ruptured vesicles and pustules with honey yellow crusts on the face, the ears, and the neck. Both Group A beta hemolytic streptococci and *Staphlococcus aureus* were cultured. The condition started with the appearance of red macules that quickly changed into thin walled vesicles and pustules. Removal of the crusts revealed a red oozing surface. The lesions responded quickly to antibiotic therapy. Hygienic care must be emphasized so that the infection does not spread to other parts of the body (through auto innoculation) or to other people.

**Differential Diagnosis:**   The differential diagnosis of impetigo includes varicella, herpes zoster, and herpes simplex infections (which also may be secondarily impetiginized) as well as allergic contact dermatitis.

**Figure 321   Herpes Zoster:**   Herpes zoster in a 12-year-old boy. Findings included a crusting vesicular rash unilaterally in the ophthalmic distribution of the trigeminal nerve (over the forehead, eye, and nose). The rash was associated with severe keratoconjunctivitis, pain, and high fever. Examination of the vesicl contents by electron microscopy revealed giant cells. The child was treated locally and systemically with vidarabine (adenine arabinoside). Infection involving the maxillary branch of the trigeminal nerve would affect the check and the ipsilateral palate; infection of the mandibular branch would affect the jaw and the ipsilateral aspect of the tongue.

**Differential Diagnosis:**   The absence of neuralgia (especially in children) does not rule out herpes zoster. Immune suppressed patients can develop a generalized zoster infection that cannot be differentiated from varicella. In cases of herpes simplex infection, the skin lesions can mimic zoster so that differentiation is possible only through serology or viral culture.

## Reference

1.   Aronson MD, et al. Successful treatment of severe herpes virus infection with vidarabine. JAMA 235:1339, 1976.

**Figure 322   Eczema Herpeticum:**   Eczema herpeticum in a 15-month-old boy with a previous history of atopic dermatitis. Numerous vesicles, which soon became pustular, ulcerated, and crusted, were found behind the ears, on the neck, and in other areas. In addition, there was high fever and regional lymphadenitis. Electron microscopy revealed intranuclear inclusion bodies (herpes simplex virus). Serum serology for herpes simplex virus was positive. Treatment is symptomatic.

The typical skin changes of eczema herpeticum not only occur on previously affected areas, but may spread widely. In cases of recurring eczema herpeticum, systemic symptoms are lacking, and the local symptoms may be mild.

**Figure 323   Filliform Warts:**   Filliform warts (verruca filiformes, a form of verruca vulgaris) on the lip of a 12-year-old girl. Of note were several white, hard, protruding lesions that varied in size. These lesions had a coarse irregular surface on a localized base. Filliform warts occur primarily on the face (eyelids lips) and on the neck. These lesions are caused by DNA viruses of the papova group. They are spread through direct contact, and autoinnoculation. Lesions located on the face can lead to infection of the oral mucous membranes.

**Differential Diagnosis:**   Filliform warts must be differentiated from common warts (verruca vulgaris), juvenile flat warts (verruca plana), plantar and palmar warts, as well as warts of the mucous membrane (condylomata acuminata). Verrucous nevi can look like verruca filiformes or digitata, but are usually arranged in a linear fashion.

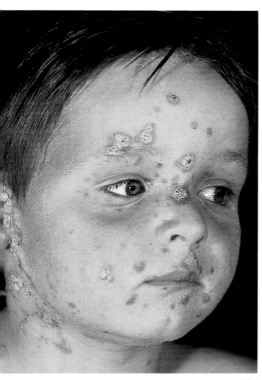

320

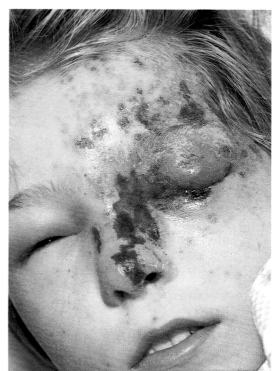

321

322

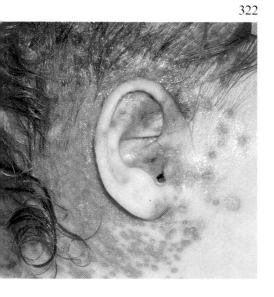

323

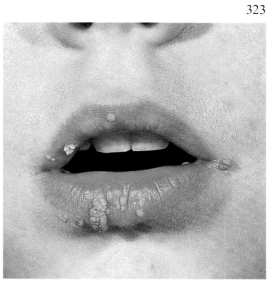

# 8. Diseases of the Skin

**Figure 324  Aphthous Stomatitis:**  Aphthous stomatitis in a 15-year-old girl. On the inner aspect of the lower lip there were several bean-sized ruptured vesicles on a large erythematous base which were covered by a grey-white membrane. Removal of the membrane demonstrated an ulcer that was very painful and slow to heal.

The cause of aphthous stomatitis is uncertain (related to psychological stress, infection, trauma). Apthous stomatitis occur more frequently in adults and may be solitary or grouped lesions (never more than three). As a rule, they are localized to the front part of the oral cavity and often reappear.

In contrast to aphthous stomatitis, the ulcers of herpes simplex virus gingivostomatitis are present in great numbers, accompanied by gingivitis, and lead to regional lymphadenitis and high fever. Bednar aphthae are usually localized to the lips and caused by trauma. In the case of solitary mucous membrane lesions, primary syphilis and tuberculous ulcerations must be ruled out. In Behçet's syndrome, ulcers can be found on all mucous membranes (eyes, mouth, oral pharynx, esophagus, stomach, intestines, genitals) and often is associated with erythema nodosum, arthritis, and central nervous system disease.

**Figure 325  Herpes Simplex:**  Herpes simplex viral infection of the perianal skin of a 12-year-old girl. Of note were several painful, ruptured vesicles covered by a grey-yellow membrane. These lesions were caused by autoinnoculation (the original site of infection was the oral mucosa). The rash was accompanied by high fever and regional lymphadenopathy.

**Differential Diagnosis:**  The differential diagnosis of herpetic lesions depends on the location. In cases of vesicular or bullous inflammation of the anogenital area, the following must be considered: juvenile pemphigoid, acrodermatitis enterpathica, impetigo, contact dermatitis, and diaper dermatitis.

## Reference

1.  Nammia AJ, Roizman B. Infection with herpes-simplex viruses 1 and 2. N Engl J Med 289:667, 1973.

**Figure 326  Herpes Simplex:**  Recurrent herpes simplex viral infection on the skin of a 14-year-old girl. Grouped vesicles with local erythema were noted on the face. The child was afebrile. The lesions resolved without scar formation after 1 week of local treatment with vidarabine.

**Differential Diagnosis:**  Similar skin lesions may be seen with impetigo (with bacteria detected on culture) and herpes zoster.

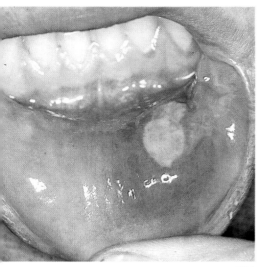

324

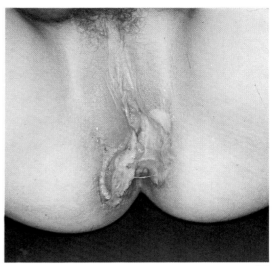

325

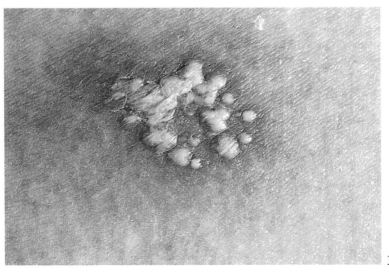

326

# 8.  Diseases of the Skin

**Figure 327  Aphthous Stomatitis:**  Aphthous stomatitis in a 4-year-old girl. Numerous ulcers (vesicle which were partially ulcerated and covered with a yellow pseudomembrane) were noted on the oral mucou membranes and the tongue. The gums were red and swollen. Fever and regional lymphadenopathy wer noted. The ulcers were painful and caused the child to refuse food and drink. The lesions resolved afte 8 to 10 days of symptomatic treatment.

**Differential Diagnosis:**  Aphthous stomatitis must be differentiated from Coxsackie viral infection (hand foot, and mouth disease), Behçet's syndrome (p 174), and Stevens-Johnson syndrome.

**Figure 328  Candida Granuloma:**  *Candida* granuloma of the lower lip of a 5-year-old boy (with cor genital immune deficiency). Findings included crusted plaques over the lips.

**Differential Diagnosis:**  *Candida* granuloma must be differentiated from various forms of cheilitis. Che litis may be caused by exposure to (lip salves, lipstick, toothpaste, and mouthwash) or may be due to allerg to foods such as oranges, artichokes, and mangoes.

**Figure 329  Impetigo Contagiosa:**  Impetigo in the mouth of a 2-year-old girl. The child had puruler vesicles around the mouth which ruptured and became scabbed and crust covered. The lesions culture staphylococcus aureus. Due to the location of the lesions, food intake was very painful and parenteral fee ing was necessary for a short period of time.

## Reference

1.   Dajani AS, et al. Natural history of impetigo II. Etiologic agents and bacterial interactions. J Clin Invest 51:2863, 197

**Figure 330  Herpes Labialis:**  Herpes labialis (recurrent herpes simplex viral infection) in a 7-year-o boy. On the lower lip, a vesicle filled with watery fluid was noted; in the left corner of the mouth, sever densely grouped vesicles erupted. The lesions resolved 3 days later.

**Differential Diagnosis:**  Cheilitis angularis (also known as perlèche) may have numerous causes inclue ing infection with *Staphylococcus aureus, Candida albicans,* or other skin diseases, such as atopic dermat tis and seborrheic dermatitis.

**Figures 331 and 332  Coxsackie Viral Infection:**  Coxsackie viral infection (hand, foot, and mouth di ease) in a 5-year-old girl. Several vesicular and ulcerative lesions were noted in the oral cavity (Figure 33 and numerous 3 to 5 mm large, pearl-grey vesicles on a narow erythematous base were noted on both fe (Figure 332) and hands. Coxsackie virus A-16 could be cultured. Fever and a generalized maculopapul. rash were associated with these findings. After 1 week, the symptoms disappeared.

Typically, the oral lesions of Coxsackie hand, foot, and mouth disease are larger than those seen cases of herpangina. The lesions are irregularly spread over the palate, the oral mucous membranes ar the tongue. The fever usually lasts only a few days. Skin changes are inconsistent. As a rule, the vesicle on the hand and feet are oval and elongated. They occur primarily on the fingers and toes (both later. and dorsal surfaces), the heels, the flexor surfaces of the fingers, and the palms and soles of the feet. Th skin lesions disappear after 2 to 3 days. In young infants, a papular or vesicular rash (either generalize or localized) can appear.

**Differential Diagnosis:**  Coxsackie infections must be differentiated from varicella, herpes simplex, papul. urticaria, and scabies.

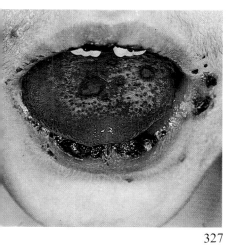

327

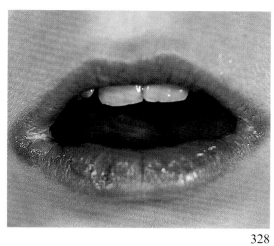

328

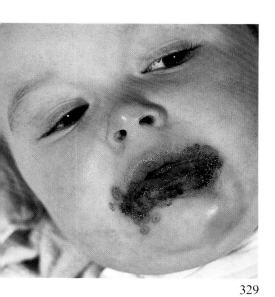

329

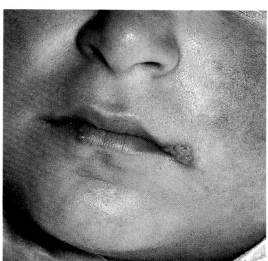

330

331

332

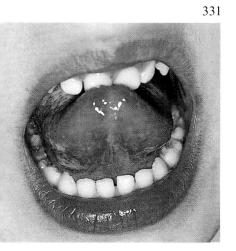

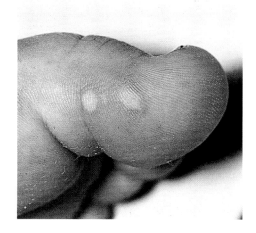

# 8. Diseases of the Skin

**Figure 333   Molluscum Contagiosum:**   Molluscum contagiosum in a 14-year-old boy. Of note were numerous 2 to 3 mm, pearl-like papules with central umbilication. These lesions were seen on the flexor surface of the arm and scattered on the face. Lateral pressure on the molluscum lesion expressed a cheesy substance that contained many infected epidermal cells with eosinophilic inclusion bodies. Microscopical ly, these can be differentiated from certain forms of warts. Molluscum contagiosum frequently affects the face, eyelids, neck, axilla, and genital area. Molluscum contagiosum rarely occurs as a solitary lesion. The lesions may vary in size from a few millimeters to approximately the size of a pea. It may be difficult to differentiate a solitary molluscum lesion from a granuloma telangiectatium (see p 146) or an epithelioma (seldom seen in children). In these cases, histological examination is required.

**Figure 334   Juvenile Xanthogranuloma:**   Juvenile xanthogranuloma in an 11-month-old girl. Of note were numerous bright red, firm nodules of various sizes, on the abdomen, and in the genital area. The lesions had been present since birth. No hyperlipidemia was noted. Biopsy of the lesions showed characteristic lipid containing histiocytes and Touton giant cells (multinucleated, vacuolated giant cells with a ring of nuclei and a rim of foamy cytoplasm at the border), which are pathognomonic. Areas frequently affected by juvenile xanthogranuloma are the scalp, the face, and the upper half of the torso. Solitary lesions are rare

**Differential Diagnosis:**   Juvenile xanthogranuloma must be differentiated from urticaria pigmentosa (papulonodular form), dermofribromas (p 148), and xanthomas associated with hyperlipidemia.

**Figures 335 and 336   Gianotti-Crosti Syndrome:**   Gianotti-Crosti syndrome (papular acrodermatitis in an 18-month-old girl. The child had been ill with rhinitis and pharyngitis 2 weeks prior to the onset of the rash. Numerous red papules approximately 2 mm in diameter appeared on the cheeks and extremi ties, but spared the torso. Areas of the rash were confluent. The eyes and mouth were not affected. Lymph adenopathy in the axilla and groin was noted; during the acute stage, there was hepatosplenomegaly. Serum transaminase, IgG and IgM were elevated and hepatitis B surface antigen was positive. After 4 weeks, the cutaneous symptoms disappeared without treatment.

Gianotti-Crosti syndrome were due to hepatitis B virus. With respect to morphology, longevity of dermal symptoms, and distribution of rash, the symptoms were characteristic. The liver is not always affected If hepatitis is noted, the infection is usually mild and the patient is anicteric, (although progressive icteri forms have been noted). Recovery from hepatitis B infections (with regards to liver findings) can take months to 4 years.

**Differential Diagnosis:**   Similar cutaneous findings may be seen in juvenile papular dermatitis. Juvenil papular dermatitis appears at age 3 to 10 years and progresses with discrete, lichenoid papules on the hand and underarms and sometimes affects the legs and torso. It has an infectious etiology and may occur in an epidemic pattern.

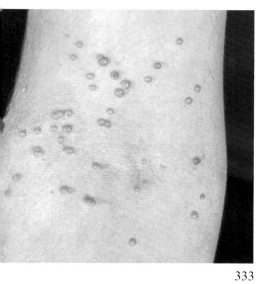

333

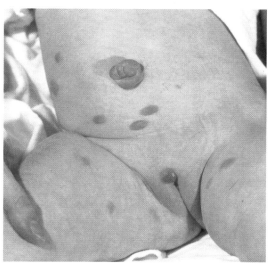

334

335

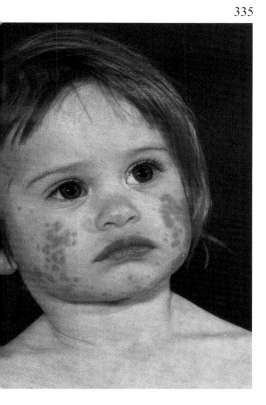

336

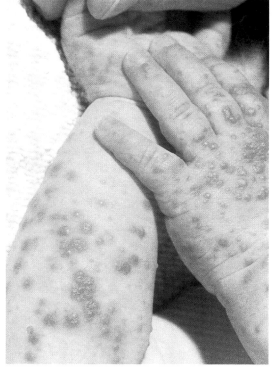

# 8. Diseases of the Skin

**Figures 337 and 338  Candida Granuloma:**  *Candida* granuloma of the face and scalp in a 10-year-c
boy. Extensive, crusted, erythematous lesions with partial scaling were noted on the face and scalp. Simil
lesions were found on the underarms and lower thighs. The boy suffered from severe combined immu
deficiency syndrome (Swiss type). Local treatment with nystatin was ineffective. Resolution followed sy
temic therapy with antifungal agents. *Candida* granuloma is an expression of chronic fungal infection a
sociated with immune suppression. The face, scalp, and other parts of the body, are frequently affecte

**Figure 339  Chronic Candidiasis:**  Chronic candidiasis of the scalp and the ears in an 8-year-old b
with congenital immune deficiency syndrome. The scalp was thickened, erythematous, and scaly. *Candi*
was identified as the causative agent through microscropic examination and fungal culture. Identificati
is important in differentiating this condition from infections caused by *Trichophyton* and *Microsporu*

**Figure 340  Tinea Corporis:**  Tinea corporis on the face of a 12-year-old boy. Numerous, sharply o
lined, partially confluent, disk-shaped, erythematous lesions with slight scaling were noted on the fac
The edge of the lesion was slightly raised and the center was beginning to heal. *Trichophyton rubrum* w
detected microscopically and through culture (obtained from the edge of the lesion). The condition resolv
after topical tolnaftate treatment of 3 weeks duration. For differential diagnosis see p 182.

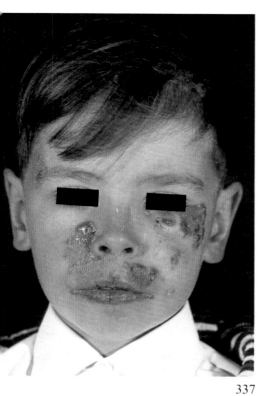

337

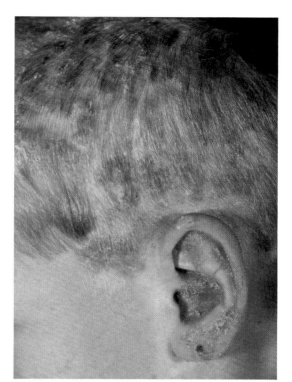

339

338

340

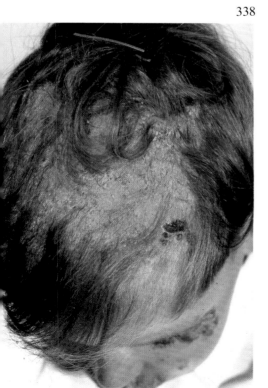

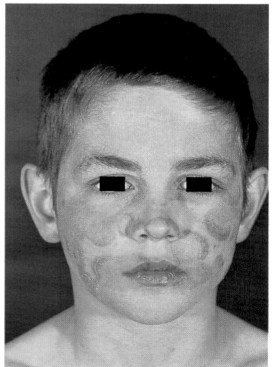

# 8. Diseases of the Skin

**Figure 341  Tinea Corporis:**  Tinea corporis in a 8-year-old boy. Ring-shaped, slightly scaling, erythematous lesions were found on the back. These lesions persisted for weeks and were caused by *Trichophyton mentagrophytes*. The specific agent causing tinea corporis cannot be identified from the skin changes alone. The most frequent agents associated with tinea corporis are *Trichophyton rubrum, Trichophyton mentagrophytes*, and *Microsporum canis*. The child apparently contracted the infection from contact with his infected brother.

**Figure 342  Tinea Corporis:**  Tinea corporis on the face of a 13-year-old girl. Dry, erythematous, scaly papules had spread centrifugally in the course of four weeks. After local treatment with miconazole nitrate the lesions healed without scar formation.

**Figure 343  Tinea Corporis:**  Tinea corporis on the chin of a 3-year-old boy. This pruritic, scaling erythematous rash was caused by *Microsporum canis* (detected by fungal culture). Tinea corporis must be distinguished from granuloma annulare (p 124), atopic dermatitis (specifically nummular eczema), psoriasis (p 154), seborrheic dermatitis, and pityriasis rosea. Initially, pityriasis rosea may look similar to tinea corporis, but pityriasis rosea has a different distribution and will heal without treatment after 6 to 9 weeks. When a fungal lesion is lichenified, it may be confused with lichen planus. Candidiasis and tinea versicolor (due to *Malassezia furfur*) must also be ruled out.

**Figure 344  Tinea Corporis:**  Tinea corporis in a 9-year-old boy. Pruritic ring-shaped, erythematous skin lesions on the neck and chest caused by *Microsporum canis* (from contact with an infected dog). Characteristic of this lesion are the disk-shaped centers with an erythematous scaly edge. The lesions resolved after local treatment with clotrimazol.

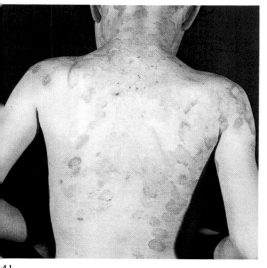

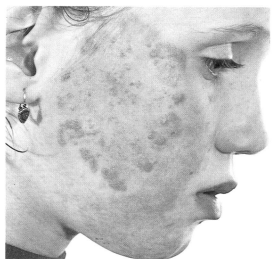

341

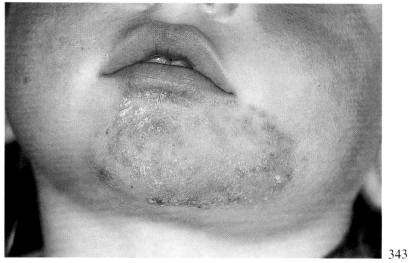

342

343

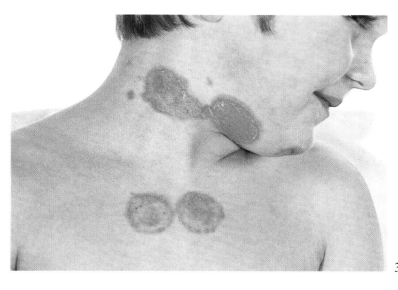

344

# 8. Diseases of the Skin

**Figure 345 Tinea Capitis:** Tinea capitis in a 5-year-old boy. Confluent centers of alopecia with areas of broken and brittle hair were observed on an erythematous, scaling scalp. There was extreme pruritis. When examined with a Wood's lamp, the affected scalp appeared green. *Microsporum audouini* was identified as the causative agent. The fungus is transmitted by contact with infected hair or epithelial cells (such as on a comb).

**Differential Diagnosis:** Hair loss with underlying skin rash can also be caused by alopecia areata (p 204), trichotillomania (p 206), Menkes' kinky hair syndrome (associated with seborrheic dermatitis), psoriasis, and impetigo (with underlying crust formation). Pityriasis simplex capitis (scaling of otherwise normal skin) can coincide with alopecia areata. Pathological scaling or hair loss exists in pityriasis amiantacea, which can appear secondarily on the scalp after bacterial dermatitis or lichen ruber planus.

## Reference

1.   Frieden IJ. Diagnosis and management of tinea capitus. Pediatr Ann 16:39, 1987.

**Figure 346 Tinea Capitis:** Tinea capitis on the scalp of a 10-year-old girl. Hair loss was noted in a 5 × 6 cm area, which was inflammed and covered with silvery scales. The remaining hair in the center of the lesion shone green in a Wood's lamp. The causative agent was *Microsporum canis.*

**Figure 347 Tinea Capitis:** Tinea capitis in a 7-year-old boy. Patchy alopecia was noted. This superficial dermatophyte infection of the scalp was caused by *Trichophyton tonsurans.* Typical of *Trichophyton tonsurans* infection were the multiple centers, which were angular rather than round, and slightly scaly. Microscopically, on KOH prep, a chain of fungal spores inside the hair shaft could be identified (endothrix). Under Wood's lamp, the hair was not fluorescent, (whereas in cases of flavus caused by *Trichophyton schoenleini* a dark green fluorescence is noted and with microsporia infections, a light green fluorescence is noted). The lesions resolved after 8 weeks therapy with systemic griseofulvin.

**Differential Diagnosis:** Discoid lupus, which can lead to localized loss of hair, should be considered.

**Figure 348 Tinea Capitis:** Tinea capitis with severe inflammatory response (kerion) in an 11-year-old boy. Of note was a palm-sized, swollen, erythematous area of scalp with pustules and a honey-yellow crusting. The hair had fallen out from this area. Microscopically, on KOH prep, one could see fungal spores distributed around the hair shaft (ectothrix). Fungal culture demonstrated an infection with *Trichophyton verrucosum.*

**Figure 349 Tinea Versicolor:** Tina versicolor in a 15-year-old girl. The skin lesions were irregularly outlined, small, red-brown macules, which were covered by fine scales. The lesions were partially confluent and nonpruritic. With a spatula, one could scrape off a thickened covering ("wood shaving" phenomenon). The lesions were located primarily on the neck, the chest, and the upper arms. The affected areas of skin did not tan when exposed to sunlight. Microscopically, in KOH prep, small, thick-walled spores and many short, thick hyphae were visible. Under a Wood's lamp, the affected hair had a golden-yellow fluorescence.

**Differential Diagnosis:** Tinea versicolor must be differentiated from seborrheic dermatitis, parapsoriasis, ichthyosis vulgaris, and other fungal infections of the skin. Erythrasma (scaling erythematous macules in the groin and axillae which has a fluorescent coral red color under a Wood's lamp) occurs in adolescents and must be ruled out. Pityriasis rosea may look similar, but differs from tinea versicolor in that it begins suddenly with a herald patch, is pruritic, and has a tendency toward lichenification.

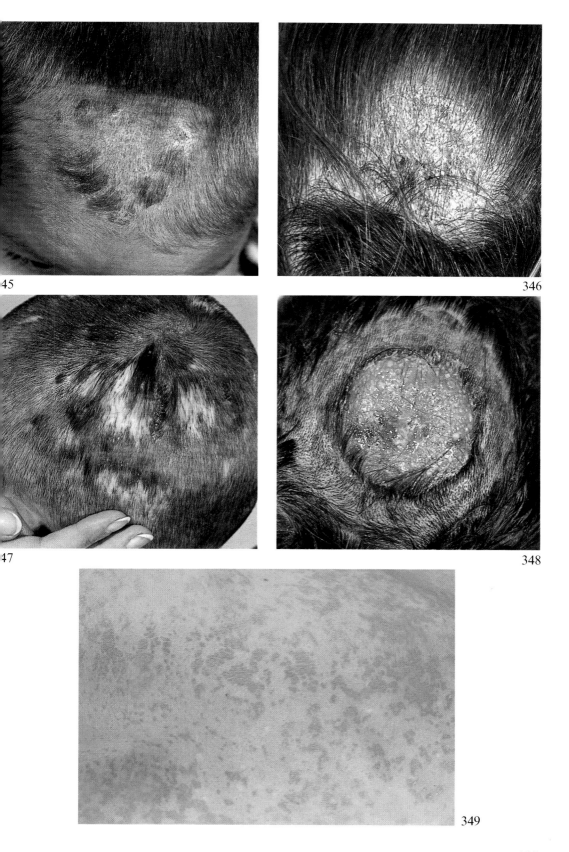

45

346

47

348

349

# 8. Diseases of the Skin

**Figure 350  Scabies:**  Scabies in a 4-month-old child. An extensive, pruritic, maculopapular, vesicula and urticarial rash on the neck and on the extremities was noted in this child. The lesions have persiste for 4 weeks. These lesions are caused by infestation with mites. Burrows, with a dark point at the entranc and light point at the blind end, were noted. The child's mother had similar lesions. Confirmation of th diagnosis was made by detecting mites microscopically (removing the mite from the burrow with a blu needle and examining under the microscope). Scabies frequently affects the flexor surfaces of the extremitie the interdigital spaces, the groin, and the axillae. In infants and small children, the hands, the soles of th feet, the neck, and the face may also be affected. Scabies frequently leads to eczematization (with vesic formation in infants and a papular rash in older children) and impetiginization (secondary bacterial infec tion causing pustules).

**Differential Diagnosis:**  The skin lesions found in scabies may also be seen in atopic dermatitis, pedicu losis and other forms of dermatitis.

## Reference

1.  Lane AT. Scabies and head lice. Pediatr Ann 16:51, 1987.

**Figure 351  Scabies:**  Scabies in a 4-year-old girl. Numerous, intensely pruritic vesicles and papules we noted over the hand with interdigital eczematization. Treatment included application of 1 percent gamm benzene hexachloride and a complete change of undergarments and linen. A short course of corticostero cream was necessary for the eczematized lesions. Despite killing the mites, pruritis can persist for son time. Concurrent reatment of infected family members is important in order to stop the spread of the infestatio

**Figure 352  Scabies:**  Scabies in a 5-month-old infant. Many pruritic maculopapular lesions with son vesicular lesions were noted. Typical burrows were seen on the dorsal side of the foot, on the sole, ar over the flexor surface of the extremities.

**Figure 353  Cutaneous Larva Migrans:**  Cutaneous larva migrans in a 16-year-old boy. Of note was 3 to 4 cm long, 2 to 3 mm wide, snake-like, erythematous band, which was located on the dorsum of th foot. The lesion was pruritic. Cutaneous larva migrans is caused by the penetration of the larva of hoo worms into the deep layers of the epidermis. The infection is usually the result of running bare foot in sar contaminated by canine feces. Eczematization and impetiginization of the rash may occur. In this case, loc treatment with thiabendazol was successful.

**Differential Diagnosis:**  Differential diagnosis should consider larva currens (caused by *Strongyloides ste coralis*) and myiasis (caused by larvae of certain *Diptera*).

**Figure 354  Tinea Pedis:**  Tinea pedis in a 15-year-old boy. Findings included extensive, painful fissur with white maceration between the third and fourth toes of the right foot. The affected areas are prurit and odorous.

Tinea pedis (Athlete's foot) is most frequently caused by *Trichophyton rubrum, Trichophyton ment grophytes,* and *Epidermophyton floccosum.* These agents may be detected microscopically (KOH prep) ( in culture. Treatment is with topical clotrimaxole or miconazole. Athlete's foot may be acquired at publ swimming pools, showers, or by the use of footwear that does not permit free flow of air. Secondary bac terial infection is possible (erysipelas due to *Streptococcus*) as well as multiple fungal infections (*Trichophyt or Candida albicans*).

**Differential Diagnosis:**  The differential diagnosis includes interdigital corns and callouses as well erythrasma (without the fissures seen in interdigital mycosis).

**Figure 355  Tinea Pedis:**  Tinea pedis in a 16-year-old girl. Maceration of the interdigital areas and extrem scaling. Fungi were detected microscopically.

**Differential Diagnosis:**  Differential diagnosis should consider contact dermatitis, atopic dermatitis, *Ca dida* dermatitis, and dyshidrotic eczema.

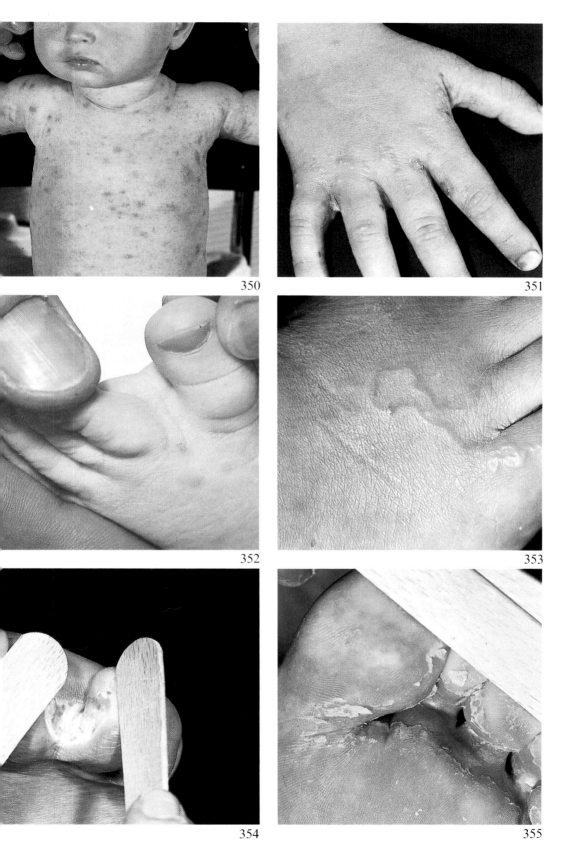

350

351

352

353

354

355

# 8. Diseases of the Skin

**Figure 356  Pili Torti:**  Pili torti (twisted hair) in a 3-year-old girl. Of note is short hair that is extremely brittle. The hair is blond colored and shiny. Microscopic examination showed that the hair shaft was twisted along the long axis, and indented and flattened at irregular intervals. These abnormalities have been noted since 2 years of age. No other family members were affected with pili torti. The mode of inheritance is variable (sporadic, autosomal dominant, or autosomal recessive).

Pili tori may be seen in Menkes' kinky hair syndrome (p 276). Menkes' syndrome is associated with retarded growth and development. The underlying cause is excessive tissue binding of copper. In this case the child's serum copper level was normal and the child's mental development was normal. Pili torti is also seen in Björnstad's syndrome (with congenital hearing defect) and Crandall's syndrome (hearing impairment with hypergonadism). Other causes of congenital hair anomalies include congenital trichorrhexis nodosa and monilethrix. Both of these conditions begin with brittle hair and may lead to partial alopecia. In case of trichorrhexis nodosa, one sees microscopic nodular swellings along the hair shaft at irregular intervals. The hair can be easily broken at these nodules. In cases of monilethrix, the scalp hair is dry, dull, and brittle. Microscopically, the hair shaft demonstrates regular ball-shaped swellings between which the hair is thinned and often breaks. Trichorrhexis nodosa occurs as an acquired disorder that is caused by trauma (inappropriate combing). Monilethrix is an autosomal dominant condition.

**Figure 357  Pediculosis Pubis:**  Nits (eggs) of pediculosis pubis (crab lice) in the eyelashes of a 7-year-old boy. There were numerous intensely pruritic macules, papules and urticarial lesions on the abdomen, upper thigh, and axilla. With the aid of a magnifying glass, not only the eggs, but also the lice, could be seen in the hairs. On the skin, crab lice look like freckles. Paraffin oil was rubbed into the eyelids twice a day for a week, during which time the nits fell out.

**Figure 358  Pediculosis Capitis:**  Grey-white nits from pediculosis capitis in the hair of a 5-year-old girl. Impetiginized bites were seen on the temples, behind the ear, and on the neck. The lesions were intensely pruritic. The nits from the head lice were oval and covered (unlike the nits from crab lice). The nits of head lice cling to the hair firmly, unlike the scales in seborrheic dermatitis or the residual from hairspray. Differentiation of the nits from the hair findings in distal trichorrhexia nodosa is possible by means of microscopic examination. The nits were removed by careful combing of the hair with vinegar water. The child was treated with a local application of a 1 percent gamma benzene hexachloride shampoo, as well as antibiotic therapy for secondary bacterial infection.

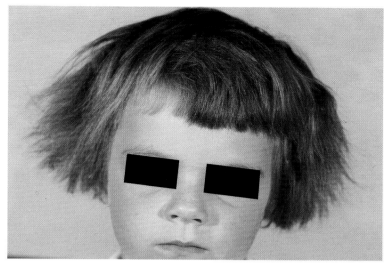

356

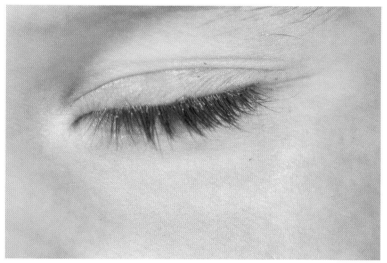

357

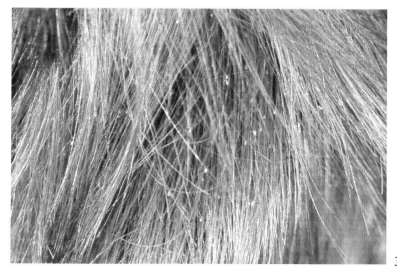

358

# 8.   Diseases of the Skin

**Figure 359   Geographic Tongue:**   Geographic tongue (lingula geographica) in a 10-year-old girl. Two large, irregularly shaped, well defined, red areas with raised, white borders were noted on the tongue. These lesions are caused by a desquamation of the filiform papillae causing the fungiform papillae to appear more prominent. Characteristically, the areas of desquamation shifted during the course of several weeks. Histology demonstrates inflammatory changes, the cause of which is uncertain. The condition may last for several months or years. Fissures of the tongue are often noted. The sensation of burning may also occur.

**Figure 360   Glossitis:**   Median rhomboid glossitis in an 18-year-old girl. Of note was a sharply outlined pea-sized, smooth, red lesion on the dorsum of the tongue (immediately anterior to the papillae vallatae). The lesion was associated with a burning sensation.

   The affected part of the tongue is usually free of papillae and has a rhombic or oval shape. The lesion are always found on the dorsal surface of the tongue and may have a bumpy surface. There may be temporary inflammation and discomfort. Median rhomboid glossitis apparently stems from a developmental anomaly (persistence of the tuberculum impar). Other theories propose that median rhomboid glossitis (which usually does not appear until adulthood) is related to a hamartoma. Biopsy (in an effort to rule out carcinoma) can lead to significant bleeding.

## Reference

1.   Goldberg MP. The oral mucosa in childhood. Pediatr Clin North Am 25:329, 1978.

**Figure 361   Mucous Retention Cysts:**   Mucous retention cysts (mucocele) of the tongue in a 2-month old boy. A taut, elastic, pea-sized growth which contain mucous was noted on the underside of the tongue. The lesion was removed surgically.

   Mucous retention cysts frequently occur as a result of trauma. Traumatic disruption of the mucous gland duct leads to retention of secretions in the tissue. A border forms, consisting of granulation tissue or connective tissue, but seldom is truly epithelialized. The cysts often have a blue color, and may be located on the lip, the floor of the mouth (ranula), the oral mucous membrane, or the tongue. Sometimes they may be mistaken for hemangiomas.

**Figure 362   Lichen Planus:**   Lichen planus of the oral mucous membrane in a 17-year-old boy. Of note was erythema of the oral mucous membrane (due to epithelial atrophy) with characteristic white papules which form a linear and reticulated network (Wickham's striae). Pruritic polygonal, flat, erythematous slightly shiny papules were also noted on the inner aspect of the upper thigh. Scratching in this area produced a linear array of papules (positive Koebner's phenomenon). The condition began suddenly and spread over the flexor surfaces of the hand and the underarm. The etiology is unclear. Diagnosis of lichen planus can be confirmed by skin biopsy. The disease can last for weeks or years, and may reappear. Local treatment of the skin with corticosteroid preparations has proven successful. Antihistamines are often prescribed for the pruritis.

**Differential Diagnosis:**   Superficial *Candida* infections of the mouth should be considered. The change in the oral mucous membranes can resemble those of systemic lupus erythematosus (which is chronic and progressive in nature). In adults, leukoplakia (white plaques which cannot be removed by rubbing) and syphilitic plaques (seen in secondary syphyilis) should also be considered.

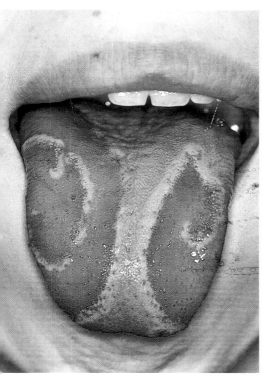

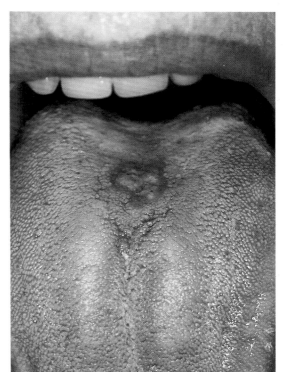

359

360

361

362

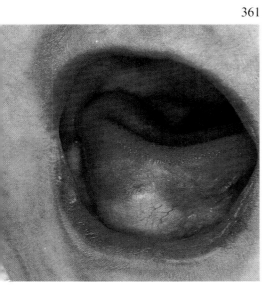

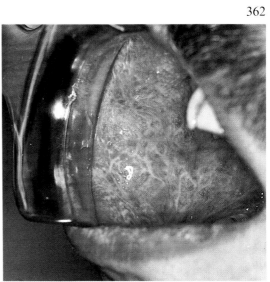

# 8. Diseases of the Skin

**Figure 363  Subcutaneous Fat Necrosis:**  Subcutaneous fat necrosis in a 12-day-old newborn. The lesion were not detected until the ninth day of life. Over the back, extensive red-purple discoloration and swelling of the skin was noted. Over the same area, the underlying tissue was diffusely hardened, but not painful.

**Differential Diagnosis:**  Subcutaneous fat necrosis must be distinguished from sclerema neonatorum and "neonatal cold injury." With sclerema neonatorum, there is progressive hardening of the subcutaneous tissue associated with serious illness in the newborn. The involved areas are hard and nonpitting. The palms and soles of the feet are spared. In cases of neonatal cold injury, the face is reddened and there is pitting edema on the body. Neonatal cold injury occurs in the newborn after prolonged cold exposure.

**Figure 364  Vitiligo:**  Extensive vitiligo (acquired pigment deficiency of the skin) on the back and on the extensor surface of the upper thigh in a 10-year-old boy. Numerous, irregularly shaped, white lesions with partially hyperpigmented borders, were noted. The lesions had recently increased in size. The areas primarily affected include the face (especially the eyes and perioral area), genitals, hands, feet, elbows knees, and chest. When the scalp is involved, hair in the affected area may loose pigment. A familial incidence has been observed. The cause of vitiligo is unclear and may be related to trauma or an autoimmune process. Vitiligo occurs more frequently in patients with hyperthyroidism, adrenal insufficiency, and diabetes mellitus. The course is variable. Spontaneous remissions are possible.

### Differential Diagnosis Includes:
1. Nevus anaemicus (congenital deficiency of terminal blood vessels in a circumscribed area).
2. Nevus achromicus (poorly defined, bright yellow skin lesions due to deficient melanin formation).
3. Multiple depigmented skin lesions associated with tuberous sclerosis (p 234).
4. Partial albinism (congenital, autosomal dominant condition with white forelock and depigmented skin on forehead).
5. Waardenburg's syndrome (cutaneous hypopigmentation, see p 206).
6. Hypomelanosis of Ito (incontinentia pigmenti achromicans—bizarre, depigmented skin pattern, present since birth, associated with ocular abnormalities and central nervous system disorders).
7. Acquired skin disorders associated with hyperpigmented macules such as pityriasis alba, tinea versicolor (p 184), scleroderma (p 114), and lichen sclerosis (p 74).

**Figure 365  Localized Lipodystrophy:**  Localized loss of adipose tissue in a 10-year-old boy. Of note was atrophy of the subcutaneous tissue at the site of injection of a corticosteroid preparation. Complete healing is possible over a substantial period of time (possibly years).

**Figure 366  Keloid:**  Keloid (after second degree burns) on the hands of an 11-year-old boy. The lesion was a 4 × 6 cm, firm, red scar with stretched shiny skin, causing restriction of finger movement.

Keloids may develop during wound healing. Frequently, keloids are located on the sternum, the neck, the face, or the ear (after ear piercing). Treatment entails surgical excision of the keloid and postoperative instillation of corticosteroids. In contrast to keloids, hypertrophic scars remain restricted to the wound area.

**Figure 367  Perniosis:**  Perniosis (skin changes caused by the inability to adjust to temperature fluctuations) in a 15-year-old girl. On the outer aspect of the lower right thigh, two silver dollar-sized, blue-red doughy, pruritic swellings were noted (erythrocyanosis crurum puellarum). Perniosis is a vascular response to cold injury. It begins suddenly, with gradual regression over the course of 2 weeks. In children, the prognosis is generally good.

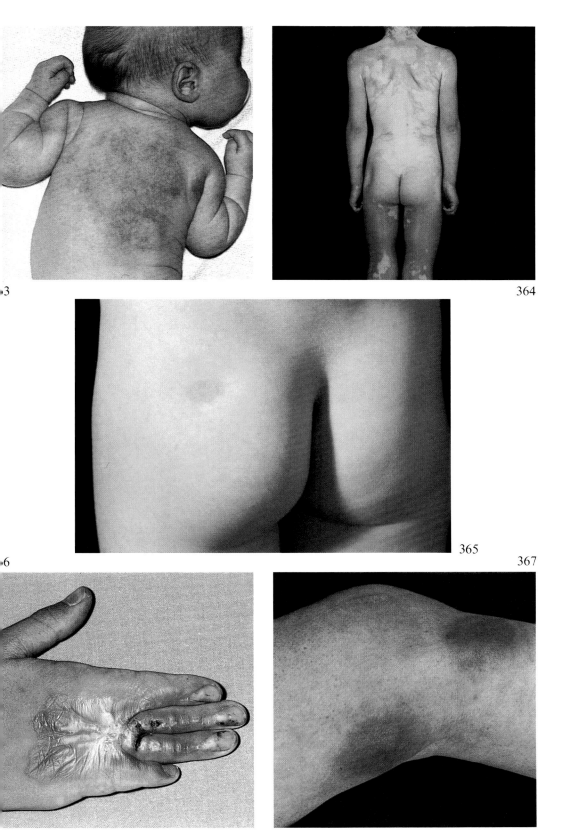

363

364

365

366

367

# 8. Diseases of the Skin

**Figure 368  Acanthosis Nigricans:**  Benign acanthosis nigricans in a 10-year-old girl. The skin had velvety texture with hyperpigmentation of the shoulders, the nape of the neck, the axilla, the groin, ar the inner aspect of the thighs and knees. Mucous membranes were not affected. Benign acanthosis nigr cans represents a congenital anomaly inherited as an autosomal dominant trait. At first, the skin is dr rough, and deeply pigmented; later, the skin is thickened and covered by small, papillomatous elevation and develops a gray-brown or black discoloration. Benign acanthosis nigricans must be differentiated fro malignant acanthosis nigricans (which occurs in conjunction with adenocarcinoma) and from pseudoacal thosis nigricans, (which occurs in obese individuals). In cases of Addison's disease, the hyperpigmentatic of the skin is not associated with changes in texture. Erythrasma, which is usually found in the joints ar is symmetrically distributed, is easily recognized by typical red fluorescence under a Wood's lamp.

**Figures 369 and 370  Pseudoxanthoma Elasticum:**  Pseudoxanthoma elasticum in a 12-year-old girl. I the skin folds of the neck, one could see numerous 1 to 3 mm, flat, yellow papules arrayed in a linea fashion. Later the lesions increased in number and gave the neck a velvety texture. Lesions are found i the axilla, the groin, and the flexor aspects of the elbows and knees. The mucous membranes (oral cavity rectum, vagina) are not affected. Pseudoxanthoma elasticum may be associated with visual disturbance or other ophthalmologic problems, as well as circulatory problems including hypertension.

The basis of this hereditary disease is unknown. Four different forms of the disorder have been described In the elastic fibers of the skin and blood vessels, degenerative changes and calcium deposition occur. Specifi therapy for this disorder is unknown. Diagnosis is confirmed through biopsy.

**Figure 371  Pseudoxanthoma Elasticum:**  Pseudoxanthoma elasticum in an 18-year-old man. Fundus copic examination of the eye revealed characteristic, yellow, vessel-like branching streaks (so-called angioi streaks) caused by the degeneration of Bruch's membrane. Vessel disease was noted in other organs (brair heart) as well as the extremities. Typical skin changes were present (yellow papules which increase in number) This is an example of the autosomally dominant inherited Type I form of the disease, which has an ur favorable prognosis.

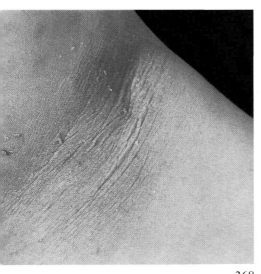

368

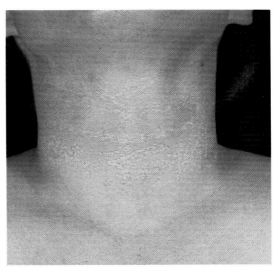

369

370

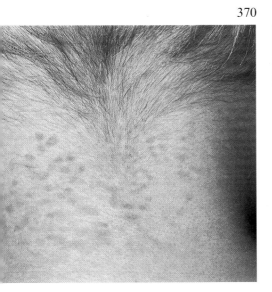

371

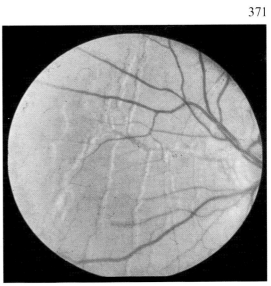

**Figure 372  Erythema Elevatum Diutinum:**  Erythema elevatum diutinum in a 13-year-old boy. Of n
were numerous, red, partly rounded, nodular lesions, with central indentation. Lesions were noted on
underarms, the hands, and the legs. The skin findings are chronic and progressive in nature, and are pro
ably related to an allergic condition.

Differential diagnosis includes granuloma annulae, hypertrophic lichen planus, and sarcoidosis.

**Figure 373  Erythema Annulare Centrifugum:**  Erythema annulare centrifugum in a 14-year-old gi
Of note were numerous erythematous and edematous lesions of varying sizes which were partly ring-shap
in form. The centers of these lesions tended to fade, and the lesions spread out centrifugally. The lesio
were located on the covered parts of the body, where one is prone to perspire lightly. Erythema annula
centrifugum (or marginatum) develops quickly and can last for weeks or months. The cause is usually u
clear. It occurs in about 10 percent of rheumatic fever cases. Since the edge of the erythematous lesi
can be slightly scaly, erythema annulare centrifugum must be distinguished from a fungal infection of t
skin (either microscopically or by culture).

**Figure 374  Erythema Annulare Centrifugum:**  Erythema annulare centrifugum in a 10-year-old bo
On the left shoulder there were several small, erythematous lesions that were slightly scaly; later the l
sions became ring- and garland-shaped.

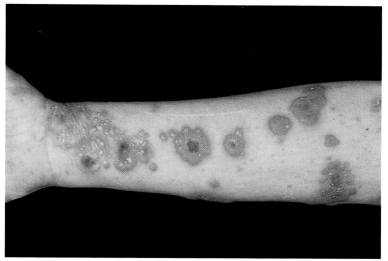

372

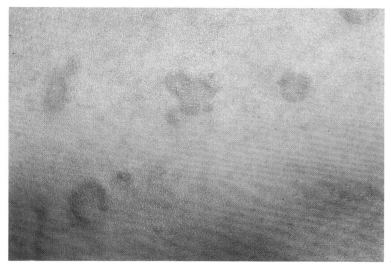

373

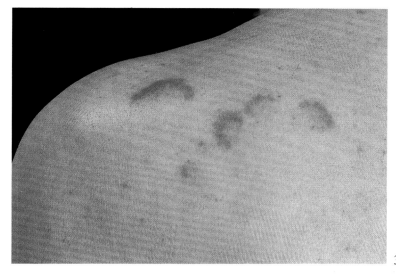

374

# 8. Diseases of the Skin

**Figure 375  Atrophoderma Vermiculatum:**  Atrophoderma vermiculatum (keratosis pilaris with resulti
atrophy) in a 2-year-old infant. On the right cheek, linear erythematous lesions with hyperkeratosis we
noted. Atrophic skin remained after the hyperkeratotic areas were removed.

**Figure 376  Keloid:**  Keloid on the neck of a 5-year-old boy. The lesion was elongated, erythemato
elevated, and sharply demarcated. The lesion limited movement of the neck. The keloid formed "spontar
ously," presumably due to exuberant reaction of the connective tissue to minimal trauma in a predispos
person. Keloids occur more frequently in the area of the sternum or the ear.

**Figure 377  Anhidrotic Ectodermal Dysplasia:**  Anhidrotic ectodermal dysplasia (Christ-Siemens-Tourai
syndrome) in a 9-year-old boy. Findings included hypoplasia of the eyelashes and eyebrows, fragile wrinkl
skin over the eyelids, hypodontia, and swelling of the lips. The hair was sparse and dry. There was a stri
ing discrepancy between the light hair on the head, and the dark pigmentation of the iris. The child al
had hypohydrosis (caused by hypoplasia of the sweat glands) with intolerance to heat and hypoplasia
the sebaceous glands. The boy's physical and mental development were normal.

Differential diagnosis includes many of the other ectodermal dysplasia syndromes.

**Figure 378  Cheilitis:**  Cheilitis granulomatosa (Miescher's cheilitis) in a 15-year-old boy. Of note w
swelling of the upper lip without involvement of the cheeks, chin, eyelids, or forehead. Initially, the swelli
would appear and resolve spontaneously; later, the lips remained swollen. In other cases, the lower lip a
one or both cheeks may be swollen. The swelling, accompanied by fever, is at first mild and brief; lat
the swelling is constant. After several years, spontaneous remission may occur. Cheilitis granulomat
may be seen in several syndromes. In Melkersson-Rosenthal syndrome, cheilitis granulomatosa occurs
conjunction with facial paralysis and fissuring of the tongue. The findings in Melkersson-Rosenthal syndro
are due to a chronic granulomatous inflammation of uncertain etiology. This syndrome may be related
Boeck's sarcoidosis. Isolated cheilitis granulomatosa is perhaps a manifestation of Melkersson-Rosent
syndrome. Cheilitis may also be mistaken for angioneurotic edema. Persistent swelling of the lip occ
in Ascher's syndrome (with abnormal lip formation, swelling of the eyelid, and thyroid enlargement).
cases of cheilitis glandularis, the lower lip is swollen and has numerous pinhead-sized openings.

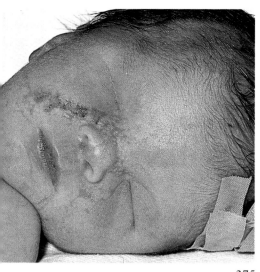

375

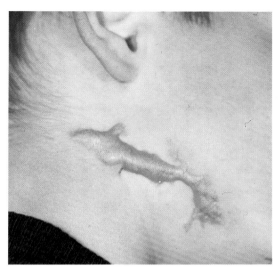

376

377

378

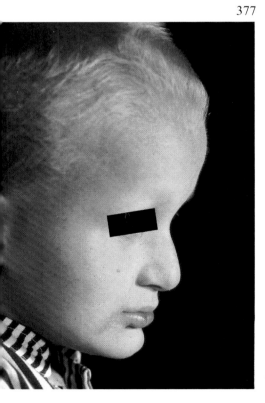

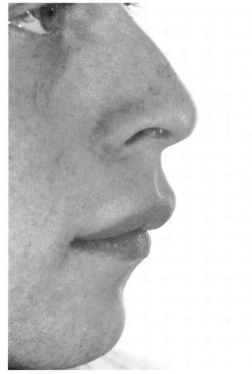

# 8.  Diseases of the Skin

**Figure 379  Panniculitis:**  Panniculitis in a 9-month-old girl who was treated with corticosteroic for infantile spasms. A 2 × 3 cm, irregularly outlined, erythematous hardening of the skin was noted ov both cheeks. Close inspection revealed several subcutaneous nodules with erythema of the overlying ski Lesions were noted 2 weeks after the end of corticosteroid treatment. These lesions are typical of post co ticosteroid panniculitis. This inflammatory reaction resolved spontaneously after 3 weeks, leaving no scarrin

In post-corticosteroid panniculitis, multiple nodules may appear on the face, arms, or torso. Durin the first year of life, panniculitis can be caused by exposure to the cold (particularly on the face). A fe hours or days after exposure to the cold, erythematous, indurated plaques may appear. Panniculitis is al seen in Weber-Christian syndrome. In Weber-Christian syndrome the lesions are 1 to 6 cm, erythematou painful nodules located on various parts of the body. The nodules are frequently accompanied by fever an arthralgia. The lesions disappear slowly over the course of several weeks, leaving behind impressions the skin (atrophy of adipose tissue).

Differential diagnosis of panniculitis includes diseases which cause granuloma formation in the su cutaneous tissue as well as certain vasculitides (such as erythema nodosum, p 112).

**Figure 380  Erythema Infectiosum:**  Erythema infectiosum in an 18-month-old girl. Findings include a butterfly-shaped erythematous rash on the face (erysipelas-like reddening with an elevated border) a companied by a garland-shaped maculopapular exanthem over the rest of the body (especially the arms The rash was not associated with fever.

**Figure 381  Adenoma Sebaceum:**  Adenoma sebaceum associated with tuberous sclerosis in a 12-yea old boy. A seizure disorder had been diagnosed since the age of 1 year. Skin changes, first appearing i adolescence, consisted of small, telangiectatic papules on the face, 1 to 3 mm in diameter, which sprea over the face. In other cases, the papules may be larger and yellow in color. Other cutaneous symptom of tuberous sclerosis include depigmented nevi and subungual fibroma of the great toe. The child was mil ly mentally retarded. Other organs (the brain, the eye, and the kidneys) were affected by the disease.

**Differential Diagnosis:**  Adenoma sebaceum may be difficult to differentiate from acne vulgaris. Acr vulgaris does not usually occur until adolescence forming comedones and pustules. In cases of benig trichoepithelioma (epithelioma adenoides cysticum), numerous, round, skin-colored papules appear on th cheeks around the time of puberty. The lesions may get larger and take on a yellow or red appearance

**Figure 382  Systemic Lupus Erythematosus:**  Systemic lupus erythematosus in a 15-year-old girl. A extensive, sharply outlined, butterfly-shaped, scaling rash was noted on both cheeks; a solitary, irregular outlined, erythematous rash was noted on the bridge of the nose and at the hairline. Associated symptom included protracted fever, arthralgia and arthritis, hepatosplenomegaly, and generalized lymphadenopath Laboratory investigations revealed antinuclear antibodies and anti-DNA antibodies; serum complement wa low. Immunohistological examination of the skin revealed immunoglobulin and complement deposition the dermoepidermal transition.

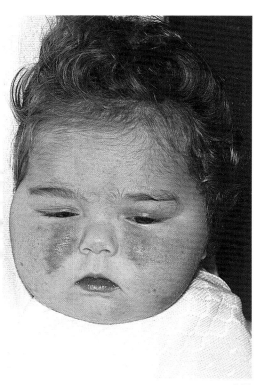

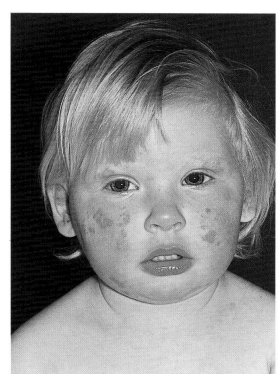

379

380

381

382

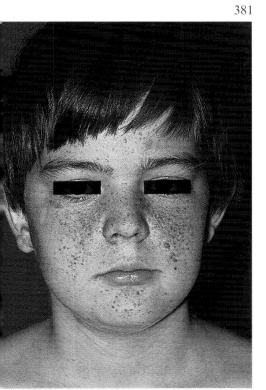

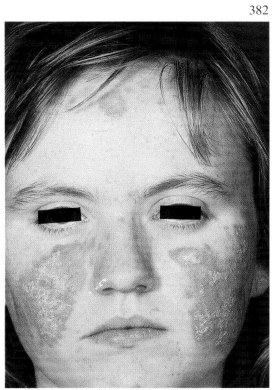

# 8. Diseases of the Skin

**Figure 383  Beckwith-Wiedemann Syndrome:**  The malformed ear of a 2-month-old boy with Beckwith‑Wiedemann syndrome is shown. The child had hypoglycemia at birth (due to hyperinsulinemia). Other physic findings including indentation of the earlobe, macrosomia, macroglossia, and visceromegaly led to the diagno‑ sis of Beckwith-Wiedemann syndrome. Omphalocele is seen in most cases. Children with Beckwith‑Wiedemann syndrome have a higher incidence of Wilm's tumor and adrenal cortical carcinoma.

**Figure 384  Microtia:**  Microtia (rudimentary ear pinna) and atresia of the external auditory canal in 2-month-old girl. The child also had nevus flammeus (port wine nevus) on the forehead just above the bridg of the nose. No abnormalities of the inner ear were noted, nor were there any other associated deformitie The cause of the deformed ear was unknown.

**Figure 385  Congenital Microcephaly:**  Congenital microcephaly and protruding ears in a 18-month-o girl. Microcephaly (OFC 28 cm at birth) and poorly formed, low set ears were noted. Mental developme was severely delayed. No other deformities were noted, and there were no signs of intrauterine infectio or chromosomal anomaly. At 3 years of age, surgery was performed to correct the ear deformity.

Microcephaly may be secondary to intrauterine infections or specific chromosomal anomalies (Dow syndrome or trisomy 13 or 18). Hereditary microcephaly (recessive mode of inheritance) may present wi findings similar to this case.

**Figure 386  Ectodermal Dysplasia:**  Ectodermal dysplasia (hypohidrotic form) in a 10-month-old bo The child was brought to the clinic because of unexplained fever and failure to thrive. Characteristic hypohidrotic ectodermal dysplasia was the sparce hair over the head and body, the absence of eyelashe thin and dry skin, decreased tearing, and decreased perspiration (detected through pilocarpine iontophor sis). Radiologic examination revealed anomalous dentition. Other findings included thick, swollen lips, hyp pigmentation of the periorbital skin, and low set ears. The child developed chronic atopic rhinitis and inte mittent hoarseness (due to hypoplasia of the mucous glands in the respiratory tract). At several times duri hospitalization, febrile episodes, without signs of infection, occurred. These temperature elevations we the result of hyperthermia from hypohydrosis. The child failed to grow normally, in part due to an intole ance to milk (weight gain improved on a diet of puréed meat). Other family members had ectodermal dy plasia. This family was an example of classic ectodermal dysplasia syndrome (Christ-Siemens-Tourai syndrome). Other forms of ectodermal dysplasia include ectrodactyly—ectodermal dysplasia clefting sy drome (EEC syndrome) and Goltz's syndrome.

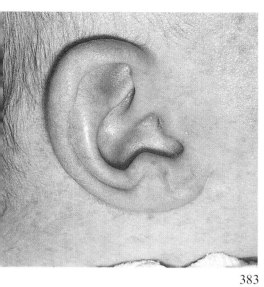

383

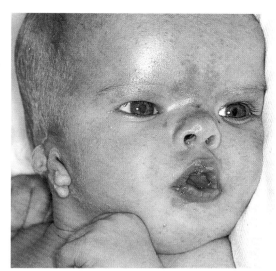

384

386

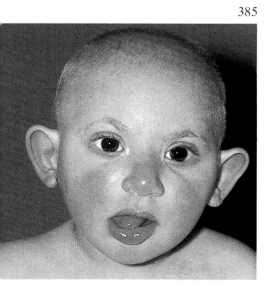

385

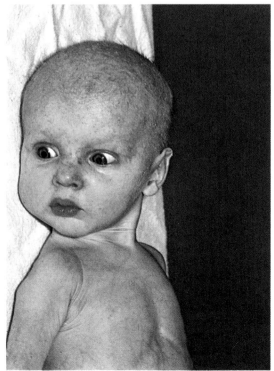

# 8.  Diseases of the Skin

**Figure 387  Alopecia Areata:**   Alopecia areata (localized hair loss) in a 6-year-old girl. The hair follicl
of the affected area were still intact. After 2 to 3 months (without specific treatment) the hair grew bac.
At first, the new hair was lighter than the rest of the scalp hair, but later the hair color was more eve
The prognosis of alopecia areata differs depending on the cause. A small number of cases will becon
alopecia totalis (loss of all scalp hair). In cases where there is scar tissue or the follicles are destroyed (
skin infection, physical damage, or ulcerating malignancy), hair loss is irreversible.

In cases of alopecia areata, the following processes must be ruled out: trichotillomania (nervou
behavior leading to hair pulling, p 206), traction alopecia (trauma from pigtails, ponytails, hair bands, an
other hair treatments), tinea capitis (p 184), severe atopic or seborrheic dermatitis, and other scalp infection

**Figure 388  Alopecia Areata:**   Alopecia areata (idiopathic form) in a 6-year-old boy. Hair loss was note
at the edge of the scalp (ophiasis) on otherwise unaffected skin. These findings occurred suddenly and t
cause is unclear. Despite local corticosteroid treatment, there was no improvement. In general, the progn
sis is unfavorable. Often, this type of alopecia areata may progress and become alopecia totalis.

**Figure 389  Alopecia Totalis:**   Alopecia totalis in a 2-year-old boy. The findings included loss of all ha
on the head (including eyebrows and some eyelashes) during a short period of time. The following caus
of diffuse hair loss must be ruled out: poisons (such as thallium), medications (chemotherapeutic agents
metabolic and endocrine disorders, severe systemic infections, central nervous system diseases (encephaliti
cranial trauma), and neoplastic diseases. Congenital alopecia totalis may occur in conjunction with a nun
ber of syndromes.

In cases of alopecia universalis, hair is lacking not only on the head, but also over the rest of the bod
Treatment of total or universal alopecia is almost always unsuccessful if no specific cause has been ident
fied. However, if a basic disease process can be identified and treated, the alopecia can be corrected
the hair follicles are not permanently damaged.

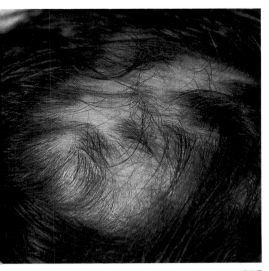

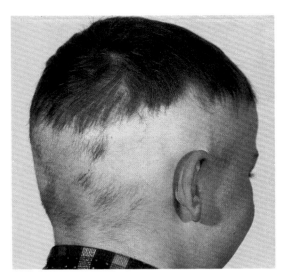

387

388

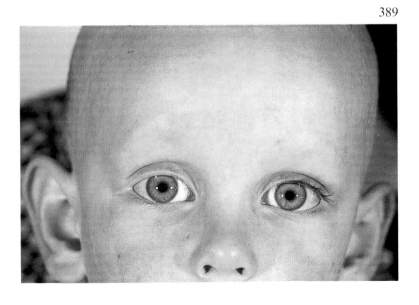

389

# 8. Diseases of the Skin

**Figures 390 and 391  Trichotillomania:**  Trichotillomania in a 14-year-old girl. Diffuse alopecia of the head resulted from the forceful tearing out of hair. Eyelashes were also missing. In certain cases, a skin biopsy is necessary to confirm the diagnosis. Findings on biopsy will demonstrate normal hair follicle juxtaposed with damaged follicles, parafollicular hemorrhage, partial atrophy of follicles, and catagen transformation of the hair.

Differential diagnosis includes tinea capitis and alopecia areata. In cases of continued trichotillomania the hair follicles can be irreversibly damaged resulting in persistent alopecia.

**Figure 392  Partial Albinism:**  Partial albinism (poliosis circumscripta) in a 6-year-old girl. A white fore lock, resulting from an abscence of melanocytes, had been noted since birth. Unlike most cases, there was no hypopigmented area of scalp where the forelock was located. In partial albinism, depigmented area of skin can occur on the torso and the extremities (with the exception of the back, hands, and feet). The term "partial" is used to describe the disease because of the distribution of the skin changes.

**Differential Diagnosis:**  Poliosis, frequently in the area of the eyebrows and eyelashes, occurs in 80 per cent of cases with Vogt-Koyanagi syndrome (uveitis, hearing difficulty, and vitiligo). With resolving alopecia areata, the hairs that grow back are often depigmented. Poliosis is also present in cases of tuberous sclerosis. Vitiligo, an acquired pigment disorder of the skin, is often first seen on areas exposed to the sun. The irregularly outlined, white macules seen in vitilgo often have hyperpigmented borders. On the affected areas of the scalp, the hairs are usually normally pigmented; only after a prolonged period do they begin to loose pigmentation. For further comments on differential diagnosis see vitiligo, p 192.

**Figure 393  Partial Albinism:**  Partial albinism (poliosis circumscripta) in a mother and child. The only anomaly was the white forelock. The other associated findings of Waardenburg's syndrome (acrocephaly, facial dysmorphism, ocular anomalies, abnormal dentation, deafness) were not noted. Isolated poliosis circum scripta, like Waardenburg's syndrome, is inherited as an autosomal dominant trait.

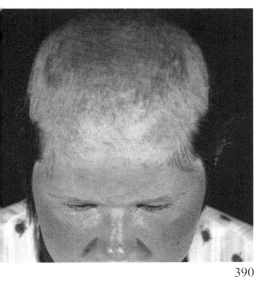

390

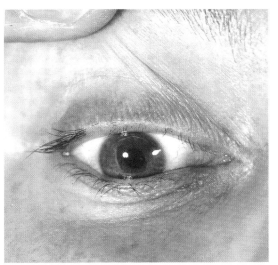

391

392

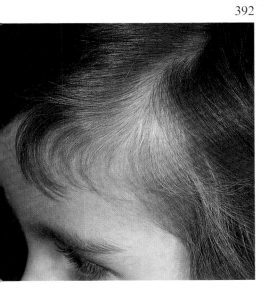

393

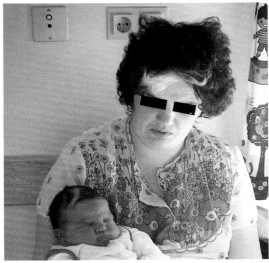

# 8.  Diseases of the Skin

**Figure 394  Verruca Vulgaris:**  Verruca vulgaris next to the fingernails of a 12-year-old boy. Of note wer numerous, painful, periungual, grey-yellow papules, with hyperkeratosis and rough surfaces that involve the nail bed. Growth of the nail can be disturbed in this area. Treatment was with topical application liquid nitrogen. These viral lesions are frequently located on the fingers, dorsum of the hand, knees, elbow and face. Both verruca vulgaris (common warts) and verruca plana (juvenile flat warts) may be found these locations. Juvenile flat warts are small (less than 3 mm), slightly raised, and red-brown in color. Fl warts are recognized by their linear arrangement along excoriations. They can be spread through the sca by combing.

**Differential Diagnosis:**  Warts involving the area near the fingernails must be distinguished from periungu fibromas, which may be seen in cases of tuberous sclerosis.

**Figure 395  Damaged Nails:**  Changes in the nails of a 5-year-old nail biter. Damage can be seen bo to the nail and to the skin surrounding the area. As a complication of this traumatic injury, paronychia an warts may occur.

Habitual nail biting is related to aggressive behavior. It occurs widely among older children and ca persist as a habit to adulthood. The first cause of nail biting to be considered is the repression of aggressiv impulses which may be unconsciously manifest in this fashion. Nail damage can also occur by consta rubbing of the finger nails, or by frequent application of particular nail cosmetics.

**Figure 396  Paronychia:**  Paronychia (purulent inflammation of the nail beds) of the thumb and secon and third fingers of the right hand in a 4-year-old boy with acute lymphocytic leukemia. The findings in cluded painful, erythematous, swelling at the base of the nail bed, and thickened elevation and brown dis coloration of the nail. The paronychia was caused by a candida infection with secondary bacterial infectio with staphylococci. The lesion healed after the infected nail was detached and the area was treated wit antifungal and antimicrobial therapy. Paronychia must be distinguished from the changes in the nail see in cases of psoriasis, dermatitis, and tinea infections.

## Reference

1.  Brooks I. Bacteriologic study of paronychia in children. Am J Surg 141:703, 1981.

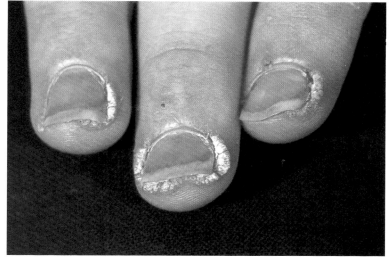

394

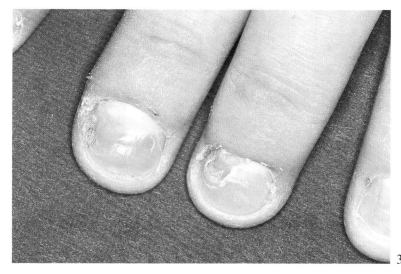

395

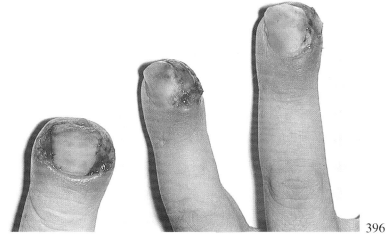

396

# 9. Pediatric Hematology

**Figure 397  Acute Nonlymphocytic Leukemia:**  Acute nonlymphocytic leukemia (ANLL) in a 6-year old boy. Of note was proptosis of the left eye due to infiltration and proliferation of myeloblasts within the orbit. Three weeks prior to these symptoms, the child had fever, bone pain and extensive cervical lymphadenopathy. This child's illness was originally thought to be due to a bacterial infection. When the symptoms failed to respond to antibiotic therapy (and proptosis developed) the child was admitted to the hospital. Peripheral blood smear and bone marrow aspirate demonstrated acute nonlymphoblastic leukemia, myeloblastic type (positive peroxidase and sudan B black stain). The child responded poorly to chemotherapy. Remission could not be achieved and the child died of sepsis two months later. For differential diagnosis of proptosis see p 34 and p 254.

## Reference

1.  Grier HE, Weinstein HJ. Acute nonlymphocytic leukemia. Pediatr Clin North Am 32:6, 1985.

**Figure 398  Acute Nonlymphocytic Leukemia:**  Acute nonlymphocytic leukemia (ANLL) in a 13-year old boy. Swelling and ulceration of the gums occurred because of leukemic infiltration. Simultaneous enlargement of the right submandibular gland was also noted. Gingival and glandular swelling regressed after an intensive two week course of chemotherapy (induction phase).
  For differential diagnosis of gingival swelling, see p 102.

**Figure 399  Acute Lymphocytic Leukemia:**  Acute lymphocytic leukemia (ALL) in a 10-year-old girl. Findings included petechial hemorrhages on the hard and soft palate (due to thrombocytopenia). In addition to petechiae, ecchymotic skin lesions were noted. In this case, the skin and mucous membrane hemorrhages were the initial symptoms that led to the diagnosis of ALL.

## Reference

1.  Poplack DG. Acute lymphoblastic leukemia in childhood. Pediatr Clin North Am 32:669, 1985.

**Figure 400  Acute Lymphocytic Leukemia:**  Acute lymphocytic leukemia (ALL) in a 10-year-old boy. A large, skin hemorrhage (suffusion) was noted over the lower thigh. Over the rest of the body, one could see ecchymoses (small, circumscribed, patchy skin hemorrhages) and petechiae. Therapy led to complete remission. After 5½ years, this boy is still in remission.

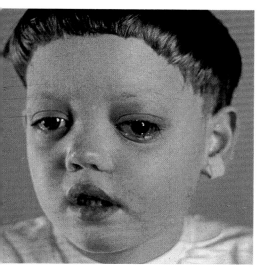

397

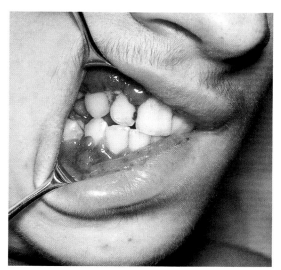

398

399

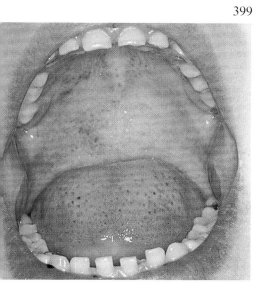

400

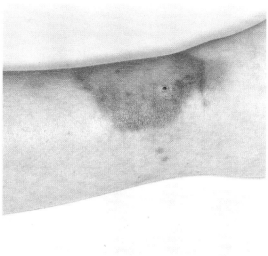

# 9.  Pediatric Hematology

**Figure 401   Acute Nonlymphocytic Leukemia:**   Acute nonlymphocytic leukemia in a 5-year-old girl. The initial symptom of disease was skin hemorrhages. Chemotherapy led to partial remission. After five months the child developed marked abdominal distension, hepatosplenomegaly, ascites, and severe anemia. Hypoproteinemia was also noted. Despite multiple blood transfusions, the child died due to persistent internal bleeding.

**Figure 402   Acute Lymphocytic Leukemia:**   Acute lymphocytic leukemia in a 7-year-old boy with chronic candidiasis. Several firm, white, irregularly shaped plaques (which were difficult to remove) were found on the tongue. *Candida albicans* was detected microscopically and by fungal culture. Lesions such as these are seen in immune suppressed individuals. The usual findings seen in cases of thrush differ in that the lesions are softer, and scraping usually results in punctate hemorrhages on an erythematous base.

**Figure 403   Acute Lymphocytic Leukemia:**   Acute lymphocytic leukemia in a 10-year-old boy with *Candida* dermatitis of the face. Round, scaly, pruritic, erythematous lesions (approximately 2 cm in diameter) were noted over the face. The child had similar skin lesions over the scalp and body. In addition, an extensive lesion that was resistent to therapy was located in the mouth. *Candida albicans* could be detected microscopically and by culture. Lesions such as these are seen in chronic mucocutaneous candidiasis. The condition is seen in immune suppressed individuals (due to a neoplastic process, chemotherapy, or an immune deficiency syndrome).

**Figure 404   Acute Lymphocytic Leukemia:**   Acute lymphocytic leukemia (ALL) in a 7-year-old girl with herpes zoster. On the right hand, groups of vesicles of various size were noted. These vesicles were either filled with a serous fluid or ulcerated and covered with a hemorrhagic crust. The illness began with a febrile period during induction chemotherapy for ALL. Within a few days, red papules developed on the hand. These papules changed to vesicles and persisted for two weeks. No other skin lesions were noted, and secondary bacterial infection did not occur. The girl previously had chicken pox (varicella) at 3 years of age.

Herpes zoster is considered to be a "second disease" caused by the herpes virus varicellae in patients who have previously had chicken pox. Virus may persist in neural tissue and reactivate when the patient is immune compromised. Herpes zoster may occur in 2 to 3 percent of patients with malignant disease undergoing chemotherapy and is of particular concern due to the danger of generalization. Relapses may occur.

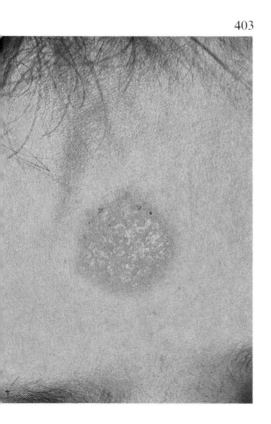

401

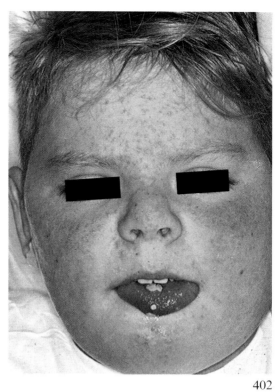

402

403

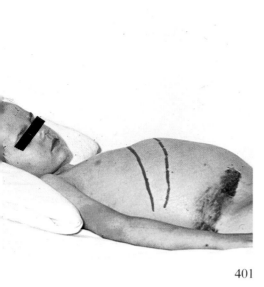

404

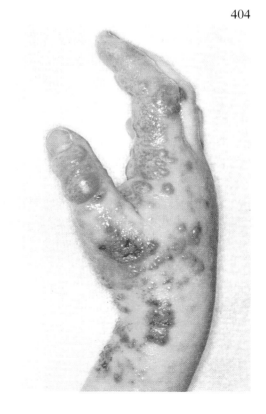

# 9. Pediatric Hematology

**Figure 405  Hemophilia:**  Hemophilia A in an 11-year-old boy. Of note was a subcutaneous hematom of the lower right thigh (after trauma). Small, superficial hemorrhages were noted over the rest of the bod The child had frequent nosebleeds, occasional hematuria, and abdominal pain. After the age of 20 year the incidence of cutaneous hemorrhage and joint hemorrhage decreased considerably despite persistent coagu lation defect.

Hemophilia A is a sex-linked coagulation disorder due to Factor VIII deficiency. Differential diagnos includes other congenital or acquired coagulation disorders such as von Willebrand's disease. Vasculit (such as Henoch-Schönlein purpura), thrombocytopenia, and thrombasthenia can be differentiated from con genital coagulation disorders by the type of hemorrhagic lesion and by laboratory evaluation.

## Reference

1.  Buchanan GR. Hemophilia. Pediatr Clin North Am 27:309, 1980.

**Figure 406  Hemophilia A:**  Hemophilia A in a 9-year-old boy. The child had severe Hemophilia A wit a Factor VIII level less than 1 percent. Of note were ecchymoses around both eyes and bruising over th forehead. Frequent hemarthrosis (particularly of the knees) occurred. In children with hemophilia, hemor rhage can occur in the eye, conjunctiva, iris, retina, and vitreous body. In order to control the bleedin manifestations of Hemophilia A, Factor VIII concentrate was given at home.

**Figure 407  Hemophilia:**  Hemophilia A with hemorrhage in the left knee joint (hemarthrosis) in a 14-year old boy. Findings included warm, fluctuant swelling of the left knee which caused restriction in movemen The child was febrile to 39° C. After administering Factor VIII and immobilizing the joint, the effusio regressed and physical therapy could begin. After this episode of hemarthrosis, a regular substituation therap was introduced in order to prevent further hemorrhage into the joint space.

For differential diagnosis of knee-joint swelling see p 110.

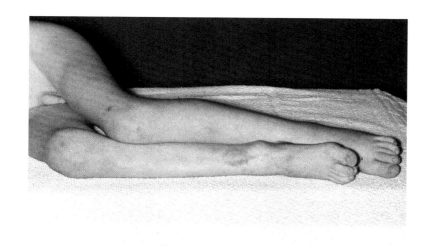

405

406

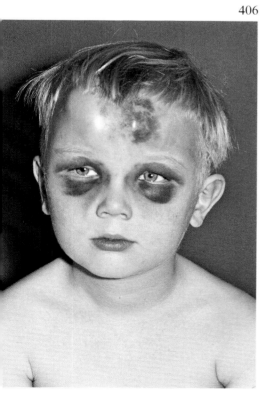

407

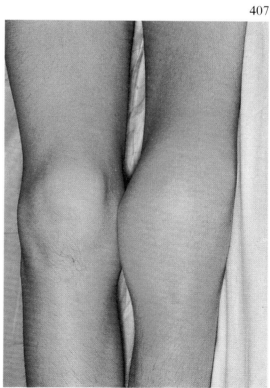

# 9. Pediatric Hematology

**Figure 408 Waterhouse-Friderichsen Syndrome:** Waterhouse-Friderichsen syndrome in a 16-year-old girl with meningococcal sepsis. Ecchymotic, purpuric and petechial lesions were noted over the body, especially on the legs. Severe circulatory collapse was also noted (cold extremities, hypotension, thready pulse, disorientation). A smear of the buffy code revealed diplococci layered in with the granulocytes. Laboratory investigations demonstrated disseminated intravascular coagulation (thrombocytopenia, decreased fibrinogen, increased fibren split products, and decreased Factor V and VIII). In septic patients, superficial skin hemorrhage can also be caused by hypoprothrombinemia (due to liver damage). Petechial and ecchymotic lesions may be seen in septic patients without consumption coagulopathy due to direct interaction of the pathogen and platelets. If only petechial lesions are seen in a septic patient, a vasculitic process should be considered.

## Reference

1. Lewis LS. Prognostic factors in acute meningococcemia. Arch Dis Child. 54:44, 1979.

**Figure 409 Idiopathic Thrombocytopenic Purpura:** Idiopathic thrombocytopenia purpura in a 3-year-old girl. Petechial skin hemorrhages were noted over the entire body, especially on the arms and legs. Ten days prior to the appearance of the petechial rash, the child had an acute upper respiratory infection and had been treated with a sulfonamide medication. Laboratory investigation revealed a platelet count of 1,000 platelets per mm³, prolonged bleeding time, and abnormal clot retraction. Bone marrow aspirate revealed an increased megakaryocyte count. The condition responded to six weeks of prednisone therapy.

**Differential Diagnosis:** Thrombocytopenic skin hemorrhages occur:
1. Associated with decreased number of megakaryocytes in the bone marrow (in cases of bone marrow aplasia or bone marrow infiltration).
2. Associated with normal number of megakaryocytes in the bone marrow (in cases of Wiskott-Aldrich syndrome).
3. Associated with normal or increased number of megakaryocytes in the bone marrow (in autoimmune disease or in consumption coagulopathy).

Petechial skin hemorrhages may also occur in disorders of platelet function such as thrombasthenia.

**Figures 410 and 411 Henoch-Schönlein Purpura:** Henoch-Schönlein purpura in a 7-year-old boy. Of note were dense, petechial lesions on the extensor surface of the upper thigh and buttocks; similar but less numerous lesions were noted on the extensor surfaces of the arms and on the face. Other manifestations of this allergic vasculitis included edema, arthralgia, hemorrhagic lesions of the intestinal mucosa, and nephritis. Laboratory evaluation revealed normal coagulation studies and platelet count.

**Differential Diagnosis:** Purpuric lesions similar to those seen in Henoch-Schönlein purpura may be caused by severe septicemia (often combined with thrombocytopenia and consumption coagulopathy) polyarteritis nodosa, idiopathic thrombocytopenic purpura, and thrombasthenia.

## Reference

1. Koskimies D, et al. Henoch-Schönlein nephritis: long term prognosis of unselected patients. Arch Dis Child 56:482, 198

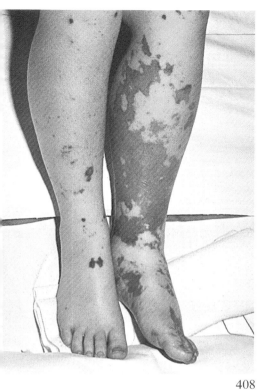

408

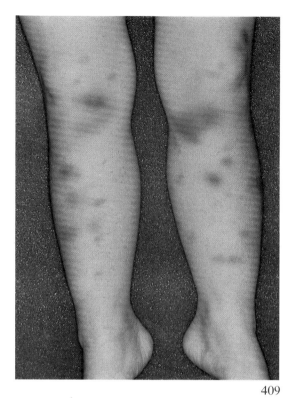

409

410

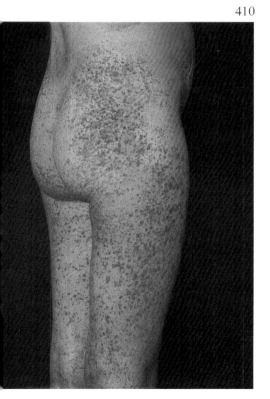

411

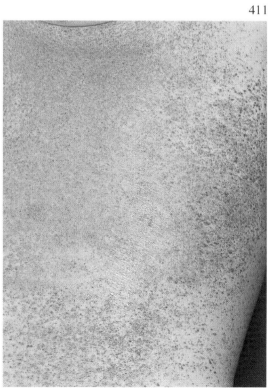

# 9. Pediatric Hematology

**Figure 412  Henoch-Schönlein Purpura:**  Henoch-Schönlein purpura in a 9-year-old boy. Ten days pri to the onset of the rash, the child had a streptococcal infection with high fever. During the days that fo lowed, joint swelling, edema, and petechial skin hemorrhages began to appear. Edematous swelling of th eyelids was noted. On the 4th day of the illness, the patient had colicky abdominal pain and bloody stool Rapid improvement followed treatment with prednisone, but a relapse occurred when steroid treatment wa stopped. After 4 weeks, the child was asymptomatic.

**Differential Diagnosis:**  Differential diagnosis includes any process which may present with petechial purpuric lesions. These include thrombocytopenia, disseminated intravascular coagulation, and various va culitic processes. Vasculitis may be due to either viral or bacterial infection, such as the hemorrhagic exa thems of measles, scarlet fever, and chicken pox. In cases of polyarteritis nodosa (an inflammatory conditi of medium and small arteries), skin changes similar to anaphylactoid purpura are present, but are usual more severe in nature. Polyarteritis nodosa includes neurologic symptoms (paraesthesia, pain, muscle wea ness) and cardiac symptoms (myocardial infarction, cardiac failure) not seen in anaphylactoid purpura. Whe the central nervous system is involved, seizures and encephalitis may result. Hepatosplenomegaly is fr quently seen. The disease is usually fatal.

**Figure 413  Polyarteritis Nodosa:**  Polyarteritis nodosa in a 14-year-old boy. Of note were petechial sk hemorrhages on the arms and legs and scattered lesions on the face and torso. The onset of disease wa sudden, with high fever and muscle aches. Later in the course, neurologic symptoms (paraesthesia) a hematuria appeared. As the disease progressed, involvement of the coronary arteries was noted. Corona arteritis lead to tachycardia, myocardial infarction, and cardiac failure. Tissue obtained from renal biop supported the diagnosis of polyarteritis nodosa.

**Figures 414 and 415  Henoch-Schönlein Purpura:**  Henoch-Schönlein purpura in an 11-year-old boy. note were urticarial lesions on the face which developed central purpuric areas. Lesions were also four elsewhere on the body, especially on the extensor surface of the extremities. Regression of the skin chang was noted after 5 days of prednisone treatment (Figure 415), but an immediate relapse was noted when thera was stopped. Prior to the appearance of the skin lesions, the child was noted to have bronchitis. Platel count and other coagulation studies were normal.

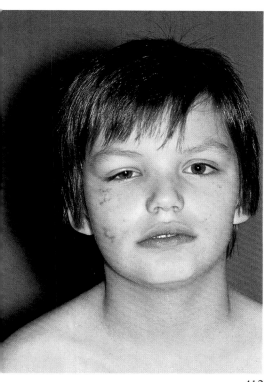

412

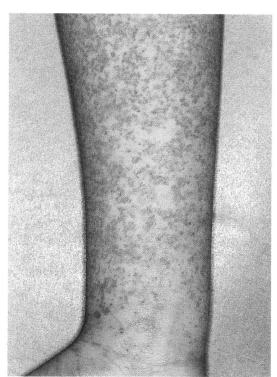

413

414

415

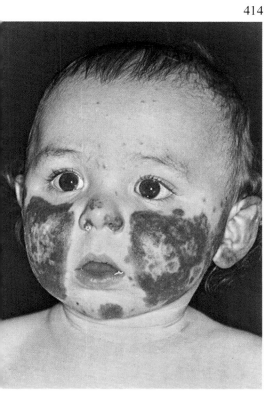

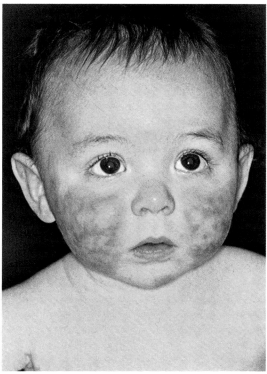

**Figure 416  Polyarteritis Nodosa:**   Gangrene of both feet, secondary to polyarteritis nodosa, in a 3-year old girl. At the onset, the child was noted to have high fever and a blue-purple discoloration of the hand and feet. The extremities were cool and peripheral pulses were diminished. Due to involvement of the coronary arteries, the child developed hypertension and severe cardiac failure (tachycardia, hepatomegaly). Laboratory evaluation revealed leukocytosis, elevated ESR, and sterile blood cultures. During the first week of hospitalization, the foot began to blacken, starting first with the toes and then spreading over the entire foot (dry gangrene). With appropriate treatment, cardiac failure began to improve and the circulatory problem in the hands also regressed. Despite therapy, the child had both feet amputated. Having ruled out other causes for the condition (embolic phenomenon, mercury posioning, other autoimmune processes), polyarteritis nodosa was suspected and prednisone treatment was begun. During the years that followed, the treatment had to be continued intermittently due to recurring circulatory problems.

**Differential Diagnosis:**   Gangrene can occur in conjunction with bacterial sepsis, disseminated intravascular coagulation, arterial emboli, systemic lupus erythematosus, scleroderma, and acrodynia (mercury poisoning).

**Figure 417  Purpura Fulminans:**   Purpura fulminans in a 12-year-old girl. Two weeks after a viral illness (stomatitis), numerous ecchymotic, and purpuric lesions were noted on both the legs and buttocks. As the condition progressed, fever and swelling and discoloration of the entire right leg (as well as vesicle formation on the foot) was noted. Laboratory evaluation revealed thrombocytopenia and decreased Factor V level. Eventually, the right foot became necrotic (dry gangrene) leading to amputation of the lower leg.

**Figure 418  Gas Gangrene:**   Gas gangrene in a 14-year-old girl. Of note was dry mummification (blackening) of the right foot and distal third of the tibia. Gas gangrene is caused by an anaerobic infection of the soft tissue. In this case, the child was infected with *Clostridium perfringens* (originating from necrotizing enteritis). Clostridia was identified on blood culture. This septic process was treated with intensive antibiotic therapy. Later, the leg had to be amputated at the thigh.

## Reference

1.   Weinstein L, Barza NA. Gas gangrene. N Engl J Med 289:1129, 1973.

**Figure 419  Urticaria Pigmentosa:**   Urticaria pigmentosa (mastocytosis) in a 2-year-old girl. The findings included numerous, poorly defined, confluent, brown nodules and vesicles over the lower leg. The lesions appeared suddenly after administration of aspirin during the course of a febrile illness. The lesions were intensely pruritic. If the lesions were rubbed, wheals would form (positive Darier sign). The child had previously been diagnosed as having urticaria pigmentosa (based on clinical presentation and tissue biopsy). The surface of the skin lesions on the legs had the typical "orange peel" texture. For differential diagnosis see p 160.

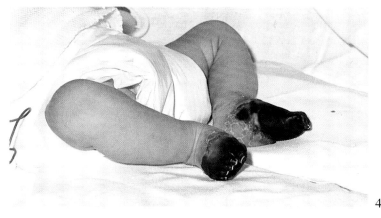

416

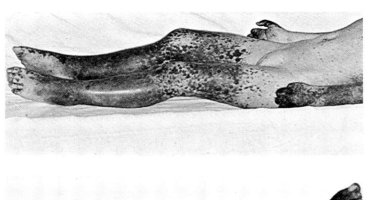

417

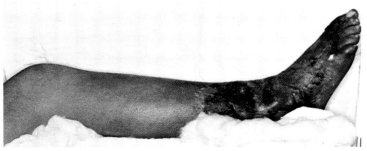

418

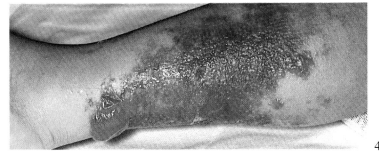

419

# 10. Pediatric Oncology

**Figure 420  Nevus Flammeus:**  Nevus flammeus in a 2-month-old boy. Of note were the extensive, i[r]regularly shaped, red skin lesions at the hair line. These findings had been present since birth. When nev[us] flammeus is located on the neck, it is commonly known as Unna's nevus.

Nevus flammeus may have varying degrees of involvement. The so-called "salmon patch" occurs i[n] 40 to 70 percent of all newborns and is a harmless anomaly (which may persist throughout life). Nev[us] flammeus found on the eyelids or at the base of the nose usually disappear in early childhood. The so-calle[d] port-wine nevus (flat hemangioma), like the nevus on the neck, usually persists. Port-wine nevi are usual[ly] asymmetric, found on the face or upper half of the torso and do not extend over the midline. Port-wi[ne] nevi may be associated with Sturge-Weber syndrome or Klippel-Trenaunay-Weber syndrome.

**Figure 421  Nevus Flammeus:**  Unilateral nevus flammeus (port–wine nevus or flat hemangioma) on th[e] upper lip of a 5-week-old boy. There was no indication of corresponding involvement of the leptomening[es] as seen in Sturge-Weber syndrome.

**Figure 422  Cavernous Hemangioma:**  A large cavernous hemangioma (strawberry nevus) in a 3-month-ol[d] boy. The nevus had grown considerably since birth, extending into the scalp and closing the right eye. Cave[r]nous hemangiomas may go through a period of growth, followed by a stationary phase and later involutio[n]. In this case, both resection and radiotherapy were deemed impossible, so no specific therapy was carrie[d] out. The decision was made to wait for spontaneous regression, which usually begins after the first yea[r]. In other cases, prednisone may be used to hasten involution.

**Figure 423  Kasabach-Merritt Syndrome:**  Kasabach-Merritt syndrome in a 3-year-old boy. Of note wa[s] a giant, cavernous hemangioma of the left thigh that reached to the scrotum and lower abdomen. Laborator[y] investigation revealed severe thrombocytopenia, fragmented erythrocytes, and consumption of coagulatio[n] factors. These findings were due to platelet entrapment in the cavernous hemangioma. Skin hemorrhag[e] or hemorrhage into internal organs did not occur. Consumption of platelets and coagulation factors spon[n]taneously improved when the blood vessels leading into the hemangioma became thrombosed.

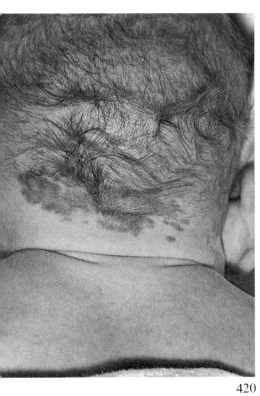

420

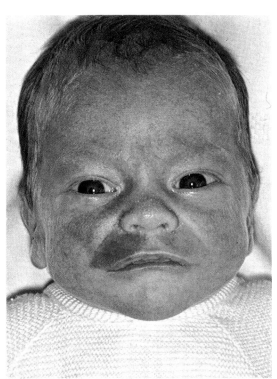

421

422

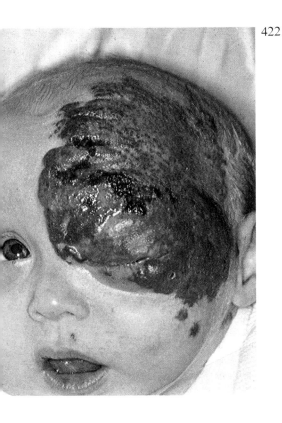

423

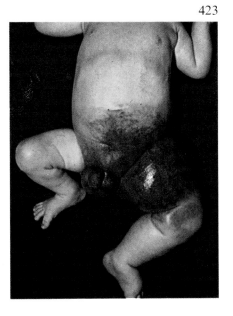

**Figure 424  Sturge-Weber Syndrome:**  Sturge-Weber syndrome (encephalotrigeminal angiomatosis) a 4-year-old boy. Of note was a unilateral nevus flammeus in the area of distribution of the maxillary branc of the trigeminal nerve. At 3 months of age, the child was operated on for glaucoma, due to choroid angie ma. To date, there have been no signs of central nervous system involvement (seizures, hemiparesis, i tracranial calcification, mental retardation).

Various oligosymptomatic forms occur (such as Milles's syndrome - facial nevus and choroid angioma In Fegeler's syndrome (post–traumatic nevus flammeus), unilateral nevus flammeus (in a trigeminal distr bution), swelling of the forehead and cheek, hyperasthesia of the affected area of the face, and ipsilater paresis of the extremities occur following trauma. In Bonnet-Dechaume-Blanc syndrome (neuroretinoangie matosis), unilateral angiomas of the retina and unilateral cerebral arteriovenous malformations may occu In Van Bogaert-Divry syndrome (corticomeningeal diffuse angiomatosis), pigmentation disorders, net-li telangiectasis, retinal angiomas, and severe central nervous system defects occur. Maffucci's syndrome characterized by multiple capillary or cavernous angiomas of the skin and internal organs, along with mul ple endochondromas and asymmetric dyschondroplasia of the bones of the extremities.

**Figure 425  Sturge-Weber Syndrome:**  Sturge-Weber syndrome in a 14-year-old boy. Of note was a n vus flammeus involving the left half of the face (stopping at the midline), the back, and the left buttoc Choroid angioma was also noted, but did not cause glaucoma. The child had serious central nervous syste involvement causing severe mental retardation and intercranial vascular calcification (in the leptomeninge of the parietooccipital area ipsilateral to the nevus flammeus). No hemiparesis was noted. Seizures, whic had been noted since the age of 3 months, were controlled with anticonvulsant medication. The facial nev faded as the child grew older.

**Figure 426  Klippel-Trenaunay-Weber Syndrome:**  Klippel-Trenaunay-Weber syndrome in a 10-year-ol boy. Findings included macrosomia of the entire left arm, enlargement of the third, fourth, and fifth fingers and ipsilateral nevus flammeus on the volar side of the hand, upper arm, and shoulder. The surface temper ature of the left arm was elevated. A vascular bruit could be appreciated over the involved areas. No othe deformities were noted. Due to multiple arteriovenous fistulas, high output cardiac failure occurred (requir ing treatment with cardiac glycosides). For differential diagnosis of macrosomia, see p 34 and 52.

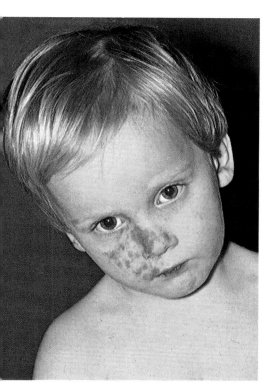

424

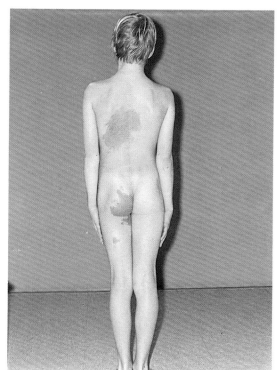

425

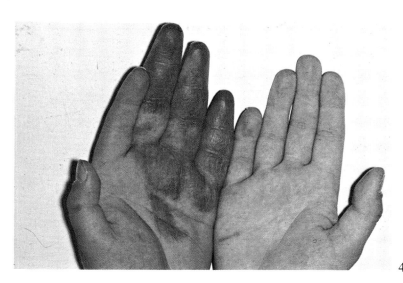

426

**Figure 427  Lymphangioma:**  Lymphangioma in a 6-day-old newborn. The findings included swellin of the cheek, without pain or erythema. The swelling was soft, diffuse, and easily impressible. At the tim of operation, this was diagnosed as a localized lymphangioma.

Localized lymphangiomas occur most frequently in the axilla, neck, upper arm, and perineum. Lymp angiomas may occur on the tongue, resulting in macroglossia, or the lips, resulting in macrocheilia. The can grow into the mediastinum and compress the trachea. Cystic lymphangiomas (cystic hygroma) can be come so large as to present difficulties at birth. They should be surgically resected as soon as possibl since spontaneous regression cannot be expected. Recurrence after complete removal is rare. At times, lymp angiomas can be difficult to differentiate from deeply located hemangiomas.

### Reference

1.  Saijo M, et al. Lymphangioma. A long-term follow-up study. Plast Reconstr Surg 56:642, 1975.

**Figure 428  Dermoid Cyst:**  Congenital dermoid cyst in a 6-week-old infant. Of note was a cherry-size smooth, round, pedunculated tumor growing from the right nostril. The cyst originated from the nasal septur The cyst was surgically removed. Histological findings confirmed the diagnosis of congenital dermoid cy (see p 22).

Dermoid cysts lie in or near the midline, and may be located in the area of the nose. Dermoid cys involving the nose may recur.

**Figure 429  Cavernous Hemangioma:**  Superficial cavernous hemangioma (strawberry nevus) in a 1-yea old child. Of note was a sharply outlined, cystic, compressible, blue-red mass on the nose. The surfac of the lesion was uneven. The growth had been present since birth, but had recently begun to increase size. The mass did not obstruct nasal breathing. No therapeutic intervention was attempted since spontane ous regression frequently occurs. Prednisone therapy can prevent further growth or cause involution of th mass.

**Figure 430  Cavernous Hemangioma:**  Deep cavernous hemangioma in a 4-month-old girl. Findings in cluded extensive swelling in the area of the hard and soft palate, extending to the right orbit. After 1 yea there was gradual regression without specific therapy.

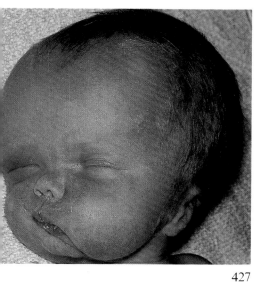

427

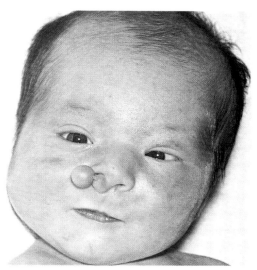

428

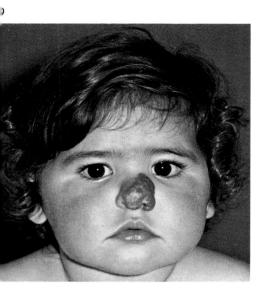

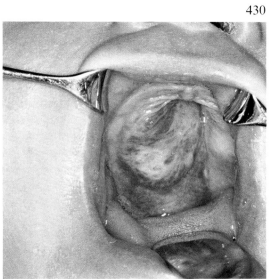

# 10. Pediatric Oncology

**Figure 431  Lipoma:**  Giant lipoma on the back of a 4-year-old boy. The findings included a soft, superficial swelling in the subcutaneous tissue above both shoulder blades and on the right side of the chest, extending down to the pelvic brim. At first, these findings were thought to be due to a lymphangioma. At the time of operation, an extensive subcutaneous lipoma was demonstrated. The lesion was removed with no recurrence.

**Figure 432  Lymphangioma:**  Lymphangioma on the right shoulder of a 2-year-old boy. This soft, fist-sized swelling was not clearly differentiated from the surrounding tissue. The mass had been present since birth and was noted to be growing during the past year. The mass caused no restriction of movement. The therapy of choice was surgical excision, which was technically difficult due to infiltration of the lymphangioma.

Simple localized lymphangioma can be differentiated from the more deeply embedded cavernous lymphangioma (see p 226). Special forms of lymphangioma include cystic hygroma (see p 230) and lymphangio hemangioma (which has vascular and lymphatic tissue). Cavernous lymphangioma and cystic hygroma are the most frequent. When localized to the mouth, pharynx, or mediastinum, lymphangioma can cause airway obstruction.

**Figure 433  Myositis Ossificans Progressiva:**  Myositis ossificans progressiva in a 6-year-old boy. Numerous, subcutaneous, bone-hard nodes were noted in the paravertebral and scapular area of the back. Involvement of the back and axilla led to restriction of movement of the right shoulder. Characteristic calcification was detected radiographically in the area of the axilla, neck, and lumbar spinal column. The condition began during the previous year, with localized painful swelling of the soft tissue of the back. After a short time these swellings turned to extensive, hard indurations. As the disease progressed, continued calcification of muscles occurred (including torticollis due to calcification of the sternocleidomastoid muscle).

**Figure 434  Myositis Ossificans Progressiva:**  Myositis ossificans progressiva in a 6-year-old boy (previously pictured in Figure 433). Myositis ossificans progressiva (progressive ossification of muscles) is frequently associated with other congenital abnormalities. The associated findings included lateral deviation of the big toe, with prominence of the first metatarsal phalangeal joint (hallux valgus). Deformities of the big toe or the thumb (brachydactyly) are frequent osseous malformations in myositis ossificans progressiva. Other anomalies include polydactyly, syndactyly, and hypodontia.

The child was followed for 7 years. During this time, there was progressive dysplasia of the connective tissue, leading to progressive ossification and restriction of movement of both the arms and the back.

**Differential Diagnosis:**  Differential diagnosis for myositis ossificans progressiva includes:
1. Localized myositis ossificans circumscripta (seen in areas of trauma).
2. Calcinosis circumscripta or universalis (see p 138).
3. Lipoid calcinosis (cholesterol accumulation, calcium deposition, and granuloma formation in the muscles).
4. Progressive scleroderma (localized or widespread calcification of soft tissue).
5. Dermatomyositis or chronic polymyositis (Wagner-Unverricht syndrome).

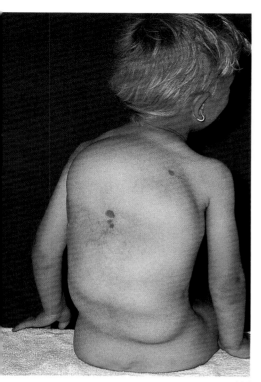

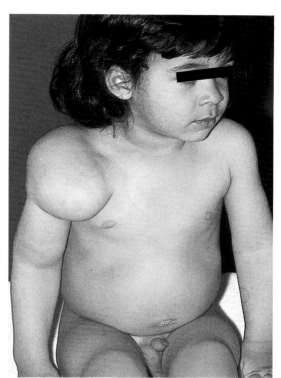

431

432

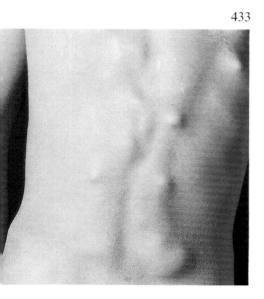

433

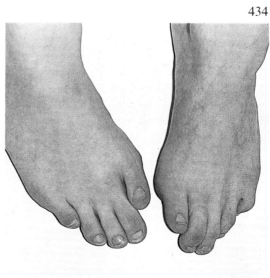

434

# 10. Pediatric Oncology

**Figure 435 Cystic Hygroma:** Cystic hygroma in a 2-month-old boy. Of note was a well defined, firm nonpainful, apple-sized swelling present since birth. At first, the mass did not appear to grow. When the operation was performed a multicystic mass with thin, transparent walls (containing amber-yellow fluid) was found. Complete removal was successful with no recurrence.

Cystic lymphangiomas can be located in the axilla, the popliteal space, the groin, or the retroperitoneum.

**Differential Diagnosis:** Cystic lymphangioma must be distinguished from cavernous and simple lymph angioma (p 226). When located in the neck, lymphangioma must be distinguished from thyroglossal duct cyst, cervical cysts, dermoid cysts, lipoma, malignant lymphoma, and tuberculous lymphadenitis.

**Figure 436 Tuberculous Lymphadenitis:** Tuberculous lymphadenitis in a 4-year-old boy. Findings included chronic cervical lymphadenitis of the left side of the neck. These lymph nodes spontaneously drained to the skin, leading to fistulous openings. Scars are noted in the submandibular area, from previous operation to remove the caseous and necrotic nodes. Lymphadenitis was caused by *Mycobacterium tuberculosis*. The primary site of involvement was probably the tonsils. Therapy included tonsillectomy, lymph node excision, and antituberculous therapy. Indolent lymphadenitis of the neck can have other causes including other acid fast bacteria (scrofula), toxoplasmosis, leukemia, and lymphoma. For other causes of neck masses see p 232.

**Figure 437 Malignant nonHodgkin's Lymphoma:** Malignant nonHodgkin's lymphoma in a 15-year old girl. Findings included numerous cherry-sized lymph nodes on both sides of the neck, particularly in the supraclavicular region. The girl also complained of fever and weakness. Biopsy of the involved lymph nodes revealed a lymphoblastic lymphoma of the convoluted cell type (T-lymphocytes). Chest radiograph detected a mediastinal mass, which caused difficulty breathing.

NonHodgkin's lymphoma of the convoluted cell type originates from the thymus and often involves the cervical lymph nodes and mediastinum. T cell lymphoblastic lymphoma may be part of a spectrum which includes T cell acute lymphocytic leukemia. In general, T cell lymphoblastic lymphoma has a worse prognosis than other malignant lymphomas.

**Differential Diagnosis:** T-cell lymphoblastic lymphoma must be differentiated from other nonHodgkin's lymphoma including undifferentiated lymphoblastic lymphoma of the Burkitt type, large cell or histiocytic lymphoma, as well as Hodgkin's lymphoma and leukemia (particularly lymphocytic leukemia).

## Reference

1. Link MP. NonHodgkin's lymphoma in children. Pediatr Clin North Am 32:699, 1985.

**Figure 438 Perimandibular Abscess:** Perimandibular abscess in a 12-year-old boy. Findings include a diffuse, fluctuant, erythematous, painful swelling in the left submandibular region. The onset of the mass was sudden. Incision and drainage revealed a purulent exudate which cultured both aerobic and anerobic organisms. The abscess was caused by an inflamed tooth, which was removed.

**Figure 439 Chronic Cervical Lymphadenitis:** Chronic cervical lymphadenitis caused by atypical myco bacteria (scrofula) in a 4-year-old girl. An egg-sized swelling of the lymph nodes and erythema of the over lying skin was noted in the submental region. Also noted was a nonpainful, movable, enlarged, preauricular lymph node. The involved lymph nodes later became fluctuant and formed fistulous tracts. Complete excision led to healing. Histologic examination of the removed nodes demonstrated granuloma formation and caseous necrosis. Culture demonstrated myobacteria resistant to several antituberculous drugs (INH, rifampin, PAS, streptomycin). Although this was an infection with an atypical mycobacteria, skin testing with old tuberculin proved positive (cross reaction).

## Reference

1. Saitz EW. Cervical lymphadenitis caused by atypical mycobacteria. Pediatr Clin North Am 28:823, 1981.

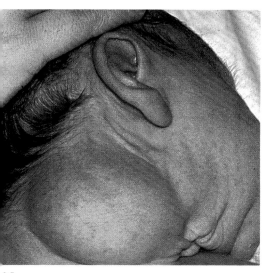

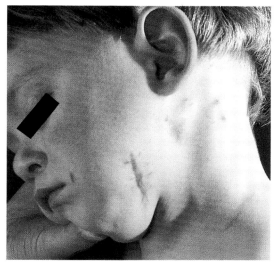

435

436

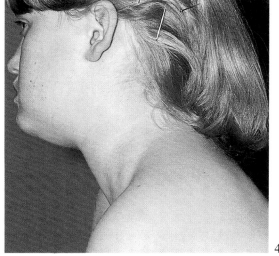

437

438

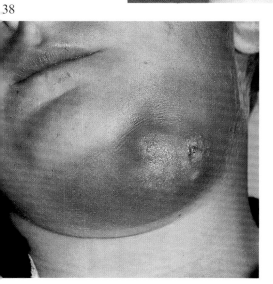

439

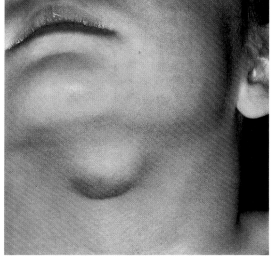

# 10. Pediatric Oncology

**Figure 440 Cavernous Hemangioma:** Deep cavernous hemangioma of the skin in a 4-day-old newborn Findings included a mandarin orange-sized, soft, movable, nonpulsatile mass of the right forehead. Radio graphic examination of the skull demonstrated that there was no bony defect (ruling out encephalocele, crania meningocele). Histologic examination of the mass revealed that this was a large cavernous hemangioma and not a malignant lesion.

**Differential Diagnosis:** Differential diagnosis includes encephalocele and meningocele, as well as othe vascular tumors, such as angiosarcoma and hemangioendothelioma.

**Figure 441 Teratoma:** Benign teratoma on the neck of a 3-month-old boy. The mass was a fist-sized sharply outlined swelling on the anterior aspect of the neck, which was present since birth. After surgica resection, examination revealed that this was a benign teratoma. During pregnancy, maternal serum alph fetoprotein was not elevated (elevated AFP is seen in two-thirds of all malignant teratomas). Radiographi examination detected calcium shadows, which corresponded to rudimentary teeth formed in the tumor

Teratomas usually occur in the midline. During the first year of life, teratomas are frequently locate in the sacrococcygeum. In early childhood, teratomas may be seen in the testicles; by school age, they ar frequently found in the ovaries. In addition, teratomas may occur in the anterior mediastinum, th retroperitoneum, the cranium (see p 100), and the neck. Other locations are rare.

## Reference

1. Ein SH, et al. Benign sacrococcygeal teratomas in infants and children: a 25 year review. Ann Surg 191:382, 1980

**Figures 442 and 443 Sacrococcygeal Teratoma:** Sacrococcygeal teratoma before resection on the fourt day of life (Figure 442), and after surgical removal on the twentieth day of life (Figure 443). The tumo was originally presumed to be benign. Surgical removal of the teratoma was accomplished without havin to remove the coccyx. After 1 month, urinary retention was noted. Radiographic examination revealed tumor in the pelvis, which compressed both ureters. A second operation was performed to remove a presacr malignant teratoma, of uncertain relation to the original lesion. After removal of the tumor, the child wa treated with both radiation and chemotherapy. The child has been free of any recurrence.

Sacrococcygeal teratoma may be either benign or malignant. The incidence of malignancy is dependen upon the patient's age. Before the fourth month of life, the malignancy rate is 6 percent; between the fourt month and the fifth year, the malignancy rate is 50 percent. Sacrococcygeal teratoma must be differentiate from other tumors of the sacrococcygeal region, such as lipoma, neuroblastoma, other neurogenic tumors cystic lymphangioma, and hemangioma. Meningocele or meningomylocele may frequently occur in th sacrococcygeal area, but can frequently be distinguished on physical examination.

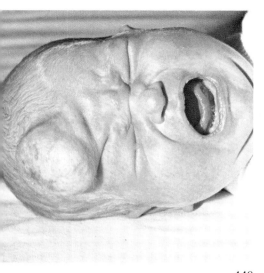

440

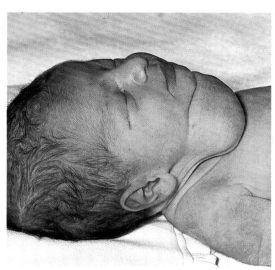

441

442

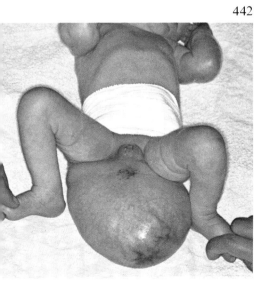

443

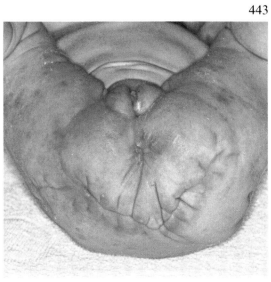

**Figure 444 Tuberous Sclerosis:** Tuberous sclerosis in a 3½-year-old girl. Pictured are multiple, hyp
pigmented macules on the upper arm. In addition, adenoma sebaceum was noted on the face and shagre
patches were noted on the leg. Computerized tomography demonstrated tumor-like nodes in the cereb
cortex along the left lateral ventricle. The course was further complicated by seizures, which began a
months of age.

There are many cutaneous changes associated with tuberous sclerosis. Hypopigmented macules (elonga
white spots 1 to 3 cm long) are easily recognized in a Wood's lamp, and are principally located on t
torso and limbs. Hypopigmented macules are an unreliable indicator for tuberous sclerosis. Cafe-au-l
spots may also occur; however, they are not as numerous as those seen in neurofibromatosis. The m
frequent skin findings in tuberous sclerosis are adenoma sebaceum (small red-brown nodules on the fac
and shagreen patches (raised indurated skin lesions).

**Figure 445 Vitiligo:** Vitiligo in a 3-week-old infant. Of note were numerous, irregular, sharply outline
depigmented macules over the back. The borders of the lesions are noted to be hyperpigmented. In t
case, the skin lesions were an incidental finding during an admission to the hospital for bronchopneumon

Vitiligo is an acquired defect in pigmentation. The cause is unknown. Hereditary factors or an autoimmu
response may play a role. The affected skin is lacking in pigment and melanocytes. Therapy is usually u
satisfactory. In black individuals, treatment with methoxypsoralen and exposure to light may be helpf
For differential diagnosis, see p 192.

**Figure 446 Tuberous Sclerosis:** Tuberous sclerosis in a 14½-year-old boy. Pictured is a periungual fibror
with resulting nail dysplasia. Periungual fibromas may not develop until puberty. They are smooth, fir
flesh colored, 5 to 10 mm large lesions. In addition to the periungual fibromas, other findings of tubero
sclerosis were present (hypopigmented macules, seizure disorder, mental retardation).

**Figure 447 Tuberous Sclerosis:** Tuberous sclerosis in a 10-year-old girl. Shagreen patches were not
over the lower back. These lesions were irregularly outlined, yellow, indurated areas of skin, with a textu
resembling that of an orange peel. The finding of shagreen patches allowed for early diagnosis of tubero
sclerosis.

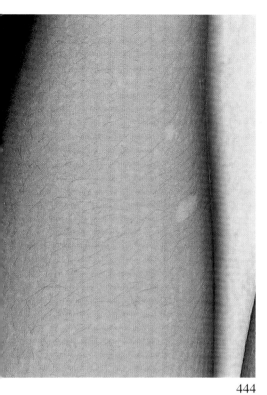

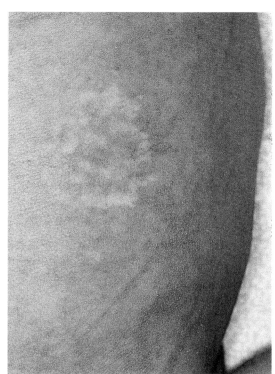

444

445

446

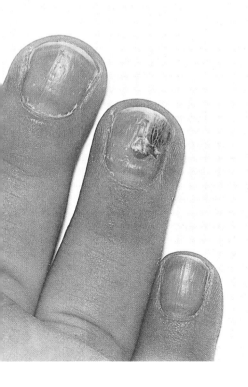

447

# 10.  Pediatric Oncology

**Figures 448 and 449  Neurofibromatosis:**  Neurofibromatosis (von Recklinghausen's disease) in a 13-year old girl. Findings included numerous cafe-au-lait spots on the torso, and cutaneous neurofibromas on the legs. These findings were first noted at approximately 11 months of age. Subcutaneous fibromas were noted along the larger peripheral nerves. In addition, there was enlargement of the right leg, due to extensive growth of neurofibromas (plexiform neuroma).

Cafe-au-lait spots are seen in 90 percent of patients with neurofibromatosis. These skin lesions are caused by hyperpigmentation of the basal epidermal cells. They develop within the first years of life. Since cafe-au-lait spots may occur in healthy children, they are considered diagnostically important only when more than six spots greater than 1.5 cm in diameter are noted. Cafe-au-lait spots may also be seen in cases of tuberous sclerosis (see p 234).

Cutaneous neurofibromas are soft, red nodes, that can attain considerable size. These nodes are sessile at first, but later the nodes become pedunculated. They are often present in great numbers. Oral mucous membranes are affected in 5 to 10 percent of the cases. These lesions may also involve the palate, the tongue, and the lips.

### Reference

1.  Burwell RG, et al. Cafe-au-lait spots in school children. Arch Dis Child 57:631, 1982.

**Figure 450  Neurofibromatosis:**  Neurofibromatosis (von Recklinghausen's disease) in a 4-year-old boy. Of note was a cherry-sized, subcutaneous fibroma of the right thigh. In addition, there were numerous cafe-au-lait spots on the body, and multiple subcutaneous nodules (arranged like a string of pearls) on the neck. The disease is inherited in an autosomal dominant fashion. In this family, both the mother and sister had neurofibromatosis.

**Figure 451  Neurofibromatosis:**  Neurofibromatosis (von Recklinghausen's disease) in a 15-year-old girl. Of note was a giant, infiltrative, brown, pigmented tumor (plexiform neuroma) on the chest and left upper arm. In addition, many cutaneous neurofibromas were noted on the torso and several cafe-au-lait spots were seen on the extremities. Histologic examination of the neuroma revealed abundant loose connective tissue with Schwann's cells and mast cells (confirming the clinical diagnosis).

Sarcomatous degeneration of neurofibromas may occur as the disease progresses (in approximately percent of patients). In addition, pheochromocytomas and optic gliomas may be observed.

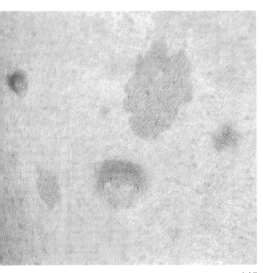

448

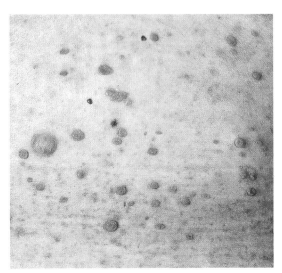

449

450

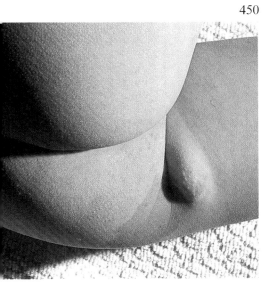

451

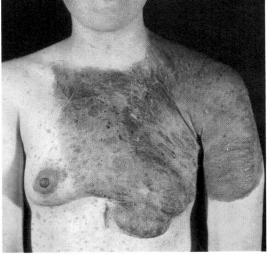

# 10. Pediatric Oncology

**Figure 452  Mucocele:**   Mucocele (mucous cyst) on the gum of a 4-week-old girl. Of note was a solitary cherry-sized, cystic protuberance of the mucous membrane, which was filled with a clear fluid. These cyst are believed to occur after traumatic rupture of a salivary duct. Treatment involves surgical excision. Reten tion cysts of the salivary glands are called mucoceles; retention cysts of the sublingual glands are calle ranula (because of the similarity to the inflated bladder of a frog's throat).

**Differential Diagnosis:**   Differential diagnosis of cysts located on the gums includes dentigerous cysts dysontogenetic cysts, epulis (see below), central glial cell growth, and "chocolate cysts" (juvenile bone cysts)

**Figure 453  Ranula:**   Ranula in a 2-week-old girl. Two bean-sized, well defined, taut, blue, mucous reten tion cysts were noted on the floor of the mouth under the tongue. These were connected with the duct of the submaxillary salivary glands. Therapy consists of surgical removal. Ranula can displace the tongue rupture easily, and lead to secondary bacterial infection.

**Differential Diagnosis:**   Differential diagnosis includes epidermoid cysts in the floor of the mouth.

**Figure 454  Epulis:**   Epulis in a 4-day-old girl. Of note was a plum-sized, pedunculated tumor, of firm consistency, originating from the gums. Recurrence after resection is possible. The cause of congenital epuli is unclear and probably not consistent.

**Figure 455  Epulis:**   Epulis in a 2-day-old newborn. Of note was an apple-sized tumor with a nodula surface. The mass was connected to the lower ridge of teeth by a pencil thick peduncle and protruded from the mouth. Surgical removal was accomplished on the same day. The diagnosis of epulis was confirme by histological examination. There was no recurrence after surgical resection.

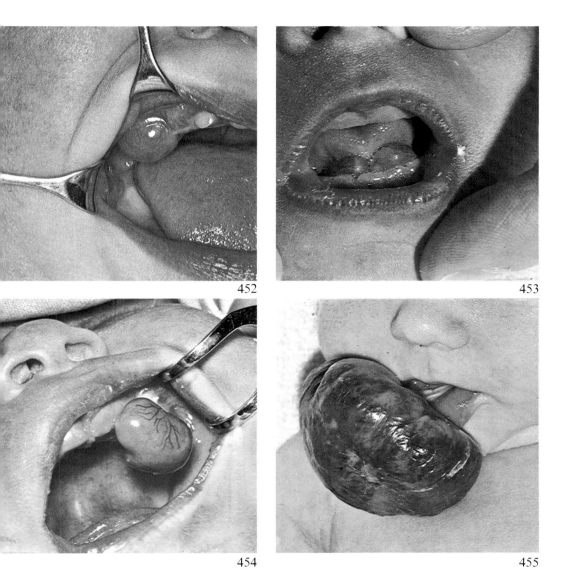

452

453

454

455

**Figure 456   Neurofibrosarcoma:**   Neurofibrosarcoma in a 15-year-old girl who had symptoms of neur
fibromatosis (von Recklinghausen's disease). The tumor had infiltrated the underlying tissue of the nerv
thereby causing the right side of the neck to be diffusely swollen. Surgical operation achieved only part
resection. Histologic examination of the tissue demonstrated that this was a neurofibrosarcoma. In cas
of neurofibrosarcoma, one must consider sarcomatous degeneration (when the nodes enlarge rapidly,
when there is pain and ulceration).

**Figure 457   Mucoepidermoid Carcinoma:**   Mucoepidermoid carcinoma of the parotid gland in a 16-yea
old boy. A nontender mass, which was difficult to distinguish from the surrounding area, was noted in t
area of the left parotid gland. Regional lymph nodes were not swollen. The tumor was completely remove
Relapse or metastasis did not occur. Histologically, mucoepidermoid tumors can be separated into w
differentiated and undifferentiated forms. Mucoepidermoid tumors can be locally invasive, but only rare
metastasize.

**Differential Diagnosis:**   Unilateral, persistent swelling in the parotid area can be caused by other parot
tumors, particularly mixed parotid tumors (pleomorphic adenomas), as well as hemangiomas and lympha
giomas. Parotid swelling can also be caused by obstruction of the duct by salivary calculus. In these case
a calcium shadow can be detected radiographically. Recurrent parotitis can be unilateral or bilateral, a
is not associated with pain. The cause of this condition is unknown; recurrent parotitis resolves after seve
al episodes without specific treatment.

**Figure 458   Parotitis:**   Parotitis (mumps) in a 15-year-old girl. Of note was painful, nonerythematou
swelling of the parotid glands. The patient complained of pain when chewing and dryness of the mout
Serum and urine amylase levels were elevated (without evidence of pancreatitis). CF antibodies were pos
tive during the second week of illness.

**Differential Diagnosis:**   Differential diagnosis for parotid swelling includes:
1.   Cervical lymphadenitis with preauricular involvement (differentiated by physical examination).
2.   Suppurative parotitis (painful, erythematous swelling of the parotid gland. Pressure on the parotid glar
     causes pus to be expressed through the duct).
3.   Recurrent parotitis (mildly painful swelling which resolves spontaneously. The etiology is possibl
     an allergic manifestation).
4.   Salivary calculus (intermittent swelling of the glands due to obstruction. Calcium can be detected radi
     graphically)
5.   Parotid tumors (unilateral chronic swelling caused by hemangiomas, lymphomas, mixed tumors).
6.   Mikulicz's disease (seen in leukemia, tuberculosis).

**Figure 459   Mastoiditis:**   Mastoiditis in a 6-year-old boy. The right ear was displaced anteriorly and i
feriorly. The area behind the ear was painful and swollen. The child originally had acute otitis media, whic
went untreated, leading to perforation of the tympanic membrane and mastoiditis. Cultures obtained fro
the periosteal abscess contain pneumococci. The child improved after systemic antibiotic therapy.

**Differential Diagnosis:**   Inflammation and swelling in the postauricular area can stem from lymphadenopath
secondary to superficial skin infection and otitis externa.

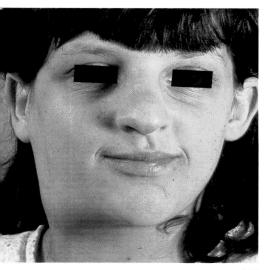

456

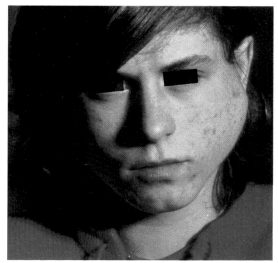

457

458

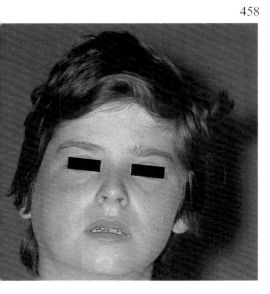

459

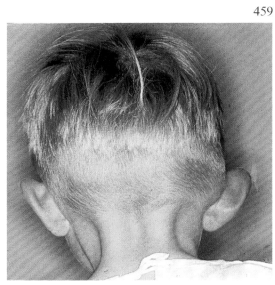

**Figure 460  Retinoblastoma:**  Retinoblastoma in a 2-year-old boy. The figure demonstrates the child after enucleation of the left eye. The first symptom of retinoblastoma was an acute increase in intraoccular pressure in the left eye. Extensive infiltration of tumor was noted in the soft tissue of the orbit, cheek, parotid gland, as well as the liver, lymph nodes, and vertebrae. The right eye was not affected. Despite surgical intervention, radiation, and chemotherapy, the child died 5 weeks later.

Although retinoblastoma can present at birth, retinoblastoma usually presents within the first or second years of life. This tumor of the posterior retina may involve one or both eyes. If the disease is bilateral, it is thought to follow an autosomal dominant pattern of inheritance. In cases of inherited retinoblastoma, other malignancies may also develop (osteogenic sarcoma).

**Differential Diagnosis:**  The differential diagnosis of childhood orbital tumors includes leukemia, teratoma, rhabdomyosarcoma, tumors of the optic nerve, malignant lymphoma, angioma, hemangioma, other vascular anomalies (arteriovenous malformation), neurofibromatosis, tubular sclerosis, histiocytosis X, oribital cysts, meningocele, and encephalocele. For discussion of pseudoglioma, see p 244.

**Figure 461  Neuroblastoma:**  Neuroblastoma in a 1-year-old child. Proptosis and ecchymosis of the orbit were due to retrobulbar metastases which involve the orbit, the sphenoid bone, and the maxillary sinus. The liver and numerous lymph nodes (in the neck and the groin) were greatly enlarged due to metastasis of the neuroblastoma. Radiologic studies demonstrated extensive metastases in the bones (especially in the long bones). On autopsy, the primary tumor was found in the right adrenal gland.

**Figure 462  Basilar Skull Fracture:**  Ecchymosis of the orbit due to basilar skull fracture in a 5-year-old boy. Bilateral ecchymoses were noted on the superior and inferior aspects of the orbits. Radiographic studies of the skull revealed basilar skull fracture. Orbital fractures, which can lead to ecchymoses of the orbit, were ruled out.

**Differential Diagnosis:**  Metastatic neuroblastoma may involve the orbit and produce unilateral or bilateral ecchymoses with proptosis. Other orbital tumors may have similar findings.

**Figure 463  Suspected Child Abuse:**  Multiple hematomas were noted on the face and body of this 3-year-old girl. There was no evidence of other bone fractures or subdural hematoma. Platelet count and coagulation studies were normal. The skin lesions could not be attributed to any disease process. Further history led to the diagnosis of suspected abuse and neglect. The child was released after investigation of the domestic situation by the social service agencies, with the diagnosis of suspected child abuse.

### Reference

1.  Bittner S, Newberger EH. Pediatric understanding of child abuse and neglect. Pediatr Rev 2:209, 1981.

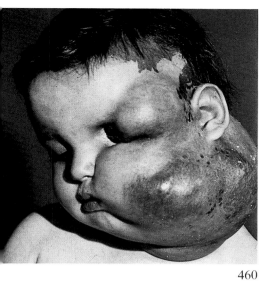

460

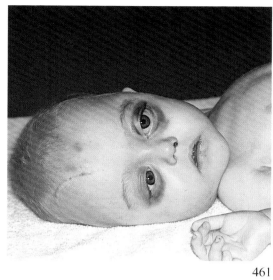

461

462

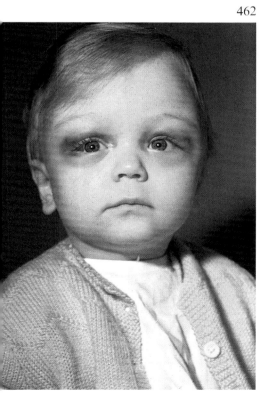

463

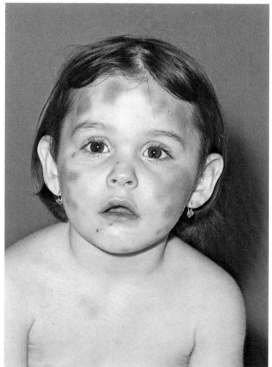

**Figure 464 Pseudoglioma (Pseudoretinoblastoma):** Pseudoglioma involving the left eye of a 2-year old child. Ophthalmologic examination revealed a circumscribed, white-yellow opacity that obliterated the red reflex. This condition stems from traumatic hemorrhage of the retina and vitreous body.

**Differential Diagnosis:** Similar opacification and loss of the red reflex may be seen in retinoblastoma, other intraocular tumors, retrolental fibroplasia, persistence of the primary vitreous body, organized purulent exudate of the vitreous body, and vascularization of the vitreous body after severe fetal uveitis. Leukocoria (white pupil) may be caused by cataracts, detached retina, and severe chorioretinal degeneration. (Photograph courtesy of University of Kiel Eye Clinic)

**Figure 465 Cavernous Hemangioma:** Deep cavernous hemangioma of the right inferior eyelid in a 6-month-old girl. Of note was an extensive, poorly defined, soft swelling of the entire inferior eyelid with blue-purple discoloration of the skin.

**Differential Diagnosis:** Differential diagnosis includes lymphangioma, lipoma of the eyelid, and dermoid cysts involving the eyelid. (Photograph courtesy of University of Kiel Eye Clinic)

**Figure 466 Dermoid Cyst:** Congenital dermoid cyst of the right superior eyelid of a 14-year-old girl. Findings included a bean-sized, poorly defined, soft swelling of the lateral corner of the eye below the brow. Histology revealed a cyst lined by keratinized squamous epithelial cells containing hair follicles and sebaceous glands. These findings confirmed the diagnosis of dermoid cyst.

**Differential Diagnosis:** Differential diagnosis includes epidermal cysts, lipoma, lymphangioma, and hemangioma. (Photograph courtesy of University of Kiel Eye Clinic)

**Figure 467 Glaucoma:** Congenital glaucoma in a 3-week-old girl. Findings included bilateral enlargement of the orbits (buphthalmos) with increased intraocular pressure, corneal opacity, and abnormal angle of the anterior chamber. In this case, optic nerve damage secondary to glaucoma had not occurred. The parent noted sensitivity to light (photophobia) and excessive tearing (epiphoria). On ophthalmologic examination a developmental anomaly of the angle of the anterior chamber was noted. Immediate surgical correction was undertaken.

Congenital and infantile glaucoma may be associated with other ocular anomalies (aniridia, spherophakia, mesodermal dysgenesis of the cornea), neurofibromatosis, Sturge-Weber syndrome, and Lowe's syndrome (oculocerebrorenal syndrome).

### Reference

1. Chew E, Morin JD. Glaucoma in children. Pediatr Clin North Am. 30:1043, 1983.

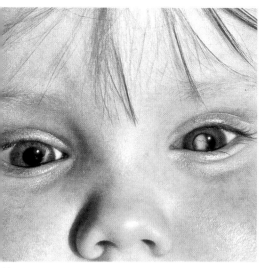

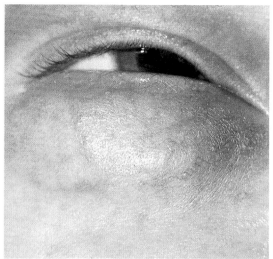

465

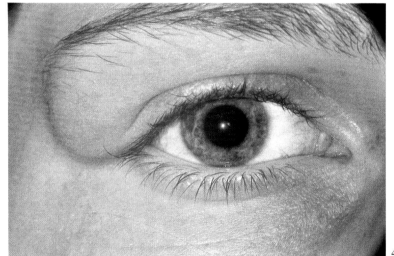

466

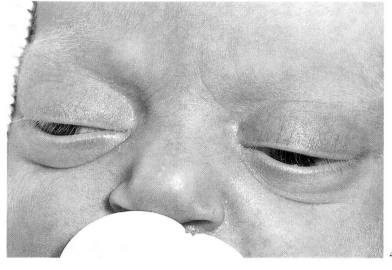

467

# 11. Diseases of the Eye

**Figure 468  Anophthalmia:**  Anophthalmia and blepharophimosis (abnormal narrowing of palpebral fissures) in a 6-week-old child. The boy developed microcephaly, mental retardation, and seizures. Examination of the eyes beyond the narrow eyelid fissures revealed only connective tissue; rudimentary orbits were not present. Later, the child was provided with ocular prostheses. No specific cause was found.

In cases of anophthalmia, the orbits are usually small, and the lids are closed and concave. Anophthalmia may occur as an isolated malformation or associated with trisomy 13 (Patau's syndrome, see p 58).

**Figure 469  Fetal Rubella Syndrome:**  Bilateral cataracts and glaucoma (as well as keratoconjunctivitis due to *Pseudomonas*) in a 5-week-old boy with fetal rubella syndrome. The infant's mother had contracted rubella during the second trimester of pregnancy. The child had many of the stigmata of fetal rubella syndrome. Shortly after birth, the child was noted to have clinical findings of patent ductus arteriosus (loud continuous murmur) and congestive heart failure. Typical radiographic changes were noted in the long bones (radiograph of the proximal tibia revealed linear radiolucencies alternating with increased density). Rubella specific immunoglobulin M was noted in the child's and mother's serum. At 6 weeks of age, the child underwent surgical ligation of the ductus arteriosus. Surgery to remove the cataract was performed at 13 months of age without complication.

In cases of fetal rubella syndrome, cataract may develop in up to 50 percent of the patients. Various forms of cataract are possible within the spectrum of fetal rubella syndrome. Other anomalies of the eye related to fetal rubella syndrome include microphthalmia, corneal opacity, strabismus, and nystagmus. Glaucoma is also associated with fetal rubella syndrome. Other prenatal infections which may cause cataract include cytomegalovirus and toxoplasmosis. For differential diagnosis of congenital cataracts, see p 152; of congenital glaucoma, see p 244 and 254.

**Figure 470  Congenital Amaurosis:**  Bilateral congenital amaurosis in an 8-month-old girl. No other symptoms were noted. Findings included pupils which were glassy when exposed to light and amaurotic nystagmus. The child was noted to rub her eyes frequently (oculodigital phenomenon). The cause of amaurosis was unclear in this case. There is no family history of partial or total visual loss.

Frequent causes of congenital blindness include microphthalmia, corneal opacification, dense lenticular opacification, atrophic chorioretinal scarring, macular colobomata, and severe hypoplasia of the optic nerve. In cases of the recessively inherited Leber's congenital retinal amaurosis, retinal degeneration may not develop until later in life (despite persistent blindness). Early diagnosis of this condition is possible with electroretinography. Often there are EEG changes, microcephaly, and other anomalies of the central nervous system.

**Figure 471  Microphthalmia:**  Unilateral microphthalmia in a 3-week-old boy. The eyeball and orbit of the right side were noted to be diminished in size since birth. This was an isolated deformity, the cause of which is unknown. Microphthalmia is frequently a bilateral defect and is often combined with other ocular anomalies including hyperopia, spherophakia, microphakia, cataract, and colobomata of the iris and the choroid membrane. Malformation of the anterior chamber may lead to glaucoma. Microphthalmia may be seen in cases of intrauterine infection (rubella, toxoplasmosis, cytomegalovirus) and thalidomide embryopathy. Certain chromosomal malformation syndromes are associated with microphthalmia (trisomy 13, see p 58). Microphthalmia is observed in the following malformation syndromes:
1. Aicardi's syndrome (agenesis of the corpus collosum)
2. Cryptophthalmos's syndrome (lack of eyelids, orbits covered by skin)
3. Ectodermal syndromes (including Hallermann-Streiff syndrome, oculodentodigital syndrome)
4. Fanconi's pancytopenia syndrome
5. Meckel-Gruber syndrome (microcephaly, genitourinary abnormalities, polydactyly)
6. Sjögren-Larsson syndrome (ichthyosis, spastic paralysis, mental retardation).

In cases of Norrie's disease (an X-linked trait), there is congenital bilateral retinal malformation and blindness, which may later lead to shrinking and wasting of the eyeball (phthisis bulbi).

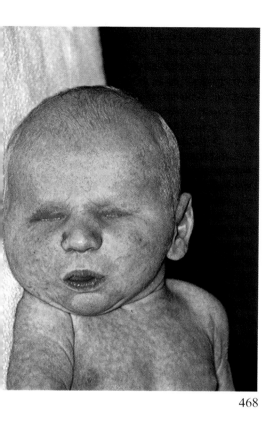

470

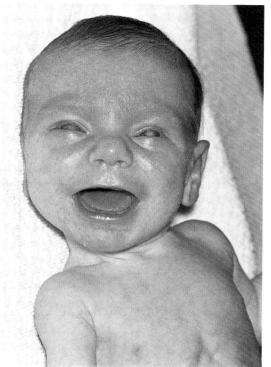

471

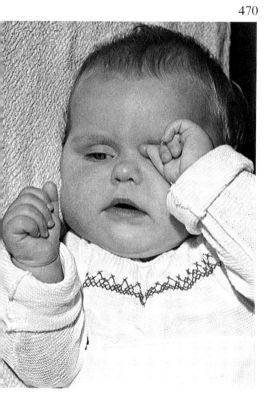

468

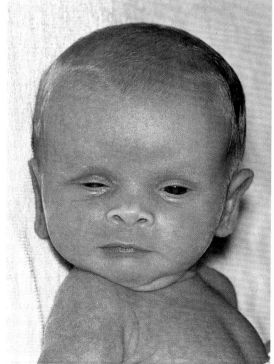

469

# 11.  Diseases of the Eye

**Figure 472  Residual Pupillary Membrane:**  Residual pupillary membrane in a 7-day-old boy. Of note were several delicate strands of tissue that extended from the iris to the capsule of the lens. Vision was not impaired.

Different grades of persistent pupillary membrane are possible. Small residual parts of the membrane are frequent in newborns. Larger residue, which may be detrimental to vision, are rare and may be combined with anterior cataracts. Residual pupillary membrane must be distinguished from posterior synechiae, which stem from an inflammatory process in the anterior section of the eye. (Photograph courtesy of University of Kiel Eye Clinic)

**Figure 473  Partial Aniridia:**  Bilateral, partial aniridia in a 7-year-old girl. The girl had poor vision and photophobia. The involved area (where the iris was absent) appeared black, like the pupil. Associated anomalies, such as glaucoma, cataract, and hypoplasia of the macula and optic nerve, were not present. Wilms' tumor, which may be associated with aniridia, was ruled out with an intravenous pyelogram. Therapy included the prescription of dark contact lenses.

Aniridia is usually bilateral and is never truly "complete." Isolated aniridia is an autosomal dominant trait with a frequency in the general population of 1:100,000. Sporadic aniridia is observed in conjunction with other anomalies (including microcephaly, renal and genital deformities, and hemihypertrophy). Neoplasms which may be associated with aniridia include Wilms' tumor, rhabdomyosarcoma, and adrenal tumors.

### Reference

1.  Shannon RS, et al. Wilms' tumor and aniridia: Clinical and cytogenetic features. Arch Dis Child 57:685, 1982.

**Figure 474  Ataxia Telangiectasia:**  Ataxia telangiectasia (Louis-Bar syndrome) in a 10-year-old girl. Symptoms, including ataxia, have been noted since the age of two years. Of note were prominent, snake-like telangiectasias of the conjunctiva, as well as telangiectasias of the superior and inferior eyelids, the pinna, and the left upper arm. In addition to truncal ataxia and ataxic gait, other extrapyramidal signs were noted (including nystagmus, dysarthria, and dementia). Serum IgA and IgE were decreased.

The differential diagnosis of conjunctival telangiectasias include nevus flammeus of the conjunctiva, Fabry's disease (deficiency of alpha galactosidase activity), lymphangiectasias of the conjunctiva, and conjunctivitis.

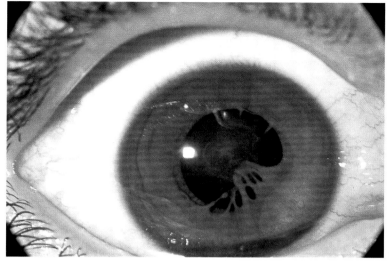

472

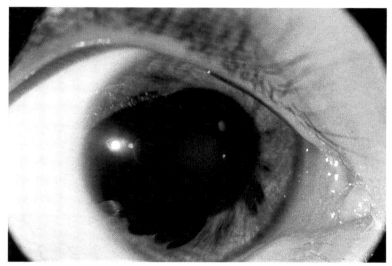

473

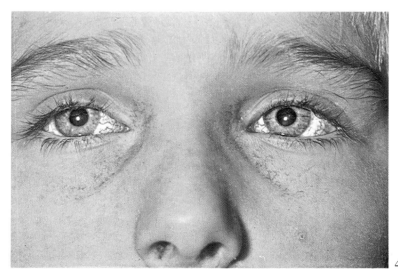

474

# 11.   Diseases of the Eye

**Figure 475   Pigment Spots of the Iris:**   Small, bilateral pigment spots of the iris in an 8-year-old bo
(without associated disease).

Pigment spots of the iris, due to an accumulation of melanocytes, occur in 50 to 60 percent of the popu
lation. Although present at birth, they become more noticeable during puberty.

**Figure 476   Conjunctival Nevus:**   Conjunctival nevus in a 12-year-old boy. Of note was a small, flat, yellow
nevus near the limbic area of the right eyelid. Pigmented nevi of the conjunctiva frequently occur. The
are usually small, slightly raised, bright yellow to brown-black colored lesions, which are first noted
early childhood and may increase in size and pigmentation during puberty. In addition to lying or the edg
of the limbus, they may also be found near the lachrimal duct or the edge of the eyelid. Malignant degener
tion is rare. (Photograph courtesy of University of Kiel Eye Clinic)

**Figure 477   Corectopia:**   Corectopia (abnormal position of the pupil) in a 6-year-old boy. This abnormali
of the pupil had been noted since birth.

Congenital corectopia may occur with dyscoria (abnormal shape of the pupil) or with discoloratio
of the lens. Acquired corectopia can occur with perforating eye injury or as a result of synechiae (inflammato
adhesions extending from the iris to the lens or the cornea).

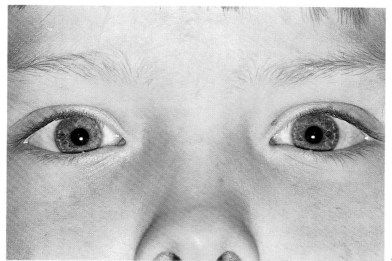

475

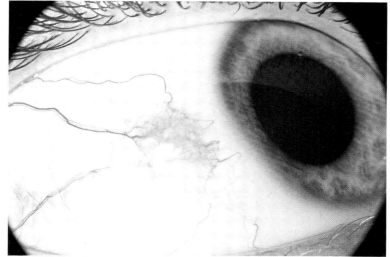

476

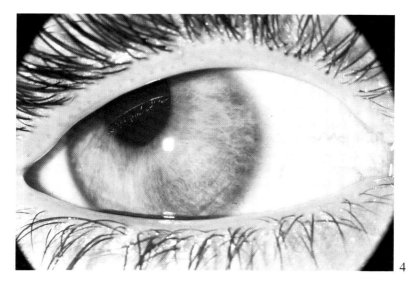

477

# 11. Diseases of the Eye

**Figure 478  Congenital Ectropion:**  Congenital ectropion (eversion of the eyelid) in a 10-month-old boy. Of note was extreme erythema of the conjunctiva of the inferior eyelid. Excessive tearing was also noted. Prolonged cases of ectropion allow for keratitis to develop. Congenital ectropion is due to poor development of the lateral canthal ligament. Other cases of ectropion may result from scar formation (after trauma, burns, or inflammation) or in conjunction with facial paralysis. Surgical correction is possible in cases of congenital ectropion.

**Figure 479  Blepharophimosis:**  Bilateral blepharophimosis (narrow palpebral fissures) in a 5-month-old boy. These findings were present since birth. Blepharophimosis is not only a congenital anomaly, but may also be an acquired disorder due to scar formation.

**Differential Diagnosis:**  Differential diagnosis includes blepharoptosis (congenital or acquired) and ankyloblepharon (fusion of the superior and inferior eyelids).

**Figures 480 and 481  Megalocornea:**  Megalocornea in a 3-month-old girl. The diameter of the cornea was 15 mm (normal range 10.5 to 12.5 mm). Intraocular pressure was not raised. This congenital, nonprogressive, enlargement of the cornea leads to refractive error. Megalocornea must be distinguished from progressive corneal enlargement due to congenital glaucoma. Glaucoma usually presents with photophobia, excessive tearing, and corneal opacity. Glaucoma requires immediate surgical treatment. Keratoconus (cone-shaped protuberance of the midcornea) or keratoglobus (ball-shaped protuberance of the cornea) usually are not seen until adolescence and can lead to visual problems.

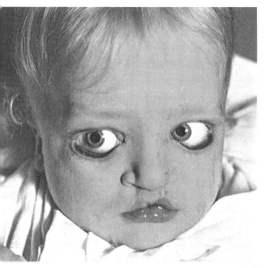

478

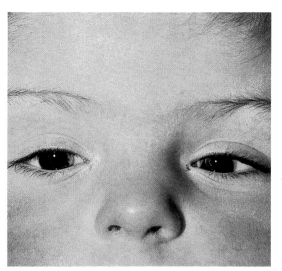

479

480

481

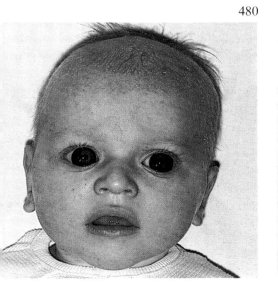

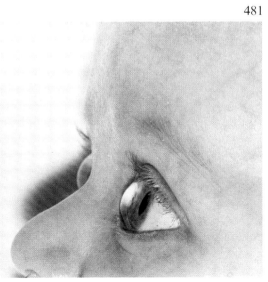

# 11. Diseases of the Eye

**Figure 482  Osteopetrosis Tarda:**  Osteopetrosis tarda (Albers-Schönberg syndrome) in a 3-month-old boy. Initial findings included bilateral exophthalmos, which was later followed by blindness and cranial nerve paralysis (due to compression of cranial foramina). The extent of the exophthalmos can be measured by an exophthalmometer. Progression of symptoms was rapid, as is seen in the autosomal recessive form of the disease.

**Differential Diagnosis:**  Bilateral exophthalmos may be due to neoplastic processes (tumors, histiocytosis X), vascular anomalies, and inflammatory processes. Exophthalmos may also be noted in hyperthyroidism and craniofacial malformations (craniosynostosis, Down syndrome).

**Figure 483  Buphthalmos:**  Unilateral enlargement of the eye (buphthalmos) secondary to glaucoma in a 7-day-old girl with Sturge-Weber syndrome (encephalotrigeminal angiomatosis). The left eye was reddened, larger, and firmer than the right eye. The wide pupil reacted only sluggishly to light. Fundoscopy revealed a cavernous hemangioma of the right choroid (ipsilateral to a nevus flammeus of the face). Surgical correction was undertaken to normalize the pressure of the eye. Glaucoma recurred, leading to iridocyclitis and eventual enucleation of the eye at 1 year of age. The child was provided with an ocular prosthesis.

   Glaucoma may lead to enlargement of the orbit during early childhood. Excessive tearing, photophobia, and blepharospasm are often the first symptoms of infantile glaucoma.

**Differential Diagnosis:**  Traumatic injury to the eye can often lead to acquired glaucoma. Other possible causes of glaucoma include megalocornea, aniridia, and other developmental disorders of the anterior chamber. Primary congenital glaucoma has an autosomal recessive pattern of inheritance and is the cause of early childhood blindness in 5 to 10 percent of the cases. (Photograph courtesy of University of Kiel Eye Clinic.)

**Figure 484  Osteogenesis Imperfecta:**  Osteogenesis imperfecta in a 3-month-old girl. Thinning of the sclera causes the uvea to become more apparent, giving the sclera a blue appearance (also seen in Marfan's syndrome and Ehlers-Danlos syndrome). Additional eye anomalies included corneal opacities, hyperopia, keratokonus, and megalocornea. Blue sclera may be normal in the first weeks of life, since the cornea is still relatively thin and transparent at this age. Confirmation of osteogenesis imperfecta is based on clinical findings (recurrent fractures, skeletal deformities) and radiologic studies of the bones.

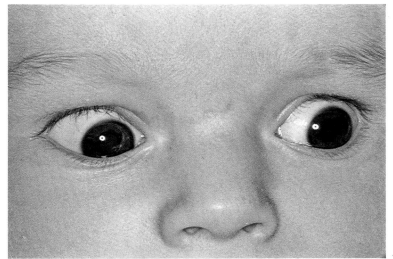

482

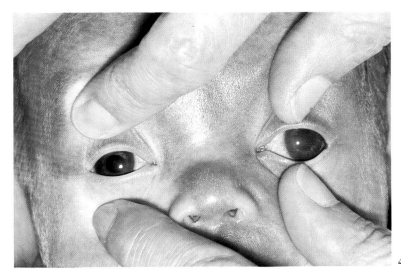

483

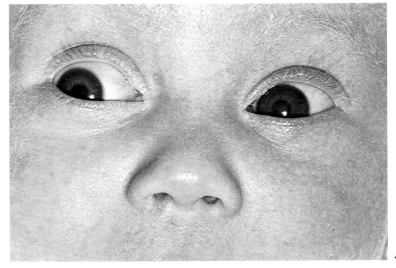

484

# 11. Diseases of the Eye

**Figure 485  Subconjunctival Hemorrhage:**  Subconjunctival hemorrhage in a 4-year-old boy with acute lymphocytic leukemia. Extensive bilateral hemorrhage was noted under the conjunctiva. In addition, vitreous hemorrhage and skin ecchymoses were noted. Laboratory investigation revealed a platelet count of less than 3,000 per cubic millimeter.

**Figure 486  Vitreous Hemorrhage:**  Resolving vitreous hemorrhage in a 16-year-old boy. Vitreous hemorrhage was the result of a perforating eye injury that led to visual impairment. Other causes of vitreous hemorrhage (which usually originates from retinal vessels) include blunt injuries to the retina, subarachnoid hemorrhage, retinal angioma, retrolental fibroblasia, retinopathy due to diabetes mellitus or hypertension, and other diseases which affect coagulation. Familial exudative vitreoretinopathy stems from a vascular anomaly of the peripheral retina, and may lead to repeated hemorrhage in the vitreous. (Photograph courtesy of the University of Kiel Eye Clinic)

**Figure 487  Cavernous Hemangioma:**  Deep cavernous hemangioma of the left superior eyelid in a 1-year-old boy. Of note was an extensive, poorly outlined, raised, blue-red hemangioma under the skin. The lesion was present since birth, but had recently grown larger. Movement of the eyelid and vision were limited because of the lesion. Differential diagnosis includes hemangioma, lymphangioma, lipoma, and dermoid cyst. (Photograph courtesy of the University of Kiel Eye Clinic)

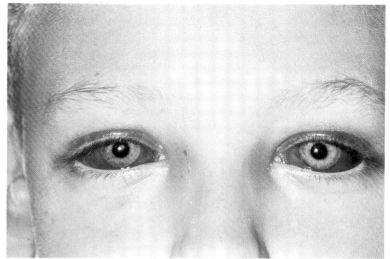

485

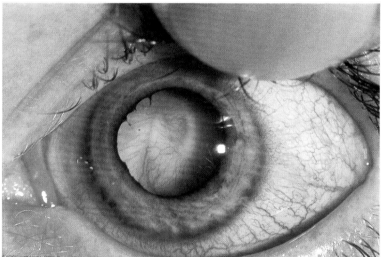

486

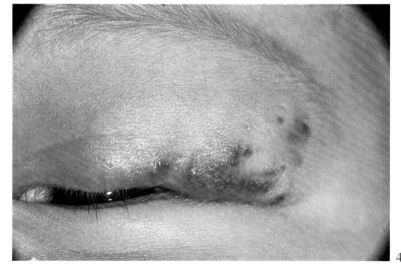

487

# 11. Diseases of the Eye

**Figure 488  Ophthalmia Neonatorum:**  Ophthalmia neonatorum (due to *Neisseria gonorrhea*) in a new born child. Of note was severe swelling of the eyelid and purulent drainage from the left eye. The corne was inflamed. The illness began on the second day of life. Transmission occurred during birth (in a mothe who was unaware of an intercurrent gonorrheal infection). The child developed opthalmia neonatorum despi prophylactic eye care with silver nitrate solution. Numerous gram-negative diplocci were found on Gra stain and in culture. The child was treated with intramuscular penicillin, gentamycin eyedrops, and compresse:

Conjunctivitis due to gonorrhea must be differentiated from other causes of purulent conjunctivitis i the newborn, including other infectious agents (staphylococci, *Pseudomonas, Haemophilus*). Conjunctiv tis can also be caused by the prophylactic eye treatment (chemical conjunctivitis). Inclusion blennorrhe of the newborn is caused by *Chlamydia* oculogenitalis. Inclusion blennorrhea does not begin until the fift to seventh day after birth, and can lead to week- or month-long purulent secretion. *Chlamydia* can be ide tified by culture. (Photograph courtesy of University of Kiel Eye Clinic)

**Figure 489  Orbital Cellulitis:**  Orbital cellulitis in a 12-year-old girl. Of note was redness and swellin of the left eyelid, proptosis, and limited movement of the eye. The child was febrile and the eye was extremel painful. In this case, orbital cellulitis was caused by an underlying ethmoid sinusitis (detected on sku radiograph). The child was treated with parenteral penicillin and gentamycin, with a rapid response to antibioti treatment. Causes of periorbital or orbital cellulitis may include purulent blepharitis, dacrocystitis, osteomye litis of the upper jaw, maxillary sinusitis, and hematogenous spread due to bacterial sepsis.

**Differential Diagnosis:**  Differential diagnosis includes cavernous sinus thrombosis, inflammation of th tear duct, and cellulitis of the eyelid.

**Figure 490  Orbital Cellulitis:**  Orbital cellulitis (due to osteomyelitis of the maxilla) in a 3-month-ol boy. Inflammation of the periorbital and intraorbital tissue was manifest by erythema and swelling of th eyelids, restricted movement of the eye, and systemic illness. In this case, antibiotic therapy and surgic drainage was required. Possible complications of orbital cellulitis include involvement of the optic nerve cavernous sinus thrombosis, meningitis, and subdural or cerebral abscess.

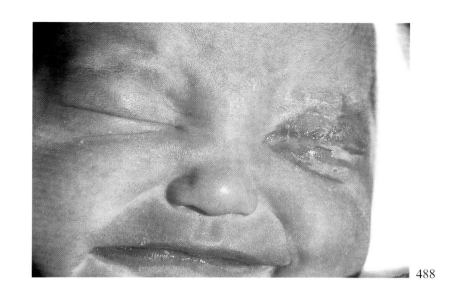

488

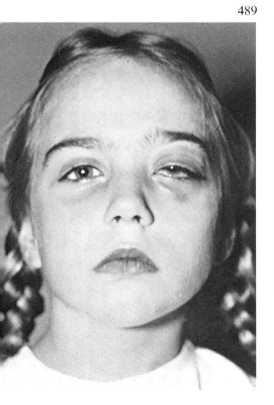

489

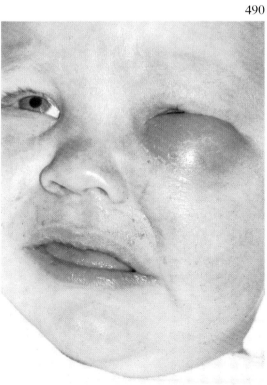

490

# 12.  Metabolic Diseases and Nutritional Disorders

**Figure 491  Obesity:**  Obesity in a 14-year-old girl. Large accumulations of adipose tissue were noted over the torso and extremities. Based on her height, the patient was 40 kg overweight. In a 6-week period (under hospital supervison), the patient lost 15 kg on a weight reduction diet. Menarche occurred at age 12; secondary sexual development was complete. Both parents were similarly obese. Pictured next to the obese girl, is a girl of the same age with normal height and weight.

**Differential Diagnosis:**  Obesity may be seen in conjunction with Fröhlich's syndrome, Cushing's syndrome, Prader-Willi syndrome, and Bardet-Biedl syndrome (associated with obesity, polydactyly, retinopathy, hypogenitalism). Obesity seen in hypothyroidism is due to both myxedema and decreased basal metabolic rate.

## Reference

1.   American Academy of Pediatrics Committe on Nutrition. Obesity in infancy and childhood. Pediatrics 68:880, 1981.

**Figure 492  Prader-Willi Syndrome:**  Prader-Willi syndrome in a 14-year-old boy. Findings included generalized obesity, hypogonadism, and cryptorchidism. The child was 12 cm shorter than average for his age. The syndrome is associated with learning disability. In the newborn period, the child had the typical muscular hypotonia which led to asphyxia. At the age of 16 years, the child developed diabetes mellitus (a frequent complication of Prader-Willi syndrome).

**Figure 493  Obesity:**  Marked obesity in a 12-year-old boy. Red "stretch" marks of the abdominal skin are noted (striae atrophicae).

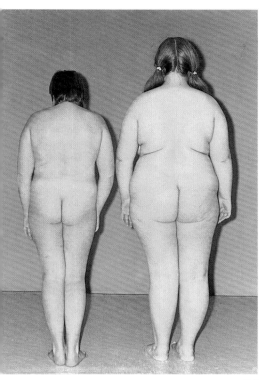

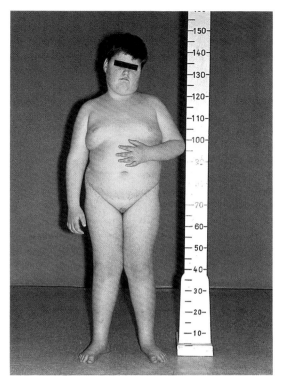

491

492

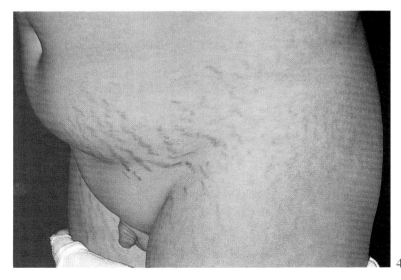

493

# 12. Metabolic Diseases and Nutritional Disorders

**Figure 494  Generalized Lipodystrophy:**  Generalized lipodystrophy in a 13-month-old boy. Since birth the child was noted to have decreased subcutaneous adipose tissue. The underlying musculature was easil apparent because of the lack of subcutaneous tissue. In addition, macrocephaly, "senile" facial expression and sparse hair were noted. Growth and mental development were extremely delayed. Feeding was difficul and could only be accomplished with the use of nasogastric feedings. Death occurred at age 15 month due to bronchopneumonia. Autopsy revealed general atrophy of adipose tissue.

**Differential Diagnosis:**  Differential diagnosis for lipodystrophy includes Seip-Lawrence syndrome (tota lipoatrophy with excessive height and hypertrichosis), Brachman-de Lange syndrome (microcephaly, ab normal facies, limb anomalies), Berardinelli's syndrome (gigantism, advanced bone age, lipodystrophy) and Simon's syndrome (progressive loss of subcutaneous adipose tissue).

**Figure 495  Failure To Thrive:**  Failure to thrive of uncertain etiology in a 6-year-old girl. Of note wa the paucity of subcutaneous adipose tissue and musculature. The child was 15 cm shorter than average an had hyperpigmented skin, cutis laxa, and extreme growth and mental retardation. The symptoms were firs noted at one month of age and have progressed since then. Despite exhaustive diagnostic investigations the cause of this growth failure remained unknown. Death of the child occurred at 8 years of age.

**Differential Diagnosis:**  Failure to thrive can occur as the result of organic disease (chronic infection neoplasm), psychiatric disease, adrenal insufficiency (Addison's disease), and hypophyseal insufficienc (panhypopituitarism). Anorexia nervosa may also occur in older children.

**Figure 496  Juvenile Generalized Fibromatosis:**  Juvenile generalized fibromatosis (Ormond's syndrome in a 10-year-old boy. The child was severely cachectic (7 kg underweight). Multiple intraperitoneal an retroperitoneal fibromas caused intestinal obstruction and displaced both ureters. In addition, there wa fibromatous involvement of the mediastinum, the pleura, and the pericardium. As a result of this generalize fibromatosis, there was edema, ascites, urinary retention, and cardiac failure. With symptomatic treatment the child initially improved, but death ensued within 5 months due to increasing cardiac failure.

In Ormond's syndrome, retroperitoneal fibrosis causes progressive compression and stenosis of the ureter which leads to hydronephrosis and, in severe cases, to uremia. Involvement of the abdominal cavity, th chest, and the mediastinum is possible (as seen in this case).

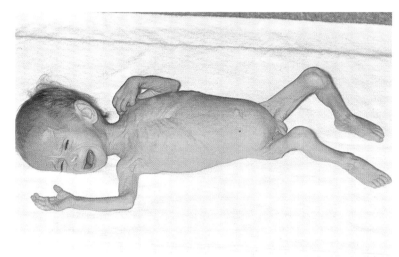

494

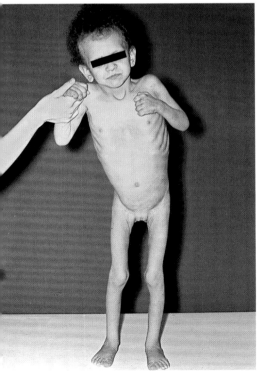

495

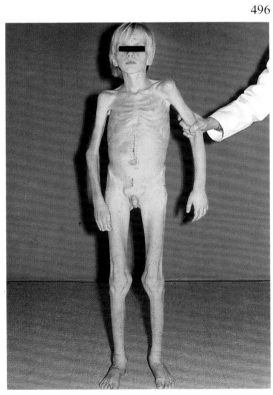

496

# 12. Metabolic Diseases and Nutritional Disorders

**Figure 497  Rickets:**  Vitamin D deficiency rickets in a 2-year-old boy. Findings included swelling of th
wrist, microsomia, and delayed motor development. Other findings included epiphyseal enlargement (lea
ing to protuberance of the malleoli), rachitic rosary, and bending of the shaft of the tibia. After 3 wee
of daily vitamin $D_3$ treatment, there was normalization of hypocalcemia and hypophosphatemia, as we
as increased calcium deposition in the bones.

**Figure 498  Rickets:**  Vitamin D deficiency rickets in a 10-month-old boy. Kyphosis of the lower thorac
spinal column was noted. When standing, there was evidence of lordosis of the lumbar spine. Joints we
hyperflexible due to relaxation of the ligaments. Therapy included vitamin D supplements and physical therap

**Figure 499  Rickets:**  Vitamin D deficiency rickets in a 14-month-old girl. Findings included bilatera
coxa vara and genu vara.

**Figure 500  Rickets:**  Vitamin D deficiency rickets in a 13-year-old Turkish girl. Of note was poor growt
(26 cm below average height) and bowing of the legs. The figure demonstrates her condition after spontaneou
fracture of the right tibia as well as fracture of the seventh and ninth ribs. Severe vitamin D deficienc
was caused by a combination of environmental factors, including poor nutrition and constant confinemer
(due to fear of being discovered as an illegal alien). Treatment included vitamin D therapy and correctiv
surgery.

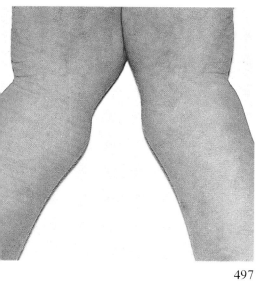

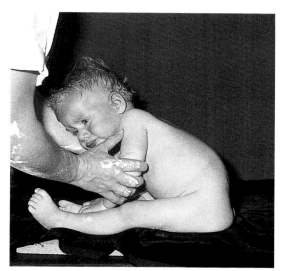

497

498

499

500

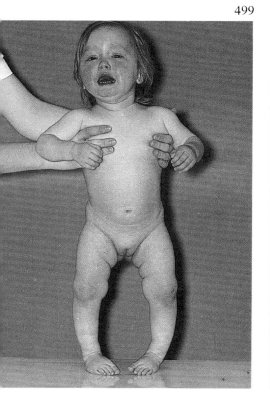

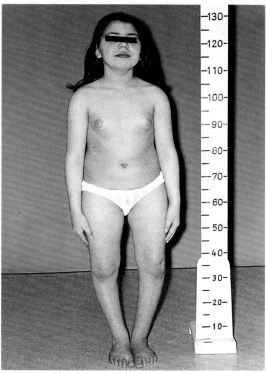

# 12. Metabolic Diseases and Nutritional Disorders

**Figure 501  Rickets:**  Vitamin D deficiency rickets in a 14-month-old boy, whose regular prophylact dose of vitamin D had been discontinued. Findings included rachitic rosary (beading of the ribs at th costochondral junction) and delayed gross motor development. The diagnosis was confirmed by radiograph studies and laboratory investigations (demonstrating a reduction in serum 25-hydroxycholecalciferol).

**Figures 502 and 503  Pseudohypoparathyroidism:**  Pseudohypoparathyroidism (hereditary osteodystroph Albright's syndrome) in an 11-year-old girl. Of note was brachydactyly and shortening of the metacarpa (particularly of the os metacarpal V with corresponding malleolus bilaterally) and metatarsal bones (partic larly of the os metarsal IV). Pseudohypoparathyroidism was first noted because of failure to thrive and d velopmental delay. Laboratory investigation revealed hypocalcemia and hyperphosphatemia. Further e aminations demonstrated an elevated parathormone level, as well as end organ resistence to parathormor (PTH did not raise the level of calcium or increase phosphate excretion in the urine). Trousseau's ar Chvostek's signs were positive, but no tetanic seizures were observed. These laboratory abnormalities ir proved after high dose vitamin D therapy and calcium supplements were given.

**Differential Diagnosis:**  Brachydactyly may be seen in 50 percent of patients with Turner's syndrom Pseudo-pseudohypoparathyroidism may be inherited as an X-linked dominant trait. Shortening of the fif finger is seen in Silver's syndrome (primoridal dwarfism with asymmetry) and in brachydactalic syndrome Brachydactyly may also appear as an isolated finding or part of other syndromes (Weill-Marchesani syndrom Biemond's syndrome, Brailsford-Morquio syndrome).

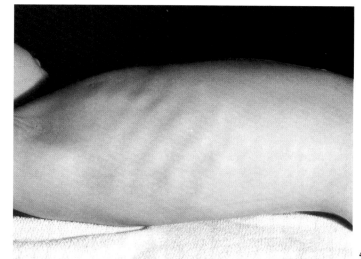

501

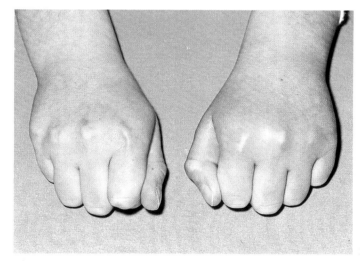

502

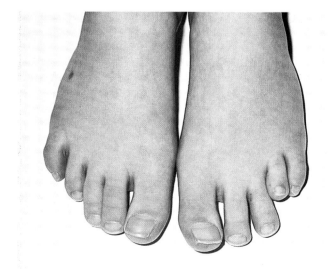

503

# 12. Metabolic Diseases and Nutritional Disorders

**Figures 504 and 505  Scurvy:**  Scurvy in an 11-month-old girl. Findings included scorbutic rosary and "frog position" posture (flexed knees and hips with external rotation—Hampelmann's phenomenon) due to malnutrition (vitamin C deficiency). Movement of the arms and legs was extremely painful due to subperiosteal hematomas (detected on skeletal radiographs). Hemorrhagic manifestations, including cutaneous and mucous membrane hemorrhage, hematuria, and melena were absent. Rumpel-Leede test was positive. Vitamin C content in plasma and leukocytes was significantly reduced, confirming the diagnosis of scurvy. The child was effectively treated with vitamin C.

**Differential Diagnosis:**  A broad range of possible diagnoses exists since the disease encompasses both skeletal abnormalities and hemorrhagic manifestations. Differential diagnosis includes arthritis, osteomyelitis, rickets, congenital syphilis, and diseases which cause cutaneous purpuric lesions (including Henoch-Schönlein purpura and thrombocytopenic purpura).

**Figure 506  Scurvy:**  Scurvy (vitamin C deficiency) in a 12-month-old boy. The child was fed a special preparation of milk lacking vitamin C, and was never given vegetables or fruit. The gums were dark red and swollen, due to bleeding of the mucous membranes. The child maintained the typical "frog position" posture (Hampelmann's phenomenon). Skeletal findings included pseudoparalysis (due to subperiosteal hematoma) and scorbutic rosary. Diagnosis of vitamin C deficiency was confirmed by radiographic studies and determination of the vitamin C content of the blood and urine (after test dose of vitamin C).

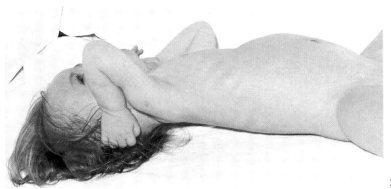

504

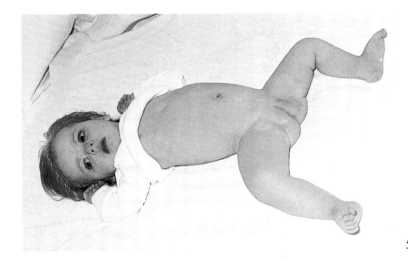

505

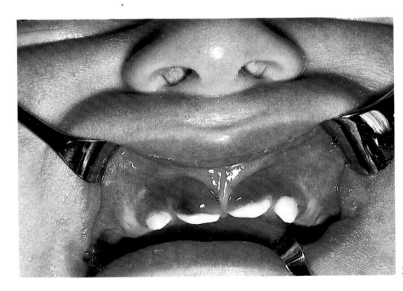

506

**Figure 507  Protoporphyria:**  Protoporphyria in an 8-year-old boy. The child routinely developed an in‑ tensely pruritic and erythematous rash on the parts of the body exposed to sunlight. Several small, atrophi‑ scars, which were the result of chronic dermatitis following repeated sunburn, were noted on the cheeks‑ Protoprophrinogen 9 was present in high concentrations in the plasma and erythrocytes.

**Differential Diagnosis:**  The differential diagnosis of photosensitivity is discussed on page 132.

**Figure 508  Insulin Fat Atrophy:**  Insulin fat atrophy in a 7-year-old boy with diabetes mellitus. Of not‑ was the loss of subcutaneous fat tissue, primarily at the sites where insulin was frequently injected (on th‑ thighs, buttocks, and upper arms). In order to prevent this condition from occurring, it was recommende‑ that the child frequently change the site of injection and use purified insulin preparations. Spontaneous regres‑ sion is possible. Some patients may develop localized lipoma-like swelling. For further discussion of cortico‑ steroid atrophy after intramuscular injection, see p 192.

**Figure 509  Hurler's Syndrome:**  Hurler's syndrome (mucopolysaccaridosis Type I-H) in a 10-year-old‑ boy. Findings included coarse facial features, enlargement of the skull, swollen lips, enlarged thick tongue,‑ coarse hair, and heavy eyebrows. The child was also noted to have microsomia, hepatosplenomegaly, corneal‑ opacities, and mental retardation. Further laboratory investigations demonstrated a decreased activity of‑ alpha-L-iduronidase in the child's leukocytes; in the urine, the excretion of dermatan sulfate and heparan‑ sulfate was increased.

**Differential Diagnosis:**  Differential diagnosis of Hurler's syndrome includes other types of mucopolysac‑ caridoses and congenital hypothyroidism (for differential diagnosis of macroglossia, see p 298).

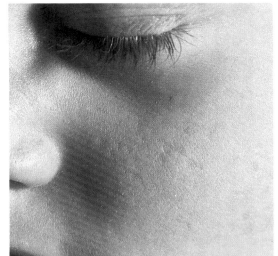

507

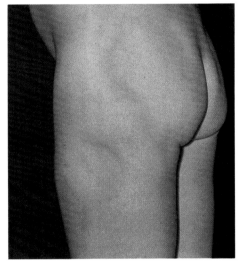

508

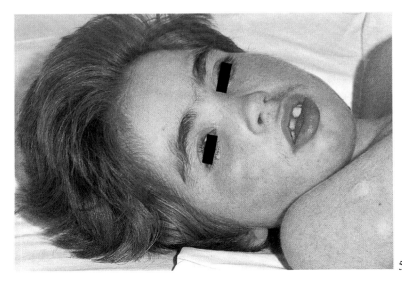

509

271

# 12. Metabolic Diseases and Nutritional Disorders

**Figure 510  Hunter's Syndrome:**  Hunter's syndrome (mucopolysaccaridosis Type II) in a 7-year-old boy. The child had the typical facial features of Hunter's syndrome: coarse facial features, depressed nasal bridge, hypertelorism, swollen lips, and enlarged tongue. Other findings included macrocephaly, microsomia, short neck, hearing impairment, hepatosplenomegaly, and dementia. No corneal opacities were noted. Laboratory investigation revealed a decreased excretion of dermatan sulfate and heparan sulfate in the urine. In fibroblast culture, L-iduronosulfate sulfatase was decreased.

Differentiation from other types of mucopolysaccaridoses can be made by specific enzyme detection. Hunter's syndrome must be differentiated from Hurler's syndrome and from Sanfilippo's syndrome (Type III A). Like Hunter's syndrome, Sanfilippo's syndrome does not include corneal opacity.

**Figure 511  Contractures Of The Fingers:**  Contractures of the fingers (claw hands) in the child from Figure 510.

**Figures 512 and 513  Mucolipidoses ML-I:**  Mucolipidoses ML-I in a 12-year-old boy. The child was first brought for medical attention at 1 year of life because of delayed psychomotor development, and was seen again at age 1½ years because of skeletal deformities. Of note was the relatively short torso, protuberance of the anterior thorax, and long extremities and hands. Movement of the joints was not restricted. The child was noted to have coarse facial features, depressed nasal bridge, and hearing difficulty. On ophthalmologic examination, a cherry-red spot was noted in the area of the macula. Corneal opacities were later noted. The liver was slightly enlarged and no splenomegaly was noted. Skeletal radiographs detected changes similar to those seen in Hurler's syndrome. Laboratory investigations demonstrated vacuolated lymphocytes on peripheral blood smear and normal excretion of mucopolysaccarides in the urine. Cells obtained in fibroblast culture demonstrated deficient sialidase activity.

**Differential Diagnosis:**  When a cherry-red spot is detected on ophthalmologic examination, the differential diagnosis includes Tay-Sachs disease, GM-I gangliosidosis, infantile Niemann-Pick disease, and metachromatic leukodystrophy. Similar skeletal changes can be seen in other mucopolysaccaridoses.

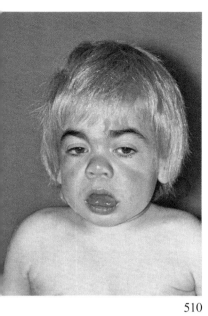

510

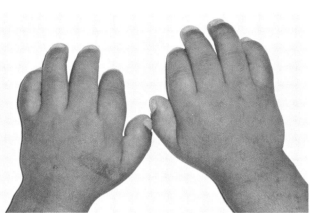

511

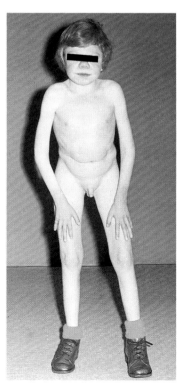

512

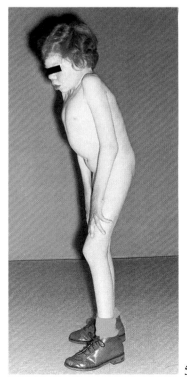

513

# 12. Metabolic Diseases and Nutritional Disorders

**Figure 514  Hyperlipoproteinemia Type IIA:**  Hyperlipoproteinemia Type IIA (familial idiopathic hyper cholesterolemia) in a 14-year-old girl. Of note was an arcus lipoides (cholesterol deposits in a gray ring around the edge of the cornea). Laboratory evaluation demonstrated increased plasma cholesterol, increased low density lipoprotein (LDL), and normal plasma triglyceride. The child's father died at age 30 years because of myocardial infarction. This child's high plasma cholesterol (700 to 1,000 mg%) indicated homozygosity, which carries an unfavorable prognosis (leading to early atherosclerosis and myocardial infarction). A diet containing low cholesterol and polyunsaturated fats was prescribed. The child was also treated with oral colestipol and nicotinic acid.

**Figure 515  Type I Hyperlipidemia:**  Type I hyperlipidemia in a 15-year-old boy. Of note were tuberous xanthomas (red-yellow nodes of varying sizes) that were found under the extensor surface of the elbow. These easily movable nodes had been noted since 3 years of age. Similar xanthomas were found on the knees and the heels. The child came for medical attention because of severe abdominal pain accompanied by fever, leukocytosis, and hepatosplenomegaly. Laboratory investigation demonstrated that the serum was cloudy, the serum triglyceride level was high, and the cholesterol content was slightly elevated. Lipoprotein electrophoresis demonstrated a wide chylomicron band. An intravenous injection of heparin did not lead to clearing of the serum, demonstrating a lack of lipoprotein lipase.

In other cases of Type I hyperlipidemia, xanthomas may be found over the face and mucous membrane (particularly the oral membranes). Xanthomas may be papular or nodular. They are often found on the extensor surfaces of the extremities near the joints.

**Differential Diagnosis:**  Differential diagnosis of xanthoma include hyperlipidemia Type II (hyper cholesterolemia), biliary cirrhosis, diabetes mellitus, Seip-Lawrence syndrome, and renal disease (including chronic renal failure and nephrotic syndrome). Xanthomas without hypercholesterolemia are seen in Letterer Siwe disease (histiocytosis X) and Niemann-Pick disease. Xanthoma dessiminatum and juvenile xanthogranu loma are not associated with hypercholesterolemia. Xanthomas may be seen Wolman's disease (primary familial xanthomatosis) in association with failure to thrive, hepatosplenomegaly, and adrenal gland calcifi cation.

## Reference

1.  Breslow JL. Pediatric aspects of hyperlipidemia. Pediatrics 62:510, 1978.

**Figure 516  Xanthelasma:**  Xanthelasma in a 35-year-old man. Findings included flat, yellow, induration of the skin caused by cholesterol deposition. Serum cholesterol and triglyceride levels were elevated. In this case, the underlying illness was biliary cirrhosis.

Xanthelasma refers to xanthomas which are localized to the eyelids. Usually they are bilateral, soft yellow, velvety nodules or plaques. Xanthelasmas also occur in healthy people, but seldom before the age of 20 years. Hyperlipoproteinemia and diabetes mellitus should be considered in the differential diagnosis (Photograph courtesy of University of Kiel Eye Clinic)

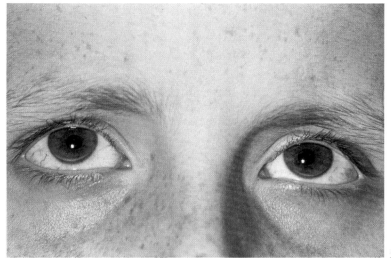

514

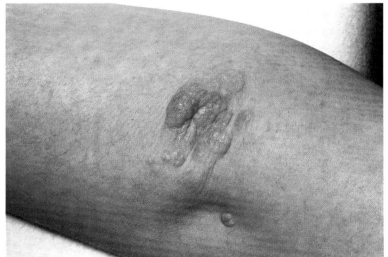

515

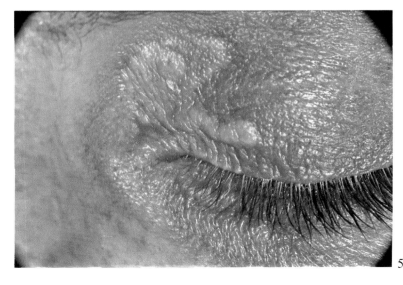

516

# 12. Metabolic Diseases and Nutritional Disorders

**Figure 517   Wilson's Disease:**   Wilson's disease (hepatolenticular degeneration) in a 17-year-old boy. Kayser-Fleischer ring of the cornea (blue-green or yellow ring on the edge of the cornea) was detected wi* a slit lamp. The diagnosis of hepatolenticular degeneration was made at the age of 11 years, when the chi* came to the clinic with hepatomegaly and jaundice. Laboratory investigation revealed decreased serum co* per and ceruloplasm levels. Liver biopsy demonstrated increased deposition of copper.

Kayser-Fleischer corneal ring is seen in the peripheral segments of the cornea, and is usually 1 to * mm wide. It can appear red, olive green, or yellow in color. These findings can regress after therapy f* Wilson's disease. Red-brown corneal discoloration has been noted in copper workers, or in cases whe* a person is exposed chronically to copper (injury with a copper containing foreign body). Ferritin deposi* may occur in the cornea of healthy people. Other heavy metals can be deposited in the cornea includi* gold (in systemic gold treatments), iron (due to intraocular blood or foreign body), and silver (due to loc* application).

## Reference

1.   Werlin SL, et al. Diagnostic dilemmas of Wilson's disease: diagnosis and treatment. Pediatrics 62:47, 1978.

**Figure 518   Wilson's Disease:**   Wilson's disease (hepatolenticular degeneration) in a 7-year-old boy. T* typical Kayser-Fleisher ring of the cornea was not visible due to copper storage in other tissues. Howeve* grey-brown hyperpigmentation of the skin and mucous membranes, evident on the gums and mucous mer* branes of the mouth, was noted.

**Differential Diagnosis:**   Differential diagnosis includes heavy metal intoxication (Burton's lines), spot* hyperpigmentation seen in some black individuals, hyperpigmentation of the mucous membranes in Addison* disease (see p 290), pigmented lesions in Peutz-Jeghers syndrome, and "amalgam" tattoo from dent* procedures.

**Figures 519 and 520   Menkes's Kinky Hair Syndrome:**   Menkes's kinky hair syndrome in a 9-mont* old boy. Of note was sparse, brittle, partially depigmented, disheveled hair. On microscopic examinatio* the hair appeared twisted and brittle (pili torti, see p 188). At first, the child's hair had appeared norma* but, as the child grew, changes in the hair were noted. Gross motor and mental development was delaye* The child was brought to clinic because of a seizure disorder, at which time the hair changes were note* Radiographs demonstrated skeletal findings similar to those seen in scurvy. Laboratory investigation demo* strated a low serum ceruloplasmin and copper level.

Menkes's kinky hair syndrome is an X-linked recessively inherited disorder of copper metabolism, whic* can lead to severe cerebellar degeneration.

## Reference

1.   Danks DM, et al. Menkes's kinky hair syndrome. Lancet 1:110, 1972.

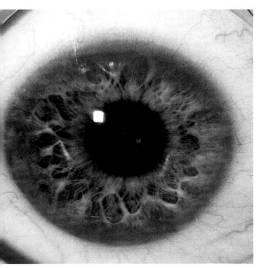

517

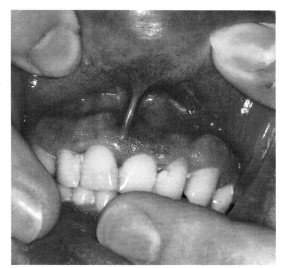

518

519

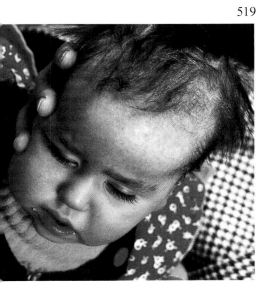

520

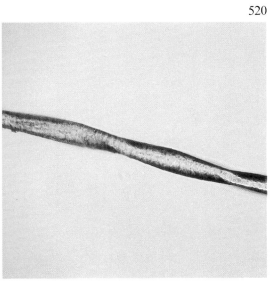

# 12.   Metabolic Diseases and Nutritional Disorders

**Figures 521 and 522   Acrodermatitis Enteropathica:**   Acrodermatitis enteropathica in a 7-month-old girl. Findings included extensive, sharply outlined, erythematous areas of skin, partially covered with crust and scales. Lesions were located in the area of the mouth, nares, anogenital region, knees, shins, and distal extremities (toes and fingers). The oral and intestinal mucosa was also involved. Of note was the symmetrical distribution of the skin lesions as well as the preference for the distal extremities. At first, the skin changes were vesicular or bullous in nature. Hair loss and nail dystrophy, which occur in acrodermatitis enteropathica, were not noted at this time. Later, the child had several severe bouts of diarrhea. Further testing revealed a low serum zinc level. Regular oral doses of zinc relieved all symptoms and prevented a relapse.

**Differential Diagnosis:**   Similar skin lesions (vesicles, scales, or crusts) must be distinguished from epidermolysis bullosa, psoriasis, and impetigo. Secondary infections with *Candida* occur frequently in cases of acrodermatitis enteropathica.

### Reference

1.   Neldner KH, Hambidge KM. Zinc deficiency of acrodermatitis enteropathic. N Engl J Med 292:879, 1975.

**Figure 523      Seborrheic Dermatitis:**   Seborrheic dermatitis in a 7-month-old girl. Of note were partly confluent, erythematous, scaly lesions of varying sizes. The lesions were nonpruritic and involved the anogenital area, the legs, and the face. The lesions had been noted during the first week of life. Despite intensive treatment, several relapses occurred. For differential diagnosis, see p 126.

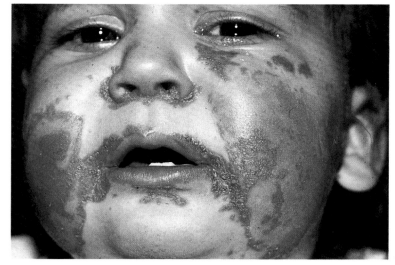

521

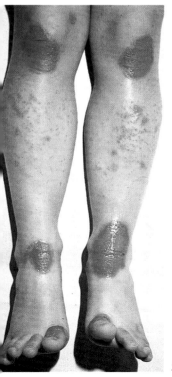

522

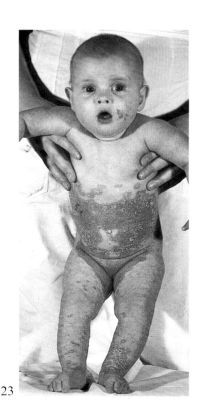

523

# 12. Metabolic Diseases and Nutritional Disorders

**Figures 524 and 525   Histiocytosis X:**   Histiocytosis X (Hand-Schüller-Christian syndrome) in a 3-year old boy. Cutaneous findings included numerous macular, papular, and nodular red-brown lesions on the face, neck, axilla, and groin. The lesions were scaly or partially covered by crusts. The child had been referred to clinic because of polydipsia and polyuria (indicating diabetes insipidis). Radiographs of the skull demonstrated numerous osteolytic centers. Skin biopsy revealed typical histiocytes (foamy histiocytes). The skin lesions of histiocytosis X must be differentiated from seborrheic dermatitis.

## Reference

1.   Osband ME, et al. Histiocytosis X. N Engl J Med 304:146, 1981.

**Figures 526 and 527   Histiocytosis X:**   Histiocytosis X (Letterer-Siwe syndrome) in a 9-month-old boy. Findings included many densely grouped maculopapular lesions on the torso, and extensive nonpruritic lesions on the lower half of the face. Petechiae and ecchymoses, which may be seen in Letterer-Siwe syndrome, were not found in this case. Two weeks before, the child presented with sudden onset of high fever and shortness of breath. Hepatosplenomegaly and generalized lymphadenopathy were noted. Chest radiograph demonstrated the pulmonary infiltrates seen in Letterer-Siwe syndrome. Bone marrow aspirate demonstrated proliferating histiocytes.

**Differential Diagnosis:**   These scaly, papular skin lesions are often mistaken for seborrheic dermatitis. Erythema and swelling of the gingiva and ulceration of the mucous membranes may be present, causing gingivostomatitis to be considered as a differential diagnosis.

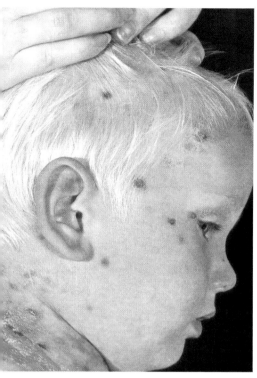

524

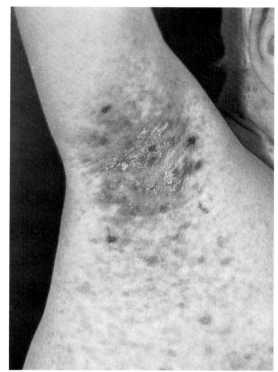

525

526

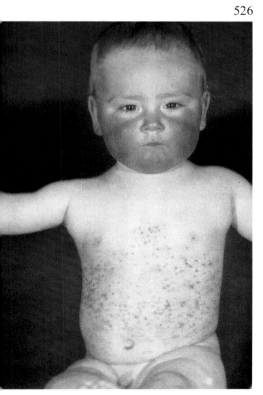

527

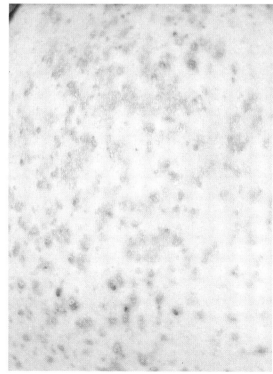

# 12. Metabolic Diseases and Nutritional Disorders

**Figure 528  Histiocytosis X:**  Histiocytosis X (eosinophilic granuloma) in a 15-year-old girl. Several groupe erythematous papules, were noted on the anterior chest wall. These lesions were originally yellow in colo but later became reddened due to hemorrhage. Because of persistent pain in her thigh, radiographs of th femur were obtained, which demonstrated the typical osteolytic areas seen in eosinophilic granuloma. Spo taneous remission can occur, and therapy is often not necessary.

**Figure 529  Histiocytosis X:**  Histiocytosis X (Hand-Schüller-Christian syndrome) in a 6-year-old gir Findings included numerous yellow, slightly scaling papules on the eyelids, the scalp, the torso, and t thighs. Exopthalmus, which occurs in 10 percent of cases, was absent in this case. Radiographs of the sku demonstrated multiple osteolytic areas. Diabetes insipidis, which is seen in 50 percent of patients with Han Schüller-Christian syndrome, developed 3 months later. The child was treated with DDAVP (for diabet insipidis), chemotherapy, and cranial radiation. Treatment led to a complete recovery.

**Figure 530  Histiocytosis X:**  Histiocytosis X (Hand-Schüller-Christian syndrome) in an 8-year-old bo Findings included elongated, red-yellow, xanthomatous plaques on the conjunctiva.

Mucous membrane lesions may be found in the oral cavity in patients with histiocytosis X (includin gingival hypertrophy, necrotizing gingivitis, and stomatitis). A wide range of cutaneous features may occ including seborrheic-like lesions on the scalp and external auditory canal, maculopapular rashes with ves cle formation, intertrigo, xanthomas, petechiae, and ecchymosis.

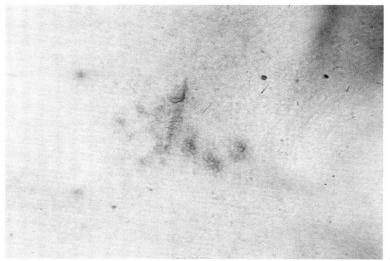

528

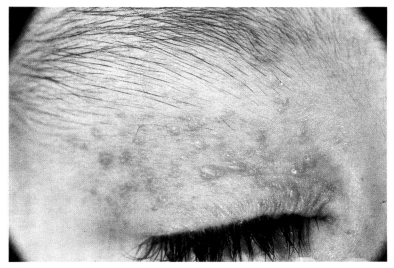

529

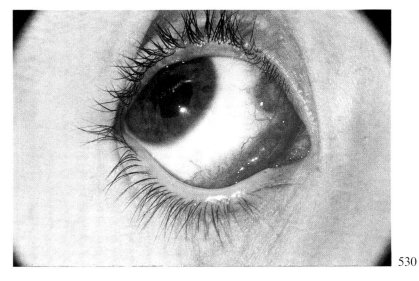

530

# 13. Diseases of the Endocrine Glands

**Figures 531 and 532  Hypothyroidism:**  Congenital primary hypothyroidism in a 4-year-old girl. Screenir tests for newborns ($T_4$, TSH) were not routinely done at the time of this child's birth. During the first ye of life, the parents noted lethargy, difficulty feeding, constipation, and delayed motor development. At years of age, the girl had significant growth delay (10 cm below average), dry bristly hair, a depressed nas bridge, and myxedema of the face and dorsum of the hand. The child's mental development appeared norm for age. Laboratory evaluation demonstrated low levels of $T_3$ and $T_4$, with elevated TSH. The child respon ed well to exogenous thyroid hormone.

**Differential Diagnosis:**  Primary congenital hypothyroidism must be distinguished from acquire hypothyroidism seen in older children (due to thyroiditis). In secondary hypothyroidism (as seen in cas of craniopharyngioma), the plasma TSH level is low.

**Figure 533  Congenital Goiter:**  Congenital goiter in a 6-week-old girl whose mother had taken potassiu iodide during pregnancy (as a treatment for bronchial asthma). The exposure to large amounts of iodic in utero caused enlargement of the child's thyroid gland and disturbed thyroid hormone synthesis leadir to hypothyroidism. The enlarged gland did not cause upper airway obstruction at birth. The symptoms grad ally regressed with thyroxine treatment.

   Congenital goiter can occur when there is a defect in the synthesis of thryroid hormone (due to fet TSH stimulation causing intrauterine growth of the thyroid gland) or in cases of maternal Grave's disea: (due to LATS antibody crossing the placenta).

## Reference

1.   Homocki J, et al. Thyroid function in term newborn infants with congenital goiter. J Pediatr 86:753, 1975.

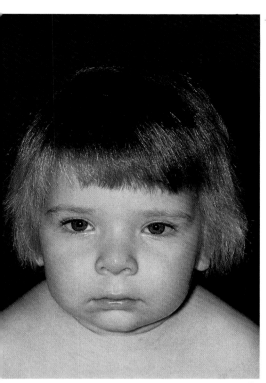

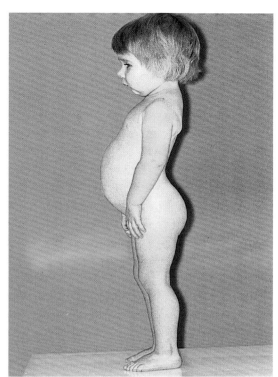

531

532

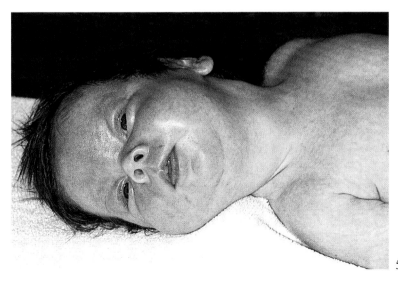

533

# 13. Diseases of the Endocrine Glands

**Figure 534  Primary Hypothyroidism:**  Primary hypothyroidism in a 1-year-old girl. Findings include coarse facial features, macroglossia, swollen lips, and nonpitting edema (myxedema) of the face, the supraclavicular area, the dorsum of the hands, and the external genitalia. Significant growth retardation (length below third percentile) and delayed gross motor development was noted. $T_3$ (triiodothyronine) and $T_4$ (thyroxin) were low. TSH (thyroid stimulating hormone) was elevated. Technetium scan demonstrated an ectopically placed thyroid gland (in a submandibular location). Biopsy of the submandibular thyroid gland (for purposes of ruling out possible malignancy) demonstrated normal thyroid tissue. Continued treatment with thyroxine led to improvement of the symptoms.

**Figure 535  Hyperthyroidism:**  Hyperthyroidism in a 10-year-old girl. Findings included diffuse goiter, exophthalmus, increased height (21 cm taller than average), sinus tachycardia, and moist skin. The child had difficulty with upward gaze and could not wrinkle her forehead (failure of the frontalis muscle to contract normally). She was brought to the clinic because of the suspicion of congenital heart disease (the symptoms being easy fatigability and systolic cardiac murmur). Laboratory evaluation demonstrated elevated $T_3$ and $T_4$. The child was treated with carbimazol with complete regression of symptoms.

Other eye symptoms seen in hyperthyroidism include retraction of the upper eyelid and infrequent blinking (Stellwag sign), convergence weakness (Möbius' sign), lagging upper eyelid (Graefe's sign), and tremor of the eyelids when closed (Rosenbach's sign). The cause of exophthalmos is uncertain, (possibly due to edema of the orbital tissue). Exophthalmos can be more pronounced on one side, or entirely unilateral. For differential diagnosis of exophthalmus, see p 34 and 254.

**Figure 536  Simple Goiter:**  Simple goiter in a 15-year-old girl. The findings included diffuse, symmetric enlargement of the thyroid gland, which began during puberty and progressed during the last few months. Thyroxine and TSH levels were normal. Technetium scan was normal. No detectable autoantibodies against thyroid tissue were noted. Thyroid hormone therapy was begun in order to prevent the goiter from increasing in size.

Simple goiter, or colloid goiter, has a familial occurrence, leading to the theory that it is caused by a genetic limitation of enzyme production. However, the increased occurrence of simple goiter in iodine deficient areas, and the low incidence of simple goiter due to the use of iodide salt, suggests that iodine deficiency may contribute to the cause of simple goiter (similar to endemic goiter). The frequent occurrence of simple goiter during puberty indicates that there is an influence of sex hormones as well as a change in iodine metabolism.

**Figure 537  Simple Goiter:**  Simple goiter in a 14-year-old girl. A goiter had been noted since 1 year of age. The goiter was diffusely enlarged, with a 2½ × 1½ cm, firm node in the right lobe of the thyroid gland. There were no clinical signs of thyroid dysfunction and laboratory evaluations of thyroid function ($T_3$, $T_4$, TSH) were normal. Technetium scan was normal. Neither carcinoma nor thyroiditis was microscopically detected on biopsy of the enlarged lobe of the thyroid gland. The goiter regressed after thyroxine was started. Simple goiter can be asymmetric or nodular. In cases of extreme nodular changes, technetium scan and biopsy are necessary in order to rule out thyroid gland carcinoma.

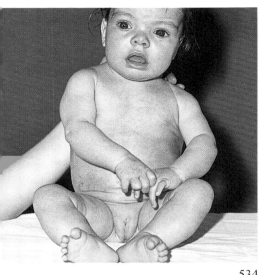

534

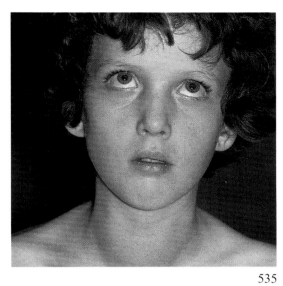

535

536

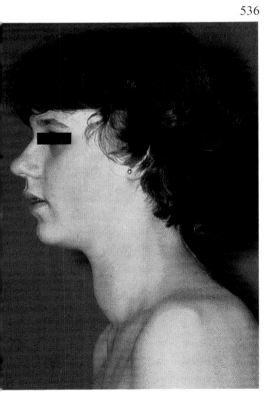

537

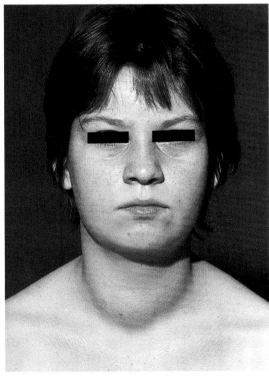

# 13. Diseases of the Endocrine Glands

**Figure 538  Cushingoid Syndrome:**  Cushingoid syndrome due to long term corticosteroid treatment for nephrotic syndrome in a 6-year-old boy. Findings included "full moon" facies and generalized obesity. The clinical manifestations are the same as those seen in Cushing's syndrome (caused by tumor or hyperplasia of the adrenal gland).

**Figure 539  Cushingoid Syndrome:**  Cushingoid syndrome in the same child. Skin atrophy and red stretch marks (striae distensae) of the thighs are demonstrated.

**Figures 540 and 541  Cushingoid Syndrome:**  Cushingoid syndrome caused by long-term corticosteroid treatment for Still's disease (juvenile rheumatoid arthritis) in a 4-year-old boy. The findings include typical "full moon" face, hirsuitism, and "buffalo hump." Hypertension was also noted.

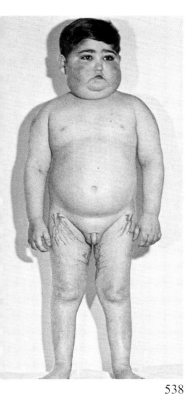

538

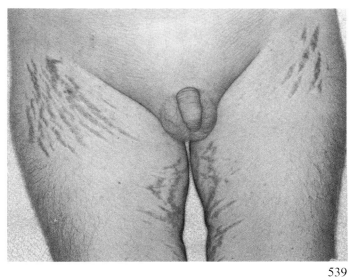

539

540

541

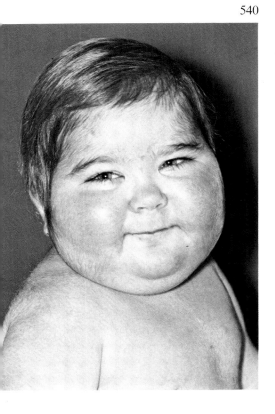

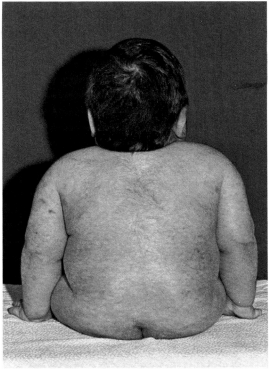

# 13. Diseases of the Endocrine Glands

**Figures 542 and 544  Addison's Disease:**  Addison's disease (adrenal insufficiency) in a 10-year-old boy. Of note was increased pigmentation of the skin (especially the face, hands, joints, anogenital region, nipples, navel, and mucous membranes). In the oral mucous membranes and on the gums, one could see brown pigment spots. The increase in pigmentation is due to increased melanocyte stimulating hormone release from the pituitary gland.

The child had experienced fatigue and weakness for some time prior to hospitalization. He came for medical attention due to an acute episode of diarrhea, vomiting, and symptoms of shock. Laboratory investigation demonstrated concurrent hyponatremia, hyperkalemia, and hypoglycemia (typical of Addisonian crisis). Plasma cortisol level was low.

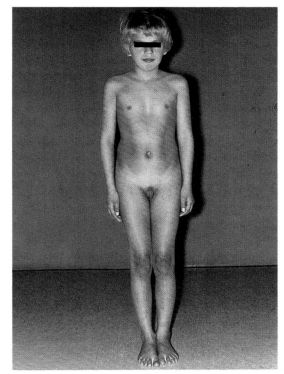

542

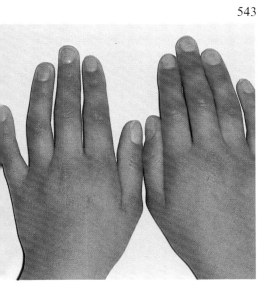

543

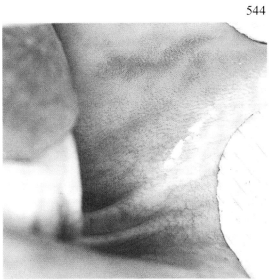

544

# 13. Diseases of the Endocrine Glands

**Figure 545   Congenital Adrenal Hyperplasia:**   Congenital adrenal hyperplasia (congenital adrenogenita syndrome) in a 14-year-old boy. The child was noted to have short stature (height 17 cm below average) Secondary sexual characteristics were fully developed. Radiographic examination of the long bones demon strated premature closure of the epiphyses (as a result of androgen overproduction in the adrenal glands) Laboratory evaluation demonstrated elevated serum levels of 17-hydroxyprogesterone (due to congenital 2 hydroxylase deficiency). Replacement therapy with hydrocortisone was instituted.

   Early diagnosis can be made in boys with congenital adrenal hyperplasia (nonsalt losing type), if th signs of premature pubertal development are noted during the course of regular medical evaluation.

**Figure 546   Congenital Adrenal Hyperplasia:**   Congenital adrenal hyperplasia in a 7-month-old girl Despite early diagnosis and treatment, the child died at 9 months of age due to acute adrenal crisis. Physica examination revealed that the clitoris was extremely enlarged, the labia majora appeared wrinkled (like th scrotum), and the vagina shared a common opening with the urethra (urogenital sinus). The autopsy demon strated hyperplasia of the adrenal cortex, as well as severe enterocolitis.

**Differential Diagnosis:**   The differential diagnosis of conditions causing clitoral hypertrophy include defect of steroid biosynthesis, carcinoma or adenoma of the adrenal cortex, administration of exogenous male hor mones during pregnancy, androgen producing ovarian or adrenocortical tumor in pregnant women, and syn dromes including Beckwith-Wiedemann syndrome (which may be associated with adrenal tumors).

**Figure 547   Adrenogenital Syndrome:**   Acquired adrenogenital syndrome due to an adenoma of the adrena gland in a 8-year-old girl. Physical findings were predominantly those associated with virilization of a fe male child. Findings had been present since 1 year of age, including hypertrophy of the clitoris, abnorma hair growth around the genitalia and underarms, deepened voice, and acne vulgaris. Premature breast de velopment was not noted. Urinary excretion of 17-ketosteroids was increased. On palpation of the uppe abdomen, one could feel a fist-sized tumor. The adenoma was surgically removed, after which no othe treatment was necessary. The voice became higher and the acne disappeared. Clitoral hypertrophy was sur gically corrected at a later date.

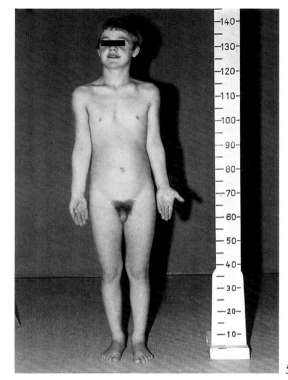

545

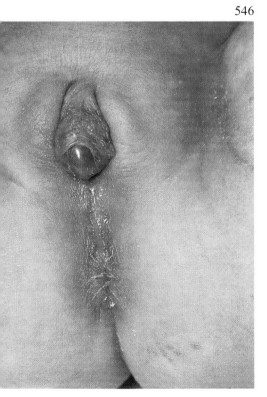

546

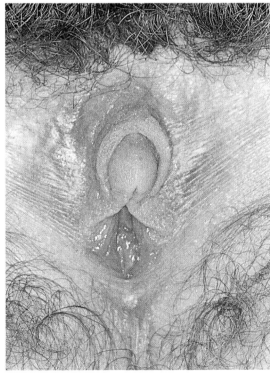

547

# 13.  Diseases of the Endocrine Glands

**Figure 548  Bardet-Biedel Syndrome:**  Bardet-Biedel syndrome in a 14-year-old boy. The findings include hypogonadism (hypoplasia of the penis) with otherwise normal secondary sexual characteristics. Other finding included poor growth, obesity, retinitis pigmentosa, polydactyly, and mental retardation.

**Differential Diagnosis:**  Differential diagnosis of hypogonadism includes Fröhlich's syndrome (prune bell syndrome), Prader-Willi syndrome, Fanconi's syndrome, and pituitary dwarfism.

**Figure 549  Hermaphroditism:**  Genuine hermaphroditism in a 6-month-old child. The genitalia were ambiguous. The karyotype was 46XX. Further examination demonstrated that there was an ovary on on side and a testicle on the other. In genuine hermaphroditism, both ovarian and testicular tissue are presen

**Figure 550  Pseudohermaphroditism:**  Male pseudohermaphroditism in a 4-month-old boy. Findings in cluded incomplete virilization of the external genitalia (underdeveloped penis and scrotum). Testicles wer present. Karyotype demonstrated the child to be of the male sex. Further laboratory investigations demonstrate elevated levels of androstendione and low levels of testosterone. Apparently, the child was deficient i 17-betahydroxysteriod dehydrogenase.

**Differential Diagnosis:**  Differential diagnosis includes other defects in the synthesis of testosterone.

**Figure 551  Pseudohermaphroditism:**  Female pseudohermaphroditism (masculinization of the externa genitalia) in a 2-month-old girl. Findings included clitoral hypertrophy and fusion of the labia majora an the urogenital sinus (common opening of the urethra and vagina). In this case, masculinization occurre due to progesterone treatment during the mother's pregnancy.

**Differential Diagnosis:**  Differential diagnosis of this condition includes other virilizing conditions such a congenital adrenal hyperplasia (due to 21-hydroxylase deficiency).

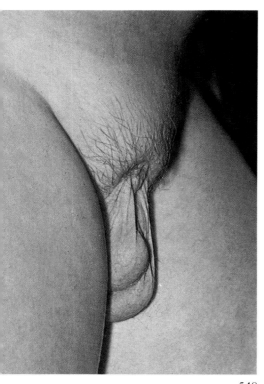

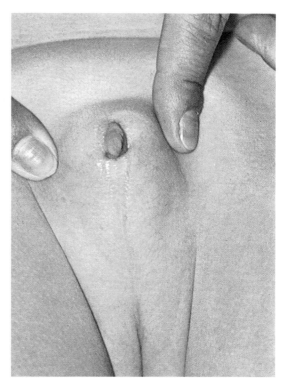

548

549

550

551

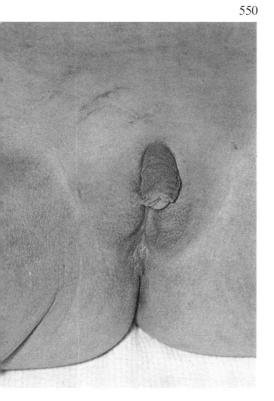

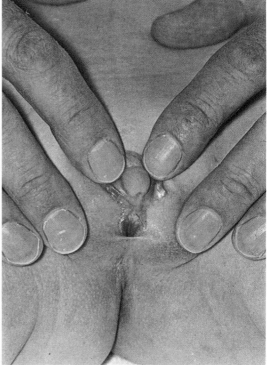

# 13. Diseases of the Endocrine Glands

**Figure 552  Premature Thelarche:**  Premature thelarche (development of the breast glands) in a 1-year old girl. The child had grown to a normal height for her age. External and internal genitalia were normal no pubic hair or axillary hair was noted. Vaginal smear demonstrated no cornification of the vaginal epithelium (normal findings at this age). Plasma FSH and LH were not elevated; urinary excretion of ketosteroids and hydroxysteroids were not increased. There was no other evidence of hypothalamic disease, CNS tumor or other tumors that could secrete gonadotropin-like substances (chorion epithelioma of the ovary). Spontaneous regression of the symptoms occurred within the year (benign form of premature thelarche). In this case, premature thelarche was probably due to the effect of small amounts of estrogen secreted by the ovary on the sensitive breast gland.

## Reference

1.   Mills JL, et al. Premature thelarche: Natural history and etiologic investigation. Am J Dis Child 135:743, 1981.

**Figure 553  Precocious Puberty:**  Precocious puberty in a 2-year-old boy. Findings included enlargement of the penis and testicles, as well as premature growth of pubic hair. Other symptoms included increased stature (16 cm taller than average), muscular build, and low voice. Plasma FSH and LH were elevated. Osseous maturation was advanced, as demonstrated by an increased bone age. After neoplastic processes and certain CNS diseases were ruled out as a cause of precocious puberty, treatment with cyproterone acetate was initiated. Cyproterone acetate (a synthetic steroid with antiandrogen and antigonadotrophic effects) not available in the United States. Usual treatment in the United States involves the use of medroxyprogesterone acetate.

**Figures 554 and 555  Gynecomastia:**  Pubertal gynecomastia, noted bilaterally in a 12-year-old boy (Figure 554), and unilaterally in a 13-year-old boy (Figure 555). Pubertal gynecomastia is a normal finding at puberty. In the mildest form, pubertal gynecomastia may occur in up to 60 percent of males between the ages 14 and 15 years. Gynecomastia may last a few months, and seldom last for more than 1 to 2 years. It caused by the decreased ratio of testosterone to estradiol in pubertal males.

**Differential Diagnosis:**  Differential diagnosis of gynecomastia includes Klinefelter's syndrome, Leydig cell tumors, feminizing adrenal gland tumors, and cirrhosis of the liver. Medications, such as ACTH and HCG (human choriogonadotropin), may also cause gynecomastia. There is also an inherited form of isolated gynecomastia.

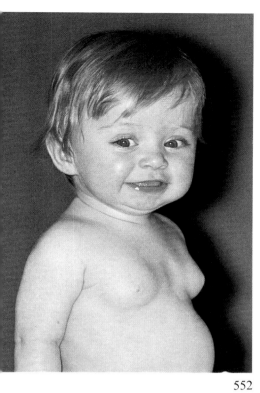

552

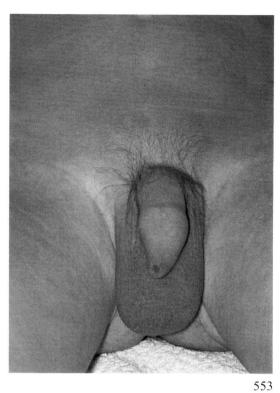

553

554

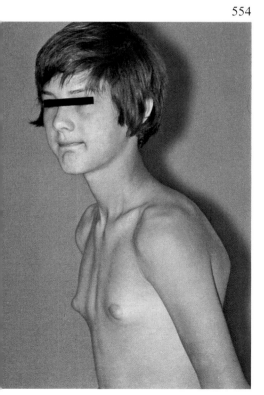

555

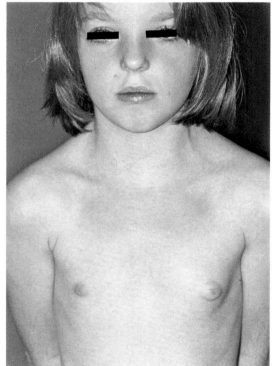

# 13. Diseases of the Endocrine Glands

**Figure 556 Precocious Puberty:** Precocious puberty in a 12-year-old boy. Findings included increased stature (height 18 cm above average), early development of secondary sexual characteristics, and deepened voice. Of particular note was the increased head circumference and widened third ventricle due to a supracellular tumor (craniopharyngioma). The craniopharyngioma required surgical excision. In addition, a ventricular shunt had to be placed for hydrocephalus. After 4 years, there were no signs of renewed growth of the craniopharyngioma, and no further endocrine disorders were noted.

**Figure 557 Acromegaly:** Acromegaly in a 19-year-old girl. Findings included coarse facial features, with enlargement of the lower jaw, the ears, the nose, and the mouth. In addition, the hands and feet appeared enlarged. The cause of these symptoms was an eosinophilic adenoma of the anterior pituitary, which led to an overproduction of growth hormone (GH). The child had the typical abnormal response to glucose load testing; hyperglycemia induced by glucose loading did not cause the normal suppression of growth hormone.

**Figure 558 Beckwith-Wiedemann Syndrome:** Beckwith-Wiedemann syndrome in a 1-week-old boy. Findings included macroglossia, visceromegaly, and macrosomia. The child was brought to the hospital because of hypoglycemic seizures. The initial therapy included intravenous glucose infusion. At a later date, the child required an operation for a large umbilical hernia.

**Differential Diagnosis:** Differential diagnosis of macroglossia includes congenital hypothyroidism, acromegaly, Down syndrome, Hurler's syndrome, glycogenosis Type II (Pompe's disease), primary amyloidosis, thyroglossal duct cyst, hemangioma, lymphoma, rhabdomyoma, and neurofibromatosis (in cases where the fibroma is localized to the tongue).

**Figure 559 Hypothyroidism:** Congenital primary hypothyroidism in a 4-month-old boy. Findings included enlarged tongue, broad nose and depressed nasal bridge. The child's growth was delayed (decreased stature, short arms and legs). The anterior fontanel was large (3×4 cm). Other signs of hypothyroidism were lacking. Thyroxine ($T_4$) was significantly reduced and TSH was elevated. Screening for hypothyroidism, which is performed today on all newborns, did not exist when this child was born.

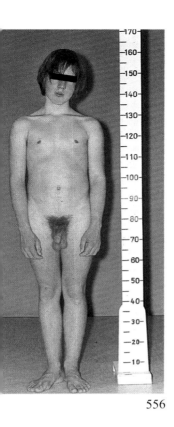

556

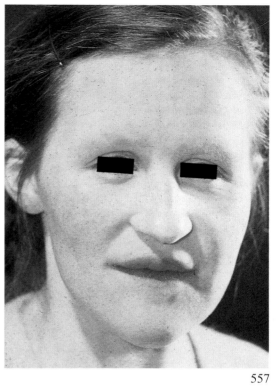

557

558

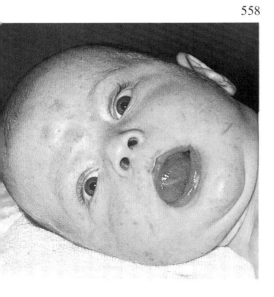

559

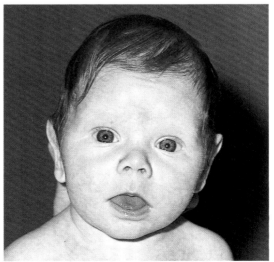

# 13. Diseases of the Endocrine Glands

**Figure 560  Pituitary Dwarfism:**  Pituitary dwarfism (due to deficiency of growth hormone) in a 5-year old girl. She is pictured standing next to a normal child of the same age. The girl is 17 cm below average height and is otherwise normally proportioned (ratio of head and torso length to the length of the legs). At birth and during the first year of life, the child's growth was noted to be normal. After the second year of life, growth was noted to slow down. Skeletal radiographs demonstrated delayed osseous maturation. The growth hormone level was low, and did not respond to insulin induced hypoglycemia or arginine infusion.

**Differential Diagnosis:**  The differential diagnosis for growth failure includes:
1. Primordial microsomia (congenital growth failure, with normal growth hormone production) and other constitutional bone diseases (achondroplasia, osteogenesis imperfecta).
2. Constitutional delayed development (body length, bone maturity, and puberty are 2 to 4 years delayed).
3. Familial microsomia (present when skeletal maturity proceeds in step with age and other famil members have short stature).
4. Hormonal diseases such as primary hypothyroidism, precocious puberty, Cushing's disease, congenita adrenal hyperplasia.
5. Chromosomal aberrations such as Turner's syndrome and Down syndrome.
6. Malnutrition and metabolic disease, such as kwashiorkor, rickets, and Hurler's syndrome.

**Figure 561  Fetal Alcohol Syndrome:**  Fetal alcohol syndrome in a 2½-year-old girl. The child's mother was an alcoholic who drank liquor every day during pregnancy. The findings included growth failure, which had been noted since birth (at birth, 8 cm shorter than average, currently 13 cm below average height), microcephaly, and typical abnormal facies (short palpebral fissures, maxillary hypoplasia, thin upper lip–see p 54). Mental development was delayed. The child exhibited behavior problems, including hyperactivity. For discussion of congenital heart disease in cases of fetal alcohol syndrome, see p 66.

**Figure 562  Diastrophic Dwarfism:**  Diastrophic dwarfism (Maroteaux-Lamy syndrome) in a 4½-year old boy. Of note was disproportionate dwarfism (abnormal shortness of the proximal segments of the limbs), club feet, and widening between the first and second toes ("sandal gap"). The big toes were abducted and the thumbs were hyperextensible and hyperabductable (hitchhiker thumbs). Mental development was normal. Radiographic examination of the long bones demonstrated spreading of the metaphyses as well as delayed closure and deformation of the epiphysis (especially of the proximal femoral epiphysis).

Diastrophic dwarfism is related to a special form of generalized osteochondrodysplasia, an autosomal recessive condition manifest at birth. It leads to severe kyphoscoliosis, which may cause significant physical handicap and require intensive orthopaedic care. Disproportionate microsomia also occurs in Down syndrome, congenital hypothyroidism, achondroplasia, and other micromelic lethal dwarfism syndromes. It occurs in cases of Hurler's syndrome, pyknodysostosis syndrome, Melnick-Needles syndrome (osteo dysplasty), and Silver's syndrome.

**Figure 563  Pituitary Dwarfism:**  Pituitary dwarfism (growth hormone deficiency) in a 4½-year-old girl. Proportionate microsomia (28 cm below average height) was noted despite growth hormone treatment since the child's second year of life. The child's height had only increased 12 cm in 3 years. No growth hormone rise was noted after insulin induced hypoglycemia or arginine infusion. Other causes were ruled out. The child's obesity is caused by growth hormone deficiency, due to inadequate lipolysis.

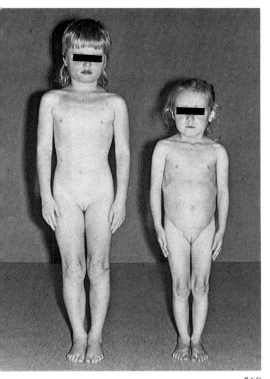

562

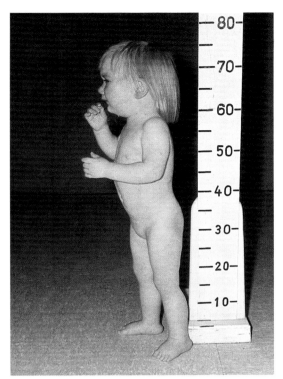

560

561

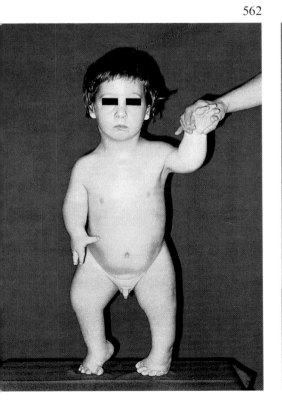

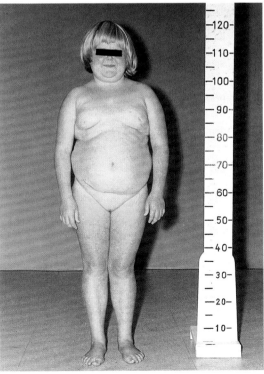

563

# 14. Infectious Diseases

**Figure 564  Measles:**  Typical measles exanthem on the face of a 3-year-old boy. The illness began with fever, rhinitis, and conjunctivitis 7 days prior to the onset of rash. The rash consisted of maculopapular lesions that were oddly shaped, irregularly outlined, and partially confluent. At first, the lesions were bright red, but later became dark red and light brown. The rash began on the head, and then spread down the torso and the extremities. The rash faded in the same sequence as it had appeared.

The rash seen in rubella spreads in a similar fashion. Maculopapular rashes appear in other viral illnesses, including Coxsackie virus, Echovirus, and adenovirus, infectious mononucleosis, and exanthem subitum. Maculopapular rashes are also seen with penicillin allergies and other drug rashes. Similar rashes may also be seen in meningococcemia, scarlet fever, congenital syphilis, and listeriosis.

**Figure 565  Measles:**  Koplik's spots seen on the inner aspect of the cheek in a 3-year-old girl. These spots were noted on the third day of illness. The lesions consisted of white spots surrounded by a red base. At first, the lesions were localized opposite the lower molars; later, the lesions were noted to spread over the remaining oral mucosa. As is typical in measles, Koplik spots were no longer detectable after the second day of the exanthem stage.

**Figure 566  Measles:**  Severe hemorrhagic measles in a 12-year-old girl. The child was unconscious due to encephalitis. Hemorrhagic change occurred in the measles lesions (black measles), and in the mucous membranes (on the palate and on the nasal mucosa).

**Figure 567  Infectious Mononucleosis:**  Pleomorphic skin rash (partially maculopapular, partially urticarial, with individual petechial hemorrhages) in a 2-year-old child with infectious mononucleosis. The clinical presentation of infectious mononucleosis included prolonged persistent fever, generalized lymphadenopathy, hepatosplenomegaly, and abdominal pain. Peripheral blood smear demonstrated the typical changes seen in mononucleosis (leukocytosis and atypical lymphocytes). A bone marrow aspirate was performed and leukemia was ruled out. The child recovered over several weeks.

**Figure 568  Penicillin Allergy:**  Penicillin allergy in a 12-year-old boy with congenital heart disease. The child had been treated with penicillin as prophylaxis for bacterial endocarditis. On the second day of penicillin treatment, the child demonstrated a generalized maculopapular rash over the entire body. The rash was pruritic. Skin test with benzylpenicilloyl-polylysine was positive. Serum benzylpenicilloyl specific IgE antibodies were detected (by RAST).

The most frequent reaction in a patient who is allergic to penicillin is an urticarial rash (see p 116). In a some cases, one can see Henoch-Schönlein purpura, Lyell's syndrome, or other drug related skin rashes.

**Figure 569  Ampicillin Rash:**  Ampicillin rash (after 9 days of treatment with antibiotics) in a 9-year-old girl with a urinary tract infection. Maculopapular nonpruritic lesions were noted over the entire body. No fever was noted. The rash disappeared after ampicillin treatment was discontinued. The child had not previously received ampicillin.

Ampicillin rashes may occur with a frequency of 5 to 10 percent. Unlike other allergic conditions, renewed exposure to ampicillin does not usually lead to exanthem. In over 90 percent of patients with infectious mononucleosis, a nonurticarial rash may appear after administration of ampicillin. If urticaria are seen in association with ampicillin, it is almost always a genuine allergic reaction. Frequently, these patients may also have an allergic response to other penicillins.

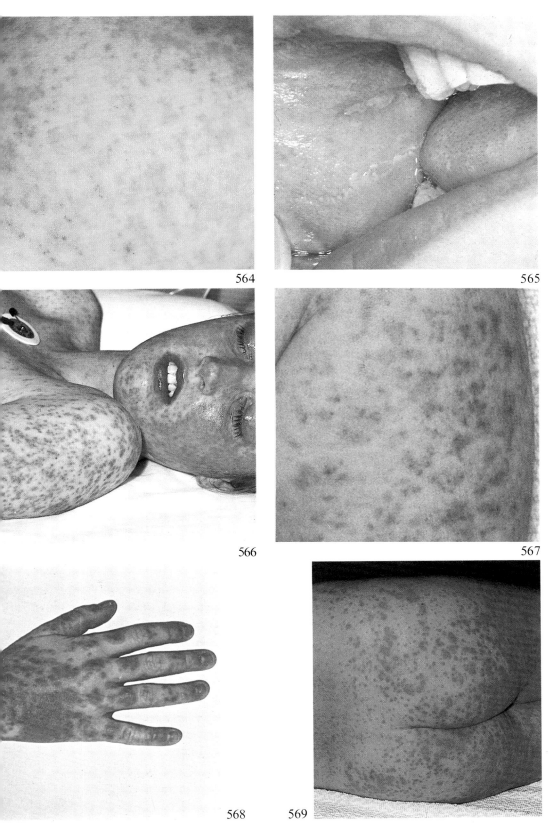

564

565

566

567

568

569

# 14. Infectious Diseases

**Figures 570 to 572  Scarlet Fever:**  Scarlet fever in a 3-year-old child. The child became acutely ill wit fever, vomiting, and pharyngitis. On the second day of illness, a diffuse erythematous rash began on th thorax (Figure 570), and quickly spread over the trunk and extremities. The rash consisted of closely groupe papules the size of pin heads, and had the appearance of sandpaper. Rash and petechial hemorrhages wer noted on the palate and palatopharyngeal arches (Figure 571). After scraping off the white coating on th tongue, one could clearly see red edematous papillae (strawberry tongue, Figure 572). The clinical diagno sis was confirmed through detection of Group A beta hemolytic streptococci on throat culture, as well a demonstrating a significant rise in serum antistreptolycine O (ASO) titer. The condition resolved after 1 days of treatment with penicillin.

**Differential Diagnosis:**  Scarlet fever must be differentiated from many other conditions including vira diseases (measles, rubella, enteroviruses, Coxsackie virus, echovirus, infectious mononucleosis), Henoch Schönlein purpura, and drug rashes.

**Figure 573  Rubella:**  Typical rash of rubella, noted behind the ears of a 1-year-old child. The rash is a measles-like, maculopapular rash, which may begin in the retoauricular area and quickly spread down the body. The prodromal phase is associated with mild symptoms compatible with an upper respiratory tract infection. This child had no prodromal symptoms. The rash appeared on the first day of illness, togethe with mild fever and painful cervical lymphadenopathy.

The rash seen in rubella fades within 2 to 3 days, more quickly than the exanthem of measles. The exanthem of measles may leave a brown discoloration as it fades.

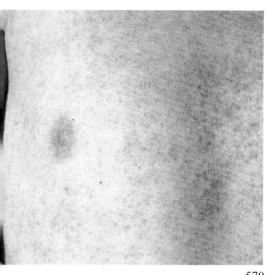

570

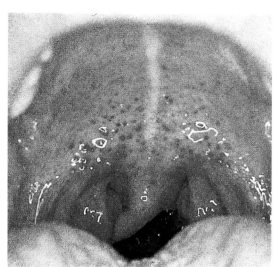

571

572

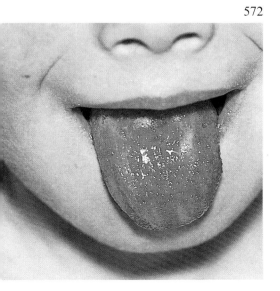

573

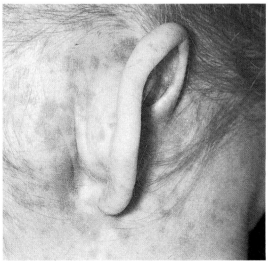

# 14. Infectious Diseases

**Figures 574 and 575  Erythema Infectiosum:**  Erythema infectiosum (Fifth disease) in a 3-year-old girl. The first sign of illness was a butterfly-shaped erythematous rash, with slightly raised edges, noted over both cheeks. The rash regressed after 2 to 3 days. Afterwards, a maculopapular, lacy, reticulated rash, which frequently changed in appearance, was noted over the torso and the extremities. The rash was nonpruritic and no fever was noted.

A butterfly-shaped facial rash can also be seen in erythema multiforme (see p 118), Gianotti-Crosti syndrome (see p 178), and systemic lupus erythematosus (see p 112).

**Figure 576  Exanthem Subitum:**  Exanthem subitum (roseola infantum) in a 10-month-old girl. After 3 days of elevated fever and no other symptoms, a bright red, maculopapular exanthem appeared over the torso, and spread to the face and extremities. The child's fever dropped with the appearance of the rash. On peripheral blood smear, neutropenia and relative lymphocytosis were noted. The rash was noted for 1 day and then disappeared.

**Differential Diagnosis:**  Differential diagnosis of exanthem subitum includes other viral diseases such as rubella and rubeola, and allergic drug reaction.

306

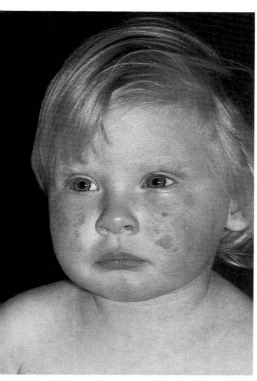

574

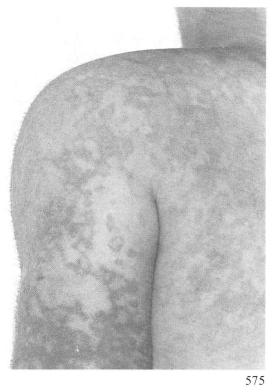

575

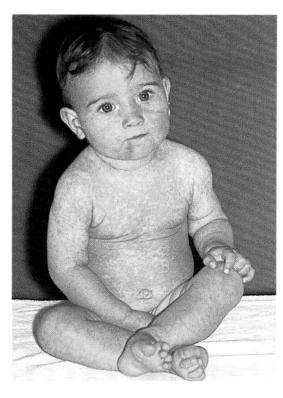

576

# 14. Infectious Diseases

**Figure 577  Varicella:**  Impetiginized varicella (chicken pox with secondary bacterial infection) in a 4-year-old boy. Findings included numerous pruritic papules and vesicles (which were partially excoriated and crusted) noted over the entire body and scalp. Many of these lesions had purulent drainage due to secondary bacterial infection. In the mouth, there were several ulcerated vesicles. The condition began on the trunk and spread to the face and extremities. To a lesser extent, the lesions involved the palmar and plantar surfaces. During the first 4 days, new lesions continued to appear (accounting for the different stages of the skin lesions).

**Differential Diagnosis:**  Differential diagnosis of varicella (chicken pox) includes herpes zoster, herpes simplex, Coxsackie hand-foot-mouth disease (see p 176), impetigo contagiosa, pemphigoid, papular urticaria (strophulus), scabies, insect bites, intercontinentia pigmenti, other vesicular dermatitides (i.e., dermatitis herpetiformis), and drug rashes.

**Figure 578  Impetigo Contagiosa:**  Impetigo contagiosa on the face of a 3½-year-old boy. Findings include small nonpruritic vesicles and pustules covered with yellow crusts. *Staphylococcus aureus* was detected on culture. For differential diagnosis see p 172.

**Figures 579 and 580  Varicella:**  Varicella in a 4-year-old boy. Findings included numerous vesicles of the mucous membranes of the mouth, as well as lesions over the torso. The rash was extremely pruritic. During this time, the child was febrile and ill. For differential diagnosis of vesicular stomatitis, see p 17

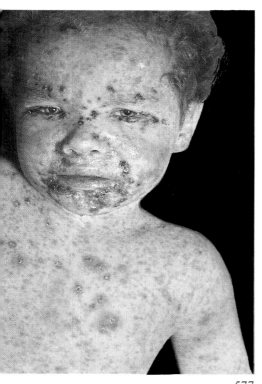

577

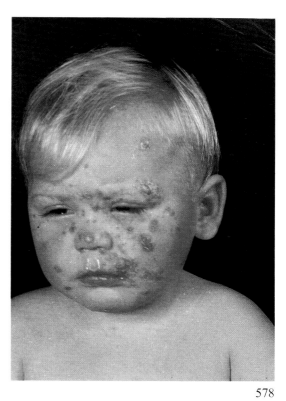

578

579

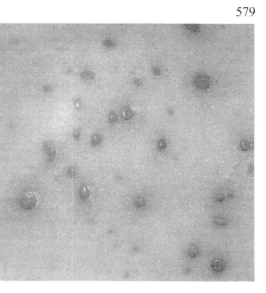

580

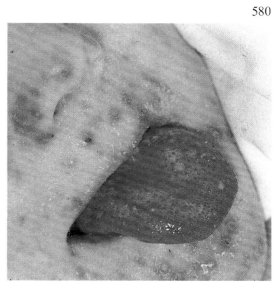

# 14. Infectious Diseases

**Figure 581  Meningococcal Sepsis:**  Meningococcal sepsis in a 3½-year-old girl. Petechial and purpuri skin lesions over the arms and legs developed while the child was ill with fever and vomiting. Peripher blood smear demonstrated leukocytosis (white cell count 38,000 per cubic millimeter). Blood culture wa positive for meningococcus. Platelet count was normal, and there was no evidence of disseminated intravas cular coagulation. The skin lesions were due to vasculitis and hypoprothrombinemia (due to hepatic dy function). These skin lesions are not pathognomonic of meningococcal infection. Similar findings are possib in sepsis due to other causes, rickettsial disease (Rocky Mountain spotted fever), and viral illnesses inclu ing Coxsackie virus and echovirus infections.

**Figure 582  Typhoid Fever:**  Typhoid fever in a 5-year-old girl. Maculopapular, erythematous skin lesion approximately 3 to 4 mm in diameter, were noted on the abdomen and lower third of the thorax. The ras appeared during the second week of illness, and disappeared after 2 days. During this time, there was hig fever, lethargy, splenomegaly, and diarrhea (pea soup-like stools). Blood culture demonstrated *Salmonel typhosa*. The child was successfully treated with Cotrim (a combination of sulfamethoxazole ar trimethoprim).

**Differential Diagnosis:**  Similar skin lesions may be seen in roseola and bacterial infections including menin gococcal sepsis, Rocky Mountain spotted fever, and brucellosis.

**Figure 583  Cutaneous Leishmaniasis:**  Cutaneous leishmaniasis (oriental sore) in a 13-year-old Gree girl. Several red nodes, 3 to 5 mm in diameter, were noted on both tibias (at the location of sandfly bites) These nodes were partially ulcerated and scab covered. The nodes later attained the size of 1 to 2 cm i diameter and healed without forming a scar. These lesions were caused by an infection of *Leishmania tropica* a protozoan seen in Mediterranean countries, Asia, Africa, and parts of South America. Human being may become infected with this protozoan through sandfly bites. The parasite may be detected microscop cally in tissue taken from the edge of the ulcer. Treatment with oral Metronidazol is effective.

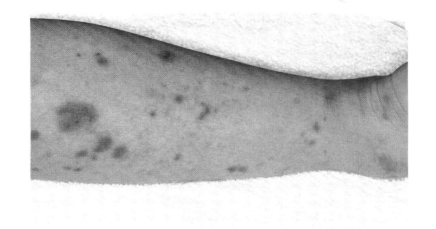

581

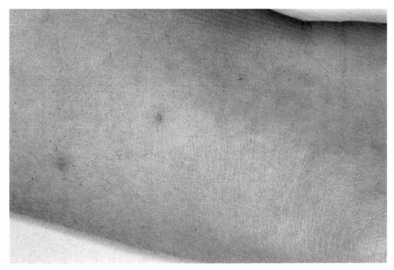

582

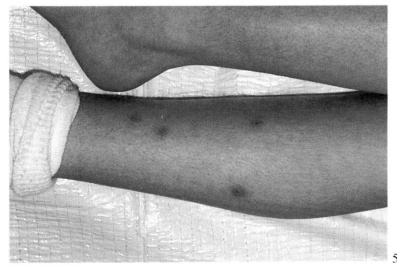

583

**Figure 584  Erysipelas:**  Erysipelas in a 15-year-old girl. Of note were extensive, painful, edematous erythematous swellings over the left half of the face, originating from two skin wounds infected with Group A betahemolytic streptococci. The child had high fever and regional lymphadenopathy. The infection responded to 7 days of penicillin treatment. Complications of this infection include nephritis, abscess formation, and septicemia. Differential diagnosis includes cellulitis and abscess from other bacterial organisms.

**Figure 585  Dog Bite:**  *Pasteurella multocida* infection caused by a dog bite in a 9-year-old boy. Findings included extensive erythema and swelling of both cheeks, with scab formation at the wound site. The pathogenic agents which cause the wound infection are almost invariably found in the oral cavities of cats and dogs. Penicillin treatment may aid in wound healing.

**Figure 586  Erysipelas:**  Erysipelas in a 12-year-old boy. An intense, erythematous, poorly demarcated swelling was noted over the dorsum of the right foot. The swelling and erythema spread to the tibia. The condition was accompanied by tenderness, regional lymphadenopathy, and high fever. The site of entry for the Group A betahemolytic streptococci was not determined. Because of the danger of abscess formation and the potential for sepsis, treatment with penicillin was immediately started.

**Figure 587  Breast Enlargement In A Neonate:**  Bilateral swelling of breast tissue in a 5-day-old boy. Palpalable and visible enlargement of breast tissue (as well as milk secretion from the mammary gland) in the newborn is caused by exposure to transplacentally acquired maternal hormones. After 1 week, the condition regressed without any treatment.

**Figure 588  Mastitis In The Newborn:**  Mastitis in a 2-week-old female child. Findings included swelling and erythema of the right breast, which did not respond to antibiotic treatment alone. After 1 week, the area had to be incised and drained, at which time a great deal of purulent material was removed. Culture of the purulent drainage revealed an infection with *Staphylococcus aureus*. The abscess resolved after incision, drainage, and antibiotic therapy.

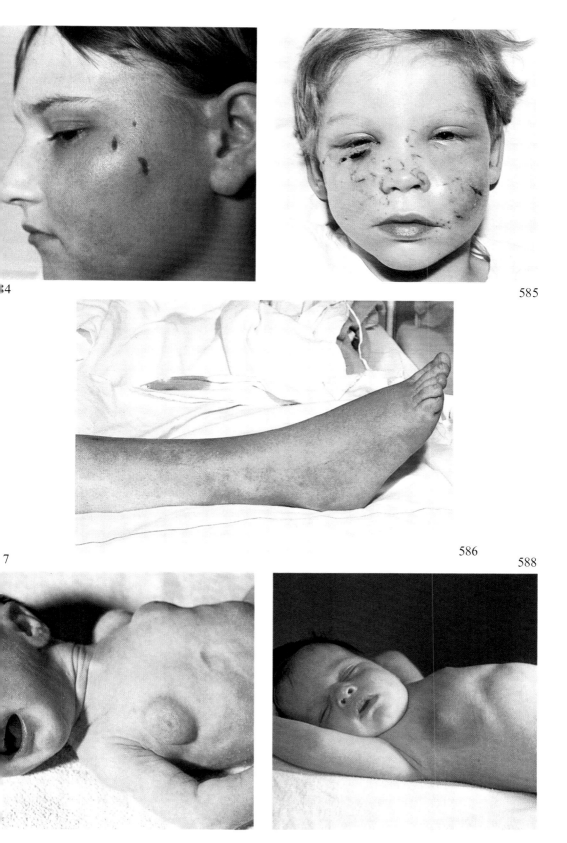

584

585

586

587

588

# 14.  Infectious Diseases

**Figure 589  Vincent's Angina (Necrotizing Ulcerative Gingivitis):**  Vincent's angina (fusobacteria infection) in a 6-year-old boy. Of note was an ulcer of the left tonsil, and painful swelling of the ipsilateral regional lymph nodes. Other findings included halitosis. The child was afebrile. Microscopically, a swab from the ulcer demonstrated abundant fusiform bacillae. The child was treated with penicillin.

**Differential Diagnosis:**  In cases of tonsillar diphtheria, a thin grey adherant exudate can be found on the tonsils (which spreads to the soft palate). In infectious mononucleosis, inflammed swollen tonsils are partially covered by grey-white, diphtheria-like exudate. The exudate is restricted to the tonsils and can easily be wiped off. With infectious mononucleosis, the peripheral blood smear demonstrates leukocytosis and atypical lymphocytes.

**Figure 590  Secondary Syphilis:**  Secondary syphilis in a 16-year-old girl. Eight weeks after the primary infection, the patient developed a generalized macular rash (primarily on the trunk) and generalized lymph adenopathy. Both tonsils were swollen and covered with many grey-white papules and plaques (mucous patches). Similar grey-white lesions were found along the buchal mucosa. The diagnosis of secondary syphilis was confirmed by detection of serum specific antibodies; a positive *Treponema pallidum* hemagglutination assay (TPHA-TP) and a positive fluorescent treponemal antibody-absorption test (FTA-ABS).

**Figure 591  Oral Thrush:**  Oral thrush (*Candida stomatitis*) in a 10-year-old boy with acute lymphocytic leukemia. Grey-white, partially confluent, firmly attached deposits were noted on the buchal mucosa and the tongue. After scraping off the thrush deposits, dot-shaped hemorrhages were noted on the inflammed base. On microscopic examination, one could detect budding cells and filaments (confirming the diagnosis of *Candida* infection).

**Figure 592  Adenoidal Hypertrophy:**  "Adenoid facies" in a 2-year-old boy, due to obstruction of nasal respiration (secondary to adenoidal hypertrophy). Findings included dry lips, dry oral mucous membranes and nasal voice. The child was noted to have loud snoring during sleep, persistent rhinitis, and recurrent otitis media with persistent middle ear infusion (causing hearing difficulty). Treatment included adenoidectomy and myringotomy.

**Differential Diagnosis:**  Obstruction of nasal respiration can be caused by foreign bodies in the nose, nasal septal deviation, intranasal polyps, and high palate.

**Figure 593  Subconjunctival Hemorrhage:**  Acute bilateral subconjunctival hemorrhage in a 9-year-old boy, caused by pertussis-like cough and bronchopneumonia. The superficial nature and intense red color were characteristic. Platelet count and coagulation studies were normal. The hemorrhage completely regressed within 2 weeks.

Subconjunctival hemorrhages often result from rupture of conjunctival vessels and, in cases less extensive than the one pictured, are sharply outlined and surrounded by normal conjunctiva. Unilateral or bilateral subconjunctival hemorrhage may be seen in cases of orbital contusions, orbital fracture, rupture of the posterior sclera, leukemia, hypertension, viral conjunctivitis (adenovirus), and from lifting heavy loads.

**Figure 594  Tuberculous Meningitis:**  Tuberculous meningitis in a 16-year-old girl with oculomotor paralysis of the left eye. With the normal right eye fixed on an object, the paralyzed left eye deviated outward due to predominance of the abducens nerve. With complete paralysis of the oculomotor nerve, one can see ptosis of the upper eyelid and paralysis of the superior rectus muscle, the medial rectus muscle, the inferior rectus muscle and the inferior oblique muscle. The pupils do not react to light or convergence

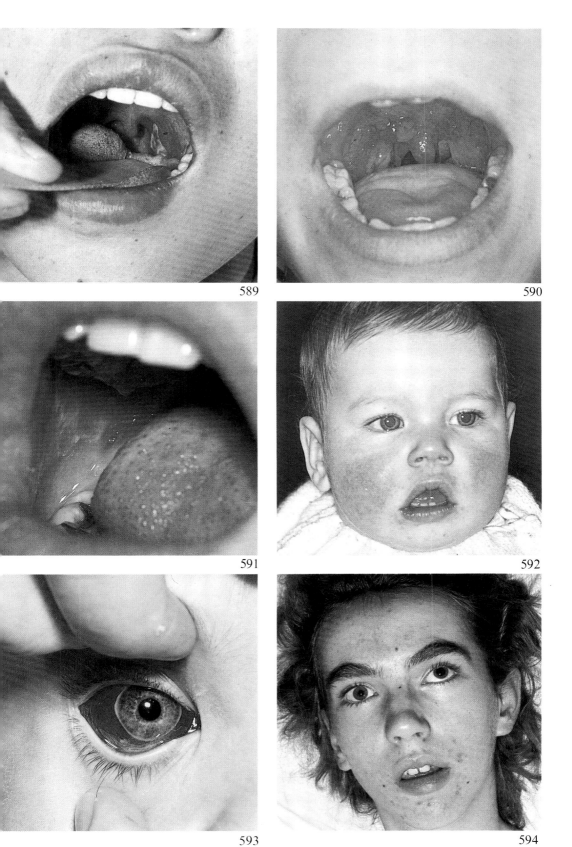

589

590

591

592

593

594

# 14. Infectious Diseases

**Figure 595  Phlyctenular Keratoconjunctivitis:**  Phlyctenular keratoconjunctivitis in an 8-year-old gi
with tuberculosis. A jelly-like mass was noted on the limbus of the eye. Small, yellow, slightly elevate
lesions were noted on the edge of the cornea (phylyctenules). The girl had continuous flow of tears an
spasms of the eyelids. In this case, ulceration of the cornea and secondary bacterial infection occurred
Phlyctenular keratoconjunctivitis is a nonspecific hypersensitivity reaction in the eye, which may be treate
topically with corticosteroids.

**Figures 596 and 597  Papulonecrotic Tuberculid:**  Papulonecrotic tuberculid in a 10-year-old girl wit
a persistent case of tuberculosis. Of note were numerous groups of blue-red papules of varying sizes. Thes
lesions had central necrosis and crust formation. Lesions were noted on the extremities and on the trunk
Skin biopsy demonstrated an area of central necrosis surrounded by an inflammatory infiltrate with epitheloi
and giant cells. Acid-fast bacteria were not detected. Skin testing to tuberculosis was strongly positive. Th
lesions healed after 2 to 3 weeks, leaving behind pigmented scars.

**Differential Diagnosis:**  Differential diagnosis includes insect bites, pityriasis lichenoides, and Much
Habermann disease (see p 156).

**Figure 598  Lupus Vulgaris:**  Lupus vulgaris in a 14-year-old boy. The lesions began as small, erythemato
papules that evolved into nodules and irregular plaques. The lesion pictured is a penny-sized, slightly scalin
brown-red plaque with central ulceration. The lesion is located on the face. The lesion had an apple-jell
color when pressure from a spatula was applied. Prominent swelling of the regional lymph nodes was note
(preauricular lymphadenopathy). Although somewhat resistent to treatment, the condition slowly respond
ed to treatment with INH, leaving an atrophic scar.

The lesions of lupus vulgaris are usually solitary and frequently located on the face and neck. Thes
lesions can be caused by cutaneous inoculation of tuberculous bacillus, or through drainage of an affecte
node. A disfiguring scar may develop, especially in older people. Today, this form of tuberculous diseas
is extremely rare.

**Differential Diagnosis:**  Depending on the stage of the infection, the following entities must be differen
tiated: lymphocytoma, juvenile melanoma, discoid lupus erythematosus, mycotic skin infection, and sa
coidosis.

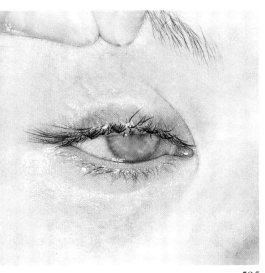

595

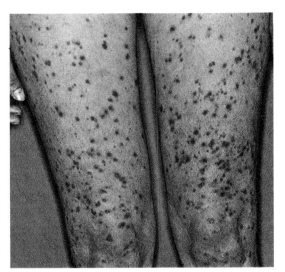

596

597

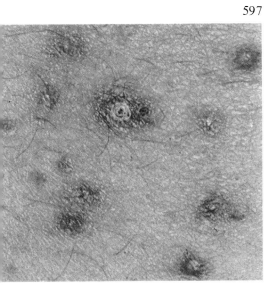

598

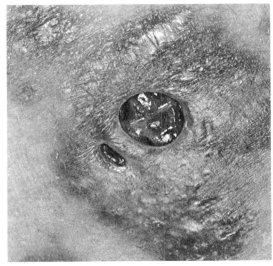

# 14. Infectious Diseases

**Figures 599 and 600  Positive Tuberculous Skin Test:**  Positive tuberculous skin test (Moro). Of note was the appearance of several red nodules 48 to 72 hours after rubbing a tuberculin salve into the skin over the chest.

**Figure 601  Positive Tuberculin Reaction:**  Positive tuberculin reaction (Mantoux test). Of note was the appearance of local inflammation (diameter 8 cm), erythema, and central necrosis after intracutaneous injection of 0.1 ml of purified protein derivative (5 tuberculin units). This reaction is typical of delayed-type hypersensitivity (greatest reaction is seen after 3 to 4 days, with resolution over 2 to 3 weeks). If the suspicion of tuberculosis infection is strong, a weak concentration of tuberculin solution should be used (1 tuberculin unit), due to the danger of severe reaction. For routine testing, 5 tuberculin units are used. In cases where the use of BCG vaccination is being considered, skin testing should first be demonstrated to be negative.

**Figure 602  Positive Tine Test:**  Tuberculosis skin testing may be accomplished with the use of the Tine test—a disposable testing unit with four small blades that have been dipped in old tuberculin concentrate. The appearance of papules, diffuse reddening, and infiltration at the site of inoculation within 48 to 72 hours is considered positive. False negatives may occur due to inadequate inoculation.

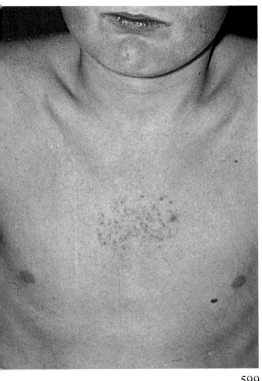

599

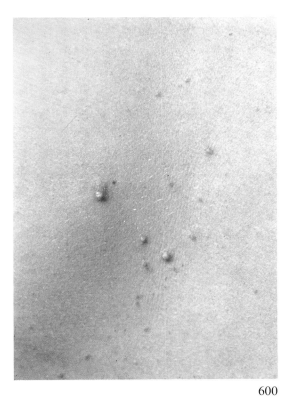

600

601

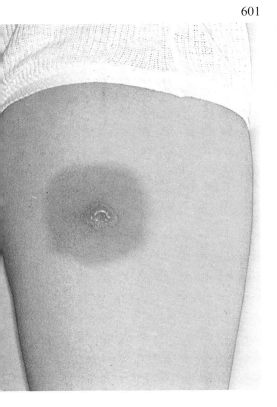

602

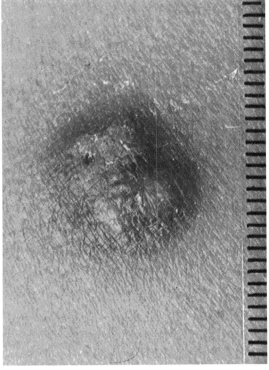

# 14.  Infectious Diseases

**Figure 603  Small Pox Vaccination:**  A 13-month-old boy 9 days after active vaccination with small pox. Grey vesicles, with central indentation and an erythematous base, are noted on the face. Some of these lesions have become partly confluent. The condition resulted from the spread of virus from the site of inoculation on the upper arm. Healing occurred without scar formation.

**Figure 604  Vaccinia Gangrenosa:**  Vaccinia gangrenosa after small pox vaccination in an 8-month-old infant. Of note were extensive palm-sized lesions on the upper right arm, with pustular formation, necrosis and early gangrene. Several pustules were also noted on the back, the axilla, and the face (due to hematogenous spread). The lesions healed leaving numerous scars.

**Figures 605 and 606  Roseola Vaccinosa:**  Roseola vaccinosa (reaction to small pox vaccination) 7 days after vaccination of a 15-month-old boy. Findings included a maculopapular, erythematous skin rash over the entire body (including the back and face). Certain individual lesions had central clearing. The lesions resolved spontaneously without treatment in the 5 days that followed. There was a normal reaction at the site of vaccination in the upper right arm.

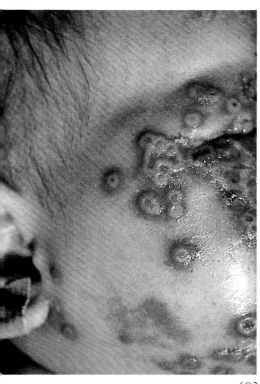

603

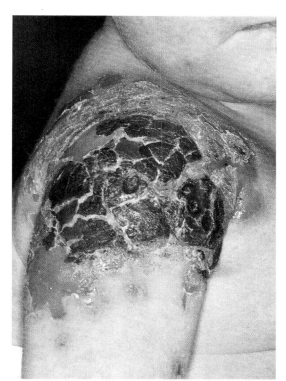

604

605

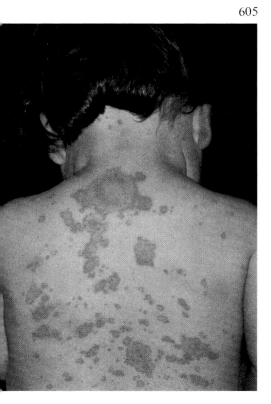

606

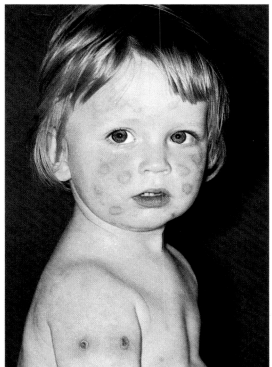

# INDEX

Strawberry nevus, 22, 222, 224, 226, 232
 of eyelid, 244, 256
"Strawberry tongue," 122, 304
Striae atrophicae, 260
Sturge-Weber syndrome, 38, 222, 224
Subconjunctival hemorrhage, 256, 314
Subcutaneous fat necrosisis, 192
Subgaleal hemorrhage, 16
Summer prurigo, 136
"Sunset" phenomenon, 94
Syphilis
 congenital, 26
 secondary, 314
Systemic lupus erythematosus, 112, 200

**T**

Talipes equinovarus, 40
Teeth, Hutchinson's, 26
Telangiectasia
 ataxia, 248
 hemorrhagic, 138
Teratocarcinoma, 100
Teratoma, 232
 sacrococcygeal, 232
Testis, hydrocele of, 78
Tetralogy of Fallot, 64
Thelarche, premature, 296
Thrombocytopenia, isoimmune, 12
Thrombocytopenic purpura, idiopathic, 216
Thrush, oral, 314
Thumb, hypoplastic, 44
Tine test, positive, 318
Tinea capitis, 184
Tinea corporis, 180, 182
Tinea pedis, 186
Tinea versicolor, 184
Toes, amputation of, 42, 46
Tongue, geographic, 190

Tongue tie (ankyloglossia), 32
Torticollis, 34
Touton giant cells, 178
Toxic epidermal necrolysis, 134
Toxoplasmosis, intrauterine, 94
Traction attempt, 90
Transfusion syndrome, feto-fetal, 10
Transposition of great vessels, 66
Trauma, birth, 12, 14
Treacher-Collins syndrome, 36
Trichotillomania, 206
Trisomy 13, 58
Trisomy 18, 60
Trisomy 21, 56
Tuberculid, papulonecrotic, 316
Tuberculin reaction, positive, 318
Tuberculin skin test, positive, 318
Tuberculous lymphadenitis, 230
Tuberculous meningitis, 314
Tuberous sclerosis, 146, 234
Tumor, umbilical cord, 14
Turner's syndrome, 4, 62, 164
Turribrachycephaly, 28
Twisted hair, 188
Typhoid fever, 310

**U**

Ulcerative gingivitis, necrotizing, 314
Umbilical cord, hematoma of, 14
Umbilical cord furrows, 14
Unna nevus, 140, 222
Urogenital tract, disease of, 72–78
Urticaria, 116
Urticaria pigmentosa, 160, 162, 220

**V**

Vaccination, small pox, 320
Vaccinia gangrenosa, 320
Van Bogaert-Divry syndrome, 224
Varicella, 308
Venereal warts, 76

Ventriculoatrial shunt, for hydrocephalus, 94, 96
Verruca filiformes, 172
Verruca plana, 208
Verruca vulgaris, 208
Vincent's angina, 314
Vitamin C deficiency, 268
Vitamin D deficinency, 264, 266
Vitiligo, 192, 234
Vitreous hemorrhage, 256
Vohwinkel's syndrome, 158
von Recklinghausen's disease, 236
Vulva, lichen sclerosus et atrophicus of, 74
Vulvovaginitis, 76

**W**

Waardenburg syndrome, 206
Warts
 common, 208
 filliform 172
 genital and venereal, 76
 juvenile flat, 208
Waterhouse-Friderischsen syndrome, 216
Weber-Christian syndrome, 200
Werdnig-Hoffman disease, 14, 92
"White pupil," 152
Wickham's striae, 190
Williams syndrome (idiopathic hypercalcemia syndrome), 38
Wilson's disease, 276
Wiskott-Aldrich syndrome, 12
"Wood shaving" phenomenon, 184

**X**

Xanthelasma, 274
Xanthogranuloma, juvenile, 178
Xeroderma pigmentosum, 136
X-linked ichthyosis, 150
XO gonadal dysgenesis, 62